ALTERNATIVE MEDICINE

Edited by **Hiroshi Sakagami**

Alternative Medicine
http://dx.doi.org/10.5772/46204
Edited by Hiroshi Sakagami

Contributors

Christina Ross, Hiroshi Sakagami, Tomohiko Matsuta, Toshikazu Yasui, Takaaki Oizumi, Madoka Kitajima, Tomoko Sugiura, Hiroshi Oizumi, Oguchi Katsuji, Daeyoun Hwang, Amirhossein Sahebkar, Seyed Ahmad Emami, Vagner Santos, Tsutomu Hatano, Xing-Tai Li, Qihe Xu, Fan Qu, Olavi Pelkonen, Akihito Yokosuka, Yoshihiro Mimaki, Shintaro Ishikawa, Masaji Yamamoto, Judy Yuen-Man Siu

Published by InTech

Janeza Trdine 9, 51000 Rijeka, Croatia

Publishing Process Manager Ana Pantar
Technical Editor InTech DTP team
Cover InTech Design team

Additional hard copies can be obtained from orders@intechopen.com

Alternative Medicine, Edited by Hiroshi Sakagami
p. cm.
ISBN 978-953-51-0903-7

Meet the editor

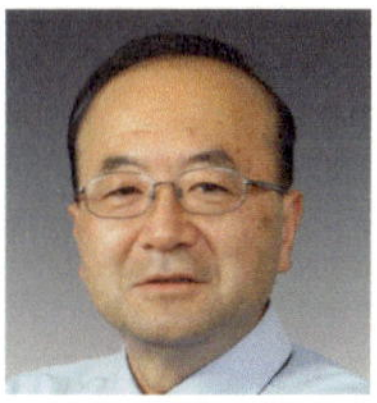

Hiroshi Sakagami received his Ph.D. from Faculty of Pharmaceutical Sciences, University of Tokyo. He worked for 17 years in the Department of Biochemistry, School of Medicine, Showa University, with a 3 year post-doctoral stay at Roswell Park Memorial Institute, Buffalo, NY. Since 1997 he has been working as a professor at the Division of Pharmacology, Meikai University School of Dentistry, and also as the director of Media Center and chairman of international exchange program. His research interest includes the structure and the biological function of lignin-carbohydrate complex (LCC), the application of LCC-containing plant extract to oral diseases, and the quest for the compounds that specifically kill oral squamous cell carcinoma.

Contents

Preface

Alternative medicine is recognized as medical products and practices that do not belong to the standard cares taken by medical doctors, doctors of osteopathy and allied health professionals. Alternative medicine includes the mind-body interventions (i.e., meditation, yoga, acupuncture, deep-breathing exercises, guided imageryAny of various techniques (such as a series of verbal suggestions) used to guide another person or oneself in imagining sensations—especially in visualizing an image in the mind—to bring about a desired physical response (such as stress reduction).hypnotherapy, progressive relaxation, tai chi), the practices based on putative energy field (also called biofield) (i.e., qi gong, healing touch) and the biologically based therapies (i.e., herbal medicines, vitamins, minerals other natural products mostly available as over the counter dietary supplements). Among them, herbs, relaxation and massage are worldwide popular. The therapeutic potential of acupuncture and herbs has been documented during the long history of human uses. Herbal medicines are used in the hospitals of Japan, Korea and China for the treatments of several diseases that are resistant to or inoperable by chemotherapeutic agents. Increasing amounts of research funds are poured into the study of alternative medicine. Furthermore, most of the medical universities in U.S. incorporate the lectures of alternative medicine. Recently developed technologies spanning through the fields of genomics, proteomics and metabolomics would surely become potential tools for the elucidation of the action mechanisms of alternative medicine. However, due to the lack of well-designed clinical trials, the safety and effectiveness of many alternative therapies are unclear. Accumulation of scientific evidence, based on the component analysis by three-dimensional high-performance liquid chromatography, pharmacokinetics-pharmacodynamics analysis and clinical trials are urgent to fill this gap.

The book Alternative Medicine consists of 12 original chapters that are divided into four parts. Part 1 describes the historical (chapter 1) and cultural perception (chapter 2) of alternative medicine. Part 2 presents the topics of structure-activity relationship of anti-bacterial tannins (chapter 3), anti-tumor steroidal glycosides (chapter 4) and anti-yeast saponins (chapter 5) purified from various plants, using the state-of-the-art analytical technologies. Part 3 reveals the therapeutic potential of energy (chapter 6), herbal (chapter 7) and over-the-counter medicines (chapter 8). Part 4 proposes the action mechanism of electroacupuncture (chapter 9), herbal medicine (chapter 10) and Qi-invigoration (chapter 11), and introduces new concept of "Network Pharmacology" that is expected to become the powerful tool for designing drugs and the estimation of therapeutic potential and side effects of alternative medicine (chapter 12).

All these chapters are written by world experts who are reviewing their original and others' research. Overall, alternative medicine has developed into a multitude of medical products and practices that significantly improve the body condition and show disease prevention actions. The content of the book does not cover all areas of alternative medicine, but provides the reader with insights into selected aspects of established and new therapies. The book will, therefore, no doubt be useful to students, clinicians, teachers and researchers who have interest in advances in alternative medicines.

Hiroshi Sakagami
Division of Pharmacology
Department of Diagnostic and Therapeutic Sciences
Meikai University School of Dentistry, Japan

Section 1

Historical and Cultural Perception

Chapter 1

Cancer and Its Treatment in Main Ancient Books of Islamic Iranian Traditional Medicine (7th to 14th Century AD)

Amirhossein Sahebkar, Nilufar Tayarani-Najaran,
Zahra Tayarani-Najaran and Seyed Ahmad Emami

Additional information is available at the end of the chapter

http://dx.doi.org/10.5772/55249

1. Introduction

Islamic medicine is a holistic and comprehensive medical school that has an antecedent over 12 centuries. By using the scientific knowledge of ancient Iran, ancient Greece, and archaic civilizations such as India and China, and adding useful and wise Islamic teachings to them, Islamic medicine has turned into a strong and permanent medical school. Islamic medicine has, for many centuries, been used for diagnosing and treating diseases of large populations that live in vast geographic areas. Some of the physicians of this school are famous worldwide and have contributed valuable services to the scientific world.

Although there is no accurate statistics as to the proportion of traditional medicine to Western medicine in Iran, it is estimated that medicinal herbs constitute around 10% of the Iranian drug market. Although this figure is low at the first look, there are two issues that need to be considered: First, the trend toward alternative medicine is increasing in Iran, and second, the reported statistics is exclusive of traditional procedures of herbal extracts on which no reliable statistics is available [1].

In this writing, we will discuss cancer and the ways to diagnose and treat it in the view of a few of the most famous physicians before the Mongolian attack who used Islamic medicine. The time course discussed is between the eighth and fourteenth centuries. The interesting point is that all of the physicians mentioned in this writing are Iranian:

- Abu Bakr Mohammad ibn Zakariya Razi known as Rhazes (251-313 A.H./865 – 925 A.D.), the renowned Iranian physician, philosopher and chemist who wrote about 250 books and treatises;
- Abu Bakr Rabi ibn Ahmad Akhaweyni Bukhaari who is one of the renowned physicians and the student of Abu al-Qassem Moqanei (a Rhazes' student). He died in 373 A.H. (983 AD);
- Ali ibn Abbas Majussi Ahwazi Arrajani who is the most noted Muslim physician after Rhazes. He was known as Haly Abbas to the westerners (338-384 A.H./948 - 994 A.D.);
- Shaykh al-Ra'is (Supreme Guide) Abu Ali Hussain ibn Abdullah ibn Sina known as Avicenna (370-427 A.H./980-1037A.D.), who is the most prestigious scholar of Iran and the world of Islam. He emerged after Ahwazi;
- Seyyed Isma'il Jorjani (434-531 A.H./ 1042-1136 A.D.) who is regarded as the most important celebrated physician after Avicenna.

Due to the vast territory of the ancient Iran, these physicians are regarded as the main icons of historical medicine in many countries of the Middle East region. The reviewed books, except Zakhireh Khaarazmshahi and Hidayat al-Muta'allimin fi al-Tibb, are written in Arabic and translated into several other languages including Persian, Turkish and Hebrew.

2. Rhazes

Al-Hawi (The Continens) (Figure 1) is Rhazes' most important and most complete book. Rhazes spent 15 years on this book. The book was translated into Latin in 1279 by Faraj ibn Salem (Farrgut) and was reprinted five times in Europe between 1488 and 1542. The Arabic text of Al-Hawi was published in Heydarabad, India, in the 7th decade of the 20th century.

Among other famous medicinal books of Rhazes one can mention:

1. Man la Yahduruhu al-Tabib (for One without Doctor), a medical advisor for the general public. Rhazes was probably the first Persian doctor to deliberately write a home medical manual (remedial) directed at the general public. The contents of this book are covered through 36 chapters.
2. Al-Mansouri that contains 10 chapters. In al-Mansouri, Rhazes has presented a description of the identification of tempers, anatomy, hygiene, orthopedics, wounds and sores, bites and a complete course of therapeutics. This book was translated into several European languages and was published many times.
3. Al-Jodari wa al-Hasbah (Smallpox and Measles) which was the first book on differential diagnosis of smallpox and measles. It was reprinted more than forty times in Europe.
4. Al-Morshed (The Guide) which includes 29 chapters and is an adaptation of one of Hippocrate's writings.

Some other of his medical books are al-Tibb al-Mlouki (Royal Medicine), Bur al-Sa'ah (Medical Emergencies), al-Taqseem wa al-Tashjir (Divisions and the Branches), al-Qarabadin al-Kabir (The Great Book of Dispensatories) and al-Shukuk al'a Jalinus (Doubts about Galen). Rhazes was the most important specialist in clinical and practical medicine in the Islamic world [2-7].

In the first section of this writing, Rhazes's view about cancer is described. In his famous book, Alhawi, he has described the views of the scientists who lived before him and in between, has also discussed and written his own opinions [8]:

Galen has quoted from Dioscorides that applying a poultice prepared from hedge mustard (*Erysimum officinale* L.) is useful for the treatment of non-ulcerative cancer. Paul of Aegina has noted that applying the aforementioned poultice is effective against parotid cancers. Galen has said that hedge mustard causes inflammation, has a taste similar to garden cress (*Lepidium sativum* L.) and is beneficial in the treatment of otitis as well as indurated swellings of breasts and testicles. According to Galen, nettle (*Urtica dioica* L.) has efficacy in the treatment of corrosive cancers which is due to the non-stinging astringent effects of this herb. Dioscorides has mentioned that applying the inner crust of walnut (*Juglans regia* L.) on ulcerative melatonic swellings is a useful therapeutic approach.

Rhazes' experience: Rubbing the lotion prepared from basic carbonate of lead is effective, chicory (*Cichorium intybus* L.) juice and a small amount of opium against ulcerative, pulsating and warm cancer with many rashes, and helps relieve its warmth and pulsation.

Rhazes' experience: Eating the cooked mixture of viper's meat, water, salt, dill (*Anethum gravolens* L.) and wine made from fragrant herbs is effective in the treatment of newly developed cancer. Viper's meat also has the same effect. In addition, poultice of water cooked pea (*Cicer arientium* L.) promotes healing of cancerous wounds. Galen and Dioscorides have mentioned that milk, either alone or in combination with analgesic drugs, could relieve the pain associated with different kinds of cancerous wounds. The best drug that could be mixed with milk for this purpose is washed zinc oxide. Galen and Dioscorides have also quoted that loferghesh has the same property and its analgesic effect is superior to that of mineral drugs. Galen has mentioned that the effect of dressings prepared from powdered lead and cold extracts is very beneficial against ulcerative cancers. Another finding of Galen is that sprinkling burnt lead, in particular in the washed form, is beneficial for the recovery of ulcerative cancers.

According to Galen, sprinkling the sifted powdered old woods of goat willow (*Salix caprea* L.) on cancerous wounds in the morning and at night is a very effective approach. Besides, washing these wounds with the decoction of oriental plane tree (*Platanus orientalis* L.) leaves is very beneficial. After washing with the aforementioned decoction, cancerous wounds should be covered with dwarf mallow (*Malva rotundifolia* L.) leaves.

Slemon has said that black bile purgatives are effective in the treatment of cancer and everything that moistens the body is implicated in the nutrition of cancer tissue. He has also pointed that administration of antidote, in particular *Electuarium Mithridatium,* is efficacious in cancer therapy. Consumption of donkey (*Equus africanus* L. subsp. *asinus* L.) milk and rubbing with non-hot-tempered emollient balm have also been suggested to be beneficial.

In his book entitled "Methods of Treatment", Galen has hypothesized cancer as a disease associated with black bile humor which is very hard to be diagnosed at early stages. In order to treat cancer, Galen has proposed that black bile should be removed from the body by means of administering an appropriate purgative, and then preventing the generation and accumulation of black bile in vessels as far as possible. If this method is not applicable, black bile should be removed from the body at regular time points. A mixture of 17.84 g clover dodder (*Cuscuta epithymum* Murr.) with cheese whey should be used for the purpose of boosting organ's function and black bile removal. Topical anti-cancer drugs should have moderate lytic activity as drugs with mild activity cannot lyse the phlegm and those with strong activity will lyse the soft parts of the phlegm and make the remaining parts tough and hard. Aside from moderate lytic activity, drugs should not be caustic because cancer is a malignant disease and is not compatible with irritant drugs. Therefore, administration of caustic and irritant medications will stimulate the disease.

Administration of the aforementioned drugs together with some black bile purgatives would lead to recovery at the early stages of disease. However, in case of advanced cancers, disease progression should be prevented. If surgery is to be performed, black bile should be removed from the body at first and as far as possible. Then, tumor should be removed in a way that no root is left behind. Bleeding should be allowed with no haste in stanching. Afterwards, adjacent vessels should be pressed in order to remove their thick blood. Then, the formed wound should be treated. Galen has also noted that the cancerous organ or other malignant non-healing ulcers should be cut.

In one of his books, Galen mentions that cancer development is due to the black bile blood. He notes the rationale for this hypothesis as follows: First, the blood in cancer tissue is black. Second, cancerous organ is not warm in physical examination. Third, vessels in the cancerous tissues are darker and have more blood content compared to tissues with warm swelling. Galen continues that cancerous tissues are more malignant if accompanied by wounds, otherwise they tend to be benign.

According to Jew (Masarjawai al-Basri al-Yahudi), cancer is frequently formed in the uterus, breast, and eyes. Galen has mentioned in the book "Purgative Drugs" that there is a possibility of treating cancer and malignant wounds by means of only administering purgatives. Sergius of Reshaina has noted that when thin blood flows from the uterus for a long period, there is the possibility of cancer formation in the mentioned organ. The reason is that in such cases the thick portion of blood will remain in the uterus and cause cancer. Likewise, flow of thin milk from breast for a long period indicates the possibility of breast cancer.

In the book entitled "Thick Substances with Abnormally High Concentrations", Galen has noted that cancer is associated with black bile humor and when the aforementioned humor is warm, it will lead to ulcerative cancer. He has also added that cancerous tissues have darker appearance and lower temperature compared to warm swellings. Besides, the vasculature of cancerous tissue is hyperemic and contains higher and darker blood content compared to other types of swelling. In case of small ulcerative cancers in non-vital organs, venesection should be performed following repeated administration of purgative drugs. Afterwards, caustic drugs should be placed to eradicate cancer. However, this method should not be performed for other types of cancer.

It has been mentioned in the "al-Fosool" book that it is better to leave latent and asymptomatic cancers untreated in order to prolong patient's life. In case of intervention in such types of cancers, there would be a possibility of death acceleration. Latent cancer refers to non-ulcerative cancers and cancers of internal organs and viscera.

Galen has noted that some types of cancers could be recovered through surgery and cauterization. Rhazes mentions that: "as far as I am aware, internal cancers are not recoverable and treatment of these cancers would accelerate patient's death. I have observed cases with palate, anal or vaginal cancers in which surgery and wound cauterization prevented wound healing and caused patient's torment till death. Apparently, if these patients were left untreated, they would have a longer life and would not undergo treatment related torments." Hence, the aforementioned types of cancer should not be treated unless they are ulcerative and have secretion. For the treatment of superficial cancers, all cancer roots, i.d. adjacent vessels that are full of dark blood, should be cut. However, many physicians have disapproved such an approach unless for cases in which cancer has irritating wounds and/or involved an organ that is possible to be cut and cauterized, as well as cases in which the patient is determined for cutting vessels. Sprinkling walnut gum on ulcerative cancer is very beneficial. Abujarih has also approved the efficacy of this remedy.

According to Athenaeus of Attalia, rubbing the mixture of whitened ash - obtained from burning an aquatic turtle - and ghee on ulcerative cancer would cleanse the wounds, accelerate their healing and prevent their relapse. The aforementioned drug is effective against all types of wounds as well as heat burns. Athenaeus has also pointed that rubbing the rennet obtained from rabbit (*Lepus capensis* L.) has wonderful effects on ulcerative cancer. In addition, he believed that rubbing the mixture of antler ash and human milk on newly formed cancer is efficacious.

In the book "al-Ayn" (the eye), Galen has mentioned that if cancer is diagnosed at its early stages, its treatment would be possible, though such types of diagnoses are scarce. After cancer progression, there would be no way except cutting the affected tissue. However, surgery and organ excision have serious problems including severe bleeding particularly in large tissues with high vessel density, severe pains in vital organs which is due to the high amount of moisture removed from dissected vessels, and impossibility of cutting or surgery for organs that are adjacent to vital organs. In contrast, cancer could be treated in its early developmental stages by administering purgatives such as clover dodder and cheese whey. Patients who suffer from these types of cancers should consume wet, soft and cool foods capable of attenuating black bile-induced burning. Some examples of these foods that could help cancer treatment or halt its progression are squarters goosefoot (*Chenopodium album* L.), pumpkin (*Cucurbita pepo* L.) and little fishes.

Antyllus has described cancer as a kind of spherical swelling with deep and hyperemic adjacent vessels that could be considered as cancer's feet. He has also mentioned that metastatic cancer has stringent and lethal pain, sensible warmth upon prolonged physical examination of the tumor and swollen and inflamed adjacent vessels. Antyllus points that cancerous wounds have inward corrosiveness, liquid and stinky pus and two thick and erythematous edges. If these wounds are deep or placed in an organ which is not possible to be cut, they should not be treated or manipulated and only pain relief should be done. If the cancer is in one of nostrils, fingers or their adjacent areas, or breast, tumor should be eradicated (if possible) and after considerable bleeding the wound should be cauterized. Otherwise, such types of cancers should not be manipulated.

In the "Methods of Treatment" book, Galen has mentioned that cancer is hard to be detected at its early stages. He has also added that newly formed cancers are curable through removal of harmful phlegms and rubbing some topical drugs. In the case of advanced cancer, the only measure is to prevent the progression. If the physician dares to operate such type of cancer, harmful phlegms must first be removed from the body. Afterwards, eradication of cancerous tumor should be attempted in a way that all tumor roots are cut. Then, adjacent vessels should be pressed in order to remove their thick blood.

Rhazes' experience implies that some hard swellings are similar to cancer. These swellings are categorized into those with and without sense. Differentiation of such swellings is based on the fact that hard swelling is usually secondary to warm swelling (such as phlegmatic or similar swellings), is dependent to other phenomena and is never formed initially. In contrast, cancer is formed primarily. Another issue is that the vessels adjacent to non-cancerous swellings are stretched and have lower temperature upon touch compared to cancerous tumors. For senseless swellings, this is the best sign of their non-cancerous nature.

In the "Semeiolgy" book it has been mentioned that cancer is primarily a small and mobile swelling similar in shape to broad bean. It could sometimes be enlarged to the size of a walnut and larger, thereby losing its mobility. Such large tumors are very sensitive and painful, with a distinctive red to yellow color and their pain is caustic and burning. Such tumors might burst spontaneously and their infectious and blood-like content becomes visible. The resulting wounds are very sensitive and could digest and spoil neighboring tissues. If potent drugs are applied on the aforementioned wounds, convulsion, fever, fainting and chills will occur and secreted pus will irritate adjacent tissues.

According to the book "Summary of Treatment Methods", for the purpose of preventing growth and progression of early cancers, black chyme should be removed from the body as far as possible. Black chyme is formed during the early stages of cancer development.

Rhazes' experience: during the initial phases of cancer, regular venesection and administration of black bile purgatives is suggested. In addition blood thinning foods with cold nature should be administered for the patient.

Masarjawai has mentioned that in the case of ulcerative cancers, the balm prepared from starch, zinc oxide, frankincense (*Boswellia carteri* Birdew.), aloe (*Aloe* spp.), red Armenian bole (*bolus armenus*) and rose oil should be dressed on the cancerous wound.

According to Aaron of Alexandria, the balm prepared from pulverized starch, sponge (*Spongia officinalis* L.), basic carbonate of lead, black nightshade (*Solanum nigrum* L.) water and rose oil should be applied for the treatment of cancerous wounds.

Paul has noted that the prevalence of cancer is higher among females which is due to their generally weaker stamina and lower tolerance to concentrated wastes. He also adds that cancer is more prevalent in some organs such as the neck, breast and nervous organs. The cancerous area should be dressed with a piece of damp cloth soaked in black nightshade extract and when the cloth becomes dried, it should be resoaked with the aforementioned extract. Poultices prepared from lettuce (*Lcatuca sativa* L.) extract, common houseleek (*Sempervivum tectorum* L.) and powdered zinc oxide are also effective. Besides, powdered red Armenian bole could be mixed with any of the aforementioned extracts and the resulting poultice could be applied on the cancerous area. Cancer patients should not consume thick foods. Instead, they should use cold and moisturizing foods such as cucumber, beer, cheese whey, sumac (*Rhus coriaria* L.), purslane (*Portulaca oleracea* L.) and young fish and bird meat. Oribasius has suggested the following remedy to be very effective against corrosive cancers:

Sumac and cassia [*Cinnamomum cassia* (L.) J.Presl] should be soaked in astringent wine for 4 days, then boiled and mixed with Mediterranean cypress (*Cupressus sempervirens* L.) wood. The mixture is then condensed and filtered followed by reboiling. When the mixture finds a honey-like viscosity, heating is stopped and the mixture should be kept in glass containers. Rubbing the above balm on corrosive wounds has an excellent effect on their healing. In addition, application of this balm is also very efficacious against progressive wounds.

According to Paul, cancer is a kind of sensitive and painful swelling which has black color, ugly and irregular appearance, and could be ulcerative. Furthermore, cancerous tissue has vessels stretched in different directions. When formed in an organ which could be cut, cancer should be eradicated and its scar be cauterized.

According to Aristoxenus, cancer is a kind of spherical swelling that, upon initiation of treatment, will start to progress. Warmth is a characteristic of cancer which could be sensed upon prolonged touch. Hyperemic vessels exist near the cancerous swelling. The main mass and inflamed areas of tumor are in its depth. In ulcerative cancers, a kind of thin, stinky and corrosive pus is secreted. The wound resulting from tumor burst has hard and red edges and the physicians do not frequently dare to cut it, unless it is situated in organs such as the nose and fingers. If cutting the tumor is applicable, it should be removed deeply and with some portions of normal adjacent tissues and then be cauterized in order to prevent its recurrence. Afterwards, some balms could be applied on the scar to eliminate the formed slough.

Rhazes' experience: In case of cancer, black bile purgatives should be administered 10 times per week and appropriate body moisturizing measures applied. If there is a large vessel near the cancerous area, it should be venesected. Afterwards, dissolvent drugs, cooling agents and damp cloth should be placed on the tumor. In case of wound formation, mild corrosive drugs such as yellow vitriol (ferric oxide) and verdigris (basic acetate of copper) should be sprinkled while care is taken not to intensify the wound's pain.

Galen and Dioscorides have mentioned that hoary stock [*Matthiola incana* (L.) W.T.Aiton] poultice is effective against non-ulcerative cancers. Galen has noted that the aforementioned poultice is greatly effective in the elimination of hard swellings especially those in the breast and testicles. Moreover, dragon wort (*Arum dracunculus* L.) seeds have a highly dry nature and are therefore effective in the treatment of chronic cancers. Galen has added that hedge mustard – a plant with leaves similar to those of rocket (*Eruca sativa* Mill.), narrow branches, yellow flowers and fine seeds – is effective against non-ulcerative cancers and all types of hard swellings. It has also been mentioned that the poultice prepared from Gundelia (*Gundelia tournefortii* L.) gum and flax (*Linum usitatissimum* L.) mucilage would eliminate cancerous swellings.

Al-Khuz (Physicians from Khuzestan) have mentioned that pea flour poultice is effective in the treatment of cancer. They have also noted that the poultice prepared from fat and burned cabbage (*Brassica oleracea* L.) roots could gradually eliminate cancer. In case of tumor irritation, chicken fat should be applied for some days until irritation is relieved. Afterwards, the treatment should be repeated. Venesection, administration of purgatives, consumption of moisturizing foods and bathing are also suggested. It has been mentioned that common plantain (*Plantago major* L.) poultice is effective against many types of cancers.

Rhazes' experience: Whenever there is a doubt about the cancerous nature of a tumor, it should be touched by hand for a long period of time and if warmth is sensed, the tumor is most likely cancerous.

Rhazes' experience: The temperature of scrofulous tumor is lower or equal to that of the body.

Qusta ibn luqa has said that aposteles' ointment treats cancer. Archigenes has noted that in the early stages of cancer, poultice prepared from equal amounts of gold or silver litharge (impure oxide) and river crab (*Liocarcinus vernalis* Risso) could be applied on the affected area. Besides, ash obtained from the river crab could be mixed with wax and oil to form a paste which could be then applied on cancerous area. In case of ulcerative cancers, application of paste from vinegar, sealing clay (*terra sigillata*) and powdered lead has been suggested. For these cancers, application of poultice obtained from black nightshade juice is also effective.

In page 73 of the 2nd volume of al-Hawi, Rhazes has mentioned points about eye cancer. Also in pages 72-75 of the 3rd volume, he has written about nose cancer and in pages 11-14 and 89-100 of the 7th volume of this book he has discussed breast cancer and liver cancer, respectively. In page 11 of the 8th volume and pages 297-314 of the 11th volume of al-Hawi some issues about intestinal and uterus cancers have been provided, respectively.

3. Akhaweyni Bukhaari

Akhaweyni dedicated his whole lifetime to medicine. He recorded his medicinal attempts in Hidayat al-Muta'allimin fi al-Tibb (An Educational Guide for Medicinal Students) (Figure 1). The book was written in an eloquent Persian language and contains three parts:

The first part includes 51 chapters on elements, tempers, humors, simple and compound organs and also descriptions on functions, souls, foods and drinks, physical movement and rest, sleep etc.

The second part, in 130 chapters, applies pathology cap-a-pie. In the third part, in 19 chapters, he has introduced various types of fevers and pulses. This book was published by Ferdowsi University of Mashhad in Iran in 1965 [3, 4, 6].

Akhaweyni has assigned a chapter of his book "Hidayat al-Muta'allimin fi al-Tibb" to cancer He states that cancer is curable during its early stages and its surgery and cutting should be performed when possible. However, incomplete cutting or cauterization of a tumor is never suggested as it might cause the patient's death.

When cancerous tumor is formed following warm swellings, treatment or stopping its progression is possible. The tumor is initially in the size of a broad bean. It will then begin to grow gradually and reaches to the size of a walnut or larger and becomes hard and a bit warm. The primary treatment measures include venesection, black bile purgation, consumption of easily digestible foods (such as chicken meat, lamb meat, fresh milk and almond oil) and application of cooling drugs such as ispaghula (*Plantago ispaghula* Roxb.), tin oxide, basic carbonate of lead, vinegar and red Armenian bole, which prevent the progression and injury of the tumor. In case of tumor injury, marsh-mallow (*Althaea officinalis* L.), or camphor [*Cinnamomum camphora* (L.) T.Nees & C.H.Eberm.] balm should be applied. The characteristic of pus secreted from ulcerative cancerous tumors is its dark color, stinky smell and black or red openings [9]. Akhaweyni has also mentioned the signs and treatment methods of uterine cancer in page 537 of his book.

4. Ahwazi

Ahwazi is the author of the valuable book Kamel al-Sina'ah al-Tibbiyah (Complete Book of the Medical Art) or al-Maliki (Figure 1). The al-Maliki is divided into 2 parts. Each part contains 10 discourses which cover the complete course of medicine. The first ten deal with the theory of medicine and its divisions and also types of tempers, elements, humors, anatomy, physiology, general principles of hygiene, diseases and their divisions, types of pulses, kinds of fevers, symptoms of diseases cap-a-pie and subjects on the period and consequences of diseases. The second ten contain topics on health and hygiene care, introductions to all kinds of therapeutic methods, treatment of different types of fevers, dermatologic ailments, all kinds of bites and poisonings, headaches and psychological diseases, respiratory diseases, heart diseases, gastrointestinal diseases, and urogenital diseases, a complete course on surgery and orthopedics, and finally a course on pharmacology and pharmaceutics. The Latin translation was published three times in Europe and the Arabic text was printed in Bulaq, Egypt [2, 3, 4, 7].

Ahwazi has described cancer as a kind of swelling that is formed by black bile and in case of progression, has no treatment and is not recoverable. If cancer has not affected a sensitive organ, it should be eradicated but if the affected organ is a sensitive and vital, one which is not possible to be cut, performing surgery will injure the tumor and change it to a non-healing wound. Manipulation and surgical operation of cancerous tumors is risky and dangerous as there may be large vessels and arteries in the affected organ which cause cancer metastasis to sensitive and vital organs. Besides, closing such vessels and arteries might cause metastasis to the sensitive organs from which these vessels have originated. Cauterization of the cancerous organ is also a dangerous action. If the cancerous swelling is diagnosed at its early developmental stages and other conditions such as age, temper and etc are favorable, the adjacent vessel should be venesected. If the patient is female, menstruation-inducing drugs should be administered before any other measure. Once the menstrual period is induced, the body should be cleaned up by means of administering black bile purgatives such as dodder and white agaric (*Polyporus officinalis* Fries) etc. An important note in this regard is that the aforementioned drugs should be administered repeatedly (not just 1-2 times) in order to cleanse the body from black bile. Black bile has a cold and dry nature and is therefore difficult to be moved in the body. One of the effective drugs for cleansing the body from black bile is the following pill:

Black myrobalan (*Terminalia chebula* Retz.) (3.34 g), dodder (4.01 g), common polypody

(*Polypodium vulgare* L.) (4.01 g), French lavender (*Lavandula stoechas* L.) (4.01 g), nafti salt (1.14 g) and black hellebore (*Helleborus niger* L.) (1.67 g) that should all be pulverized, pasted and then formed into a pill. A portion equivalent to 10.02-13.36 g of the above pill should be used. After complete cleansing of the body from black bile, appropriate measures (with moderate to wet nature) should be taken to relieve the violence and pungency of black bile until proper blood is produced in the body. In addition, the patient should live in regions with moderate climate and use foods with good chyme such as blite (*Amaranthus blitum* L.) and pumpkin. Consumption of beer, cheese whey and black bile purgative powders is also suggested.

As for topical medications, the first measure that should be taken before black bile vomit is the application of moderate drugs such as black nightshade, chicory juice, bladder cherry (*Physalis alkekengi* L.), and similar drugs on the cancerous organ. After cleansing the body from black bile, especially if cheese whey or dodder were used, drugs with moderate lytic activity should be applied. One such a drug is zinc oxide which has the following formula:

Equal amounts of powdered and washed Kermanian zinc oxide, litharge of lead and lead basic carbonate are mixed, gently pulverized and filtered through a silk cloth. The oil part of the balm is prepared by melting wax in rose oil (1:4 ratio). Then, the powder and oil phase are mixed to obtain the balm.

Yellow vitriol balm, cinnabar (mercuric sulphide) balm and apostles' ointment are other topical medications that could be used for the treatment of cancer and other indurated swellings. Drugs with mild lytic activity are not effective against black bile as this bile is very thick. On the other hand, drugs with high lytic activity would lyse weak phlegms. Therefore, thick phlegms would remain, become hard, and form a stone that could not be lysed.

In case of tumor injury, application of the following balm is suggested: equal portions of basic carbonate of lead and washed zinc oxide should be mixed with a mixture of rose oil and black nightshade juice [blite juice or coriander (*Coriandrum sativum* L.) juice could be used, alternatively]. The resulting balm should be applied on the cancerous tumor. Application of the above balm on unwounded cancerous swelling prevents it from being wounded.

http://dx.doi.org/10.5772/55249

Another topical anti-cancer drug is prepared as follows: pulverize red Armenian bole and sealing clay with the mixture of water and vinegar (or yoghurt) using lead mortar and pestle until the mixture becomes black. The resulting balm should be rubbed on the cancerous tumor. It is better to pulverize common houseleek and rose oil along with the above components [10].

In some parts of his book, Ahwazi has discussed about eye (Vol. 1, P. 340) and uterine (Vol. 1, PP. 86-87) cancer.

5. Avicenna

Avicenna was not only a physician but a great dignity in philosophy as well. The witness for this claim is his books: al-Shifa (The Recovery), al-Esharat wa al-Tanbihat (Remarks and admonitions), al-Naajat (Book of Salvation), Uyun al-Hikmah (Principles of Wisdom) and Daneshnameh-e-Alaii (Alaii's Encyclopaedia). Avicenna further wrote about 61 books and treaties in medical science including al-Adawiyah al-Qalbiyah (Cardiac Drugs), al-Orjozah fi al-Tibb (A Poethical Book in Medicine), al-Tashrih (Anatomy), al-Vasayah (Testament), and Resaleh Judiyah. Avicenna's masterpiece is the book of "al-Qanun fi al-Tibb" (The Canon of Medicine) (Figure 1) which is the mother book of medicine in the eastern and western worlds [2-7]. Canon comprises 5 major books each divided into some arts, tuitions, sentences and chapters.

The first book of Canon discusses the concept of medicine, particularly the medicine extent and its subjects and also topics around humors, tempers, elements, organs, spirits, functions, and powers. Themes on diseases and their etiology, hygiene, and finally general guides to treatment are also mentioned.

The second book is assigned to simple drugs and includes about 800 mineral, herbal, and animal based medicinal materials. The drugs are ordered alphabetically (Abjad), and in each drug monograph, the manner, characteristics, the best type of drugs, nature, application, properties and indication are mentioned.

The third book of Canon elaborates diseases cap-a-pie in 22 arts. Each art comprises several articles. In fact, this part acts as a complete review of pathology.

The fourth book offers ways to cure general diseases such as fevers and edema, and also includes orthopedics, toxicology, and cosmetic and hygienic products

The fifth and final book which is allocated to compound drugs is called Qarabadin and represents properties and recipes to make all kinds of pills, mixtures, powders, syrups, suppositories, tablets, and so on.

There have been numerous expositions of whole Canon or its parts and it has been summarized many times. The book has been translated into European, Hebrew and Persian languages and it has been reprinted frequently.

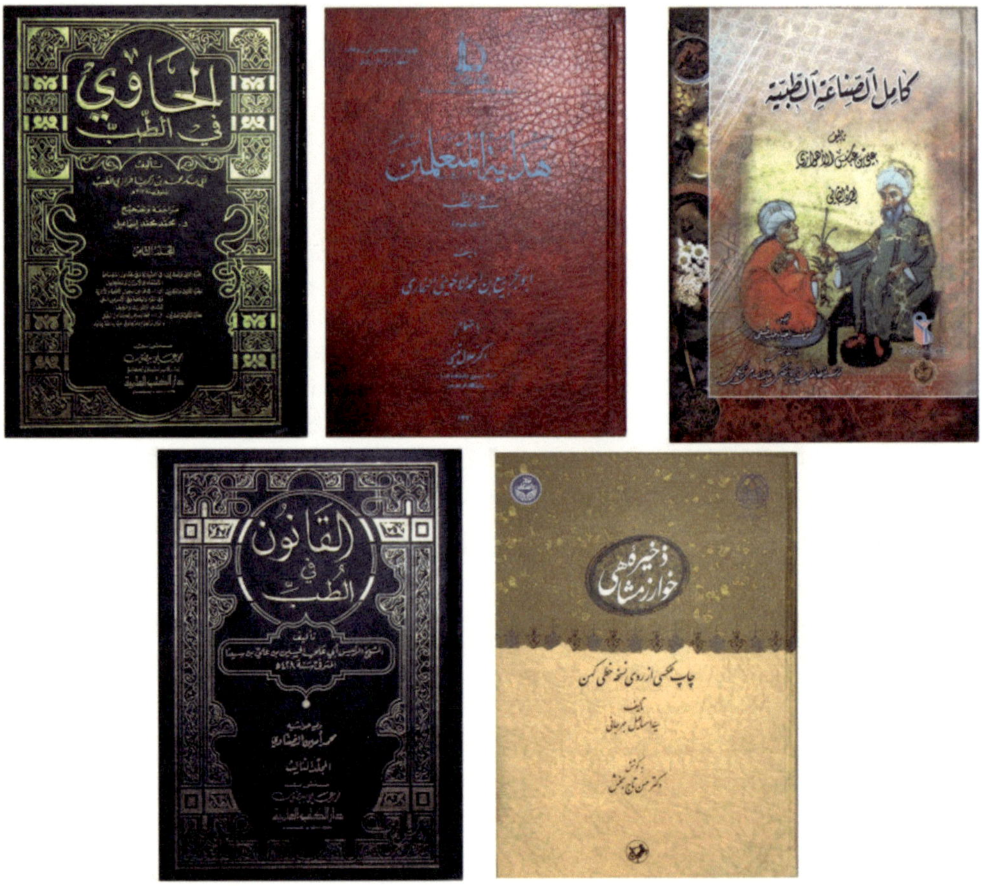

Figure 1. Cover image of main ancient Islamic Iranian traditional medicine books discussed in the present article. From left to right: al-Hawi fi al-Tibb, Hidayat-al-Muta'allimin fi al-Tibbe, Kamel al-Sina'ah al-Tibbiyah (upper row), and al-Qanun fi al-Tibb and Zakhireh Khaarazmshahi (lower row).

Avicenna has assigned a chapter of Canon to cancer [11]. From his point of view, cancer is a kind of black bile swelling, which is caused by the black bile resulting from burning of the yellow bile. After mentioning differential characteristics of cancer and scirrhus, he adds that cancer frequently affects hollow organs and for this reason, its prevalence is higher among

http://dx.doi.org/10.5772/55249

females. Highly innervated organs are more prone to cancer. At early stages, cancer growth is covert and latent. After progression, treatment of cancer would be difficult. Initially, cancer is the size of a broad bean or smaller, hard, spherical, dark and slightly warm. Some types of cancer are accompanied by severe pain, while others have mild pain, and some are painless. Some cancers are prone to ulceration but in some cases, ulcerative cancer could become non-ulcerative. In some occasions, manipulation of a tumor may lead to its ulceration. Naming of this disease as cancer (crab) might be due to the similarity between the shape of a cancerous tumor affecting an organ and a crab with its prey. The appellation may be also due to the sphericity and darkness of tumor and origination of vessels from its surroundings which resembles crab's feet.

An important point in the treatment of cancer is that the progression and ulceration of cancerous tumor should be prevented as far as possible. Although some types of cancer could be treated during early stages of development, there is no possibility for the treatment of advanced cancers. In most occasions, cancer grows in viscera in a latent manner. In these cases, as Hippocrates mentions, its irritation should be strictly avoided as it might lead to death. In contrast, when left untreated, the patient would have a longer life, especially if appropriate foods such as beer, soft-boiled egg yolk, and small river fishes are consumed.

When the cancerous tumor is small, its cutting is possible. If so, the tumor should be eradicated and some parts of adjacent normal tissues should also be excised in order to cut all tumor-feeding vessels. After cutting the cancerous tumor, bleeding should be allowed until large blood volumes come out of the body. Of course, purgation and venesection should have already been performed to cleanse the body from carcinogenic substances. Body cleansing should be performed by using proper foods (from both qualitative and quantitative aspects) in order to prepare the organ for cutting. In some occasions, it may be necessary to cauterize the scar. However, if the cancerous tumor has come close to sensitive and vital organs, cauterization may be very dangerous. It has been quoted that a physician excised the cancerous breast of a woman but after a short time, her other breast became cancerous. For the purpose of purgation, either the mixture of dodder (18.75 g) and cheese whey or honey syrup, or decoction of dodder in oxymel should be administered once every few days. If the patient has good stamina, potion of black hellebore could be administered.

Administration of topical anti-cancer drugs is performed to achieve the following 4 goals: 1. Complete eradication of cancer. This goal is very difficult to achieve; 2. Preventing growth and progression of cancer; 3. Preventing ulceration of the cancerous tumor; and 4. Treatment of cancerous wounds.

Drugs that are used for the eradication of cancer should be able to lyse the carcinogen and facilitate excretion of the lysed carcinogen present in the cancerous organ. These drugs should not be strong or irritant because strong drugs increase cancer's malignancy. Another requisite for these drugs is lack of caustic and irritant effects and lack of caustic taste. From the above points, it appears that washed mineral drugs are the best option. An example is washed zinc oxide mixed with oils such as *Cheiranthus cheiri* L. oil. In order to prevent growth and progression of cancer, the drug should reach the tumor's body. On the other hand, modification of food and organ strengthening should be performed to prevent cancer progression. For this latter purpose, topical application of the following drugs is very beneficial: powdered grinding stone or knife grinder stone, liquid obtained from pulverization of lead in rose oil or coriander juice, and salving with unripe grape powder. Drugs that are administered for the prevention of tumor ulceration are also effective in halting tumor progression provided that they do not cause irritation. These drugs are especially effective if administered in combination with the liquid obtained from lead pulverization. The aforementioned drugs include sealing clay, red Armenian bole, unripe olive oil, common houseleek juice, basic carbonate of lead with *L. sativa* extract and psyllium (*Plantago psyllium* L.) mucilage. Another drug for this purpose, which is among the best ones, is the poultice prepared from mashed fresh caught river crab especially with litharge of gold or silver. Treatment methods that are employed for the healing of cancerous wounds include: 1. Dressing with a cotton cloth soaked in black nightshade juice. When dried, the cloth should be moistened with the mentioned water; 2. A mixture of wheat kernel (3.34 g), frankincense (3.34 g), basic carbonate of lead (3.34 g), sealing clay (6.68 g), red Armenian bole (6.68 g), and washed aloe solid extract (6.68 g) should be prepared and pulverized. If the cancerous wound is wet, the powder should be sprinkled but if the wound is dry, the powder should be mixed with rose oil and converted to balm before application. Topical application of the mixture prepared from crab ash and ghiroty (mixture of wax and rose oil) is also useful. Likewise, topical application of drug prepared from washed zinc oxide and *P. oleracea* water (or *P. psyllium*) is beneficial.

6. Jorjani

Jorjani wrote valuable books in medicine during his lifetime. His biggest treasure is the detailed book of Zakhireh Khaarazmshahi (Treasure of Khaarazmshah) (Figure 1). Zakhireh is the most important medical book in Persian. The book contains nine main books and two appendices on simple and compound drugs.

The first book of Zakhireh is about medical science, identifying types of humors and temperaments, and also general aspects of anatomy.

The second book discusses health and diseases and also types of pulses, sweating, urine and feces.

The third book includes a complete course on maintaining health.

The forth book is allocated to ways of diagnosing disease and disease duration.

The fifth book is on identifying different types of fevers and methods to cure them.

The sixth book is assigned to methods of curing diseases cap a pie.

The seventh book describes types of inflammation, wounds, and fractures, and the ways to treat them.

The eighth book includes cosmetics and beautification.

http://dx.doi.org/10.5772/55249

The ninth book is assigned to types of poisons, antidotes, bites, venerations, and their treatments.

The final section explains simple and compound drugs in detail.

In fact, the mentioned book is an encyclopaedia fraught with pure Persian medico- pharmaceutical terms. Zakhireh is also noticeable in literary.

The complete text of Zakhireh was photo-printed in 1976 by the Iranian Culture Foundation. Some of the book volumes were published incompletely. Due to its importance, Zakhireh was translated into Hebrew and Turkish.

Jorjani wrote a summary of the Zakhireh named al-Aqraz al-Tibbiah wa al-Mabaheth al-Alaiah (Medical Goals and Alaaiyeh's Discussions). This collection contains five books. The first offers an introduction to medicine, the second book is about public health, the third one discusses disease treatment cap-a-pie, the forth book comprises simple drugs and finally the fifth book is assigned to evaluation of compound drugs. The photo-print of al-Aqraz al- Tibbiah was published in 1966 by the Iranian Culture Foundation. Fortunately, this book was edited by Professor H. Tadjbakhsh and published by Tehran University press in 2006.

The third book of Jorjani in medicine is named "Khofi Alaii" (Alaaii's hidden book), which is an abbreviated medical text and has two parts. The first part includes the theoretical aspects of medicine and has two articles. The second is a scientific medical knowledge and comprises seven articles. The book was lithographed in Kanpur in India in 1891. It was also published with valuable footnotes and descriptions by Etela'at Institute located in Tehran.

The forth book of Jorjani namely "Yadegar" (The Keepsake) is an extract text and codified in five parts. The first part has 17 chapters, the second includes 30 chapters, the third contains 2 chapters, the forth is comprised of 11 chapters and finally the fifth is inclusive of 3 chapters. Yadegar was edited by Professor M. Mohaghegh and published by the Institute of Islamic Studies in Tehran in 2003.

One of Jorjani's essays is "Zobdat al-Tibb" (Selected Topics in Medicine). The book was written in Arabic, and its context was ordered in numerous tables. This book has not been printed yet [3, 4, 6, 7].

Jorjani has assigned part of Zakhireh to cancer [12]. In his point of view, cancer is a kind of black bile swelling which is, unlike scirrhus, accompanied by pain, pulsation, inflammation and angiogenesis. These characteristics could be applied for the differential diagnosis of cancer from scirrhus. In addition, vessels of cancerous tissue have a dark green color. Cancer is frequently formed in soft and porous organs and for this reason, it mainly affects breast and innervated organs (such as uterus) in females, and throat, larynx, testicles and penis in males. Intestine is another organ which is prone to cancer. Diagnosis of cancer in the early stages is difficult. On the other hand, upon progression and appearance of clinical manifestations, treatment of cancer would be difficult. Cancerous tumor is initially hard, dark colored, slightly warm and in the size of a broad bean or smaller. In some cases, cancer is accompanied by severe or mild pain. Some cancerous tumors are easily ulcerated but some other are not. In some occasions, application of appropriate drugs would prevent the ulceration of susceptible tumors. In contrast, some cancerous tumors that are not prone to ulceration would be ulcerated following the administration of some drugs.

Jorjani has mentioned that stabilization and prevention of cancer progression should be attempted. In addition, ulceration of cancerous tumor should also be avoided. If treatment is started during early stages of cancer development, recovery is possible but advanced cancers are not treatable. In most cases, development and progression of cancer in visceral organs is a gradual process. For such cases, manipulation and treatment of tumor should be avoided as these may cause irritation and progression of the disease and eventually lead to the shortening of the patient's life. Conversely, lack of manipulation, using appropriate diets and timely evacuation would increase the longevity of patients. For these patients, foods like beer, almond oil, soft-boiled egg yolk, vetch (*Phaseolus mungo* L.), spinach (*Spinacia oleracea* L.), and pumpkin are administered. In cases with high temperature, administration of fresh cow's dough (prepared after isolation of butter) is beneficial. Such dough should be consumed before becoming sour. In some occasions, small cancerous tumors which are distant from vital organs may be removed via surgery. If so, the tumor should be cut from its origin and some parts of adjacent normal tissues should be cut as well. In addition, bleeding should be allowed until large blood volumes come out. Afterwards, the injured site should be salved. In some cases, the organ is cauterized after cutting the tumor. It must be noted that cutting the tumor may be perilous in the majority of cases.

To treat the aforementioned complication, the body must first be cleansed from black bile. For this purpose, 13.36 g of dodder in cheese whey or honey syrup is administered once every few days. Among mineral drugs, washed zinc oxide is beneficial especially if rubbed with rose oil on the tumor. Likewise, rubbing the liquid obtained from pulverization of lead pieces in chicory juice, coriander juice or lettuce extract on tumor could prevent its enlargement and ulceration. Other useful medications include poultices of basic lead carbonate, aloe, red Armenian bole, sealing clay, common houseleek extract and ispaghula mucilage.

In another part (PP. 562-563) of his book, Jorjani has explained the signs and treatment methods of uterine cancer as well as effective drugs against this type of cancer.

7. Conclusions

The common point of all assessed books in the present review is the pivotal role of black bile in the development of cancer. Therefore, all listed physicians have insisted on the prominent impact of black bile purgatives in cancer therapy. All evaluated medical books implied that in case of advanced cancers with progression (metastasis) to other tissues, organectomy is the only therapeutic measure, followed by eradication of all cancer roots and adjacent vessels. Finally, all physicians mentioned in the present review consistently relied on the use of herbal medicine for the treatment of cancer or halting its progression (Table 1). It is greatly recommended that further research be undertaken to explore the contents of modern scientific literature on the ant-cancer properties of medicinal plants mentioned in the major books of Islamic traditional medicine (Figure 2).

Scientific name	Arabic common name	English common name	Family	Application
Aloe spp.	Sabr	Aloe	Liliaceae	Healing of cancerous wounds
Althaea officinalis L.	Khatmi	Marsh-mallow	Malvaceae	Healing of tumor injury
Amaranthus blitum L.	al-Baghlah al-yamaanieh	Blite	Amaranthaceae	Black bile purgative; healing of tumor injury
Anethum gravolens L.	Shabath	Dill	Apiaceae	Newly developed cancers
Arum dracunculus L.	al-Luff	Dragon wort	Araceae	treatment of chronic cancers
Boswellia carteri Birdew.	Kondor	Frankincense	Burseraceae	Healing of cancerous wounds
Brassica oleracea L.	al-Karnab al-nabti	Cabbage	Brassicaceae	treatment of cancer
Cheirantus cheiri L.	al-Khiri	Aegean wallflower	Brassicaceae	Facilitating lysis and excretion of carcinogen
Chenopodium album L.	al-Sarmagh	Squarters goosefoot	Chenopodiaceae	Cancer treatment or halting its progression
Cicer arientium L.	al-Hems	Pea	Fabaceae	Healing of cancerous wounds
Cichorium intybus L.	al-Hindeba	Chicory	Asteraceae	ulcerative, pulsating and warm cancers; cleansing the body from black bile
Cinnamomum camphora (L.) T.Nees & C.H.Eberm.	Kafur	Camphor	Luraceae	Healing of tumor injury
Cinnamomum cassia (L.) J.Presl	Salikhah	Cassia	Luraceae	Healing of corrosive cancerous wounds
Coriandrum sativum L.	al-Kozborah	Coriander	Apiaceae	Healing of tumor injury
Cucurbita pepo L.	al-Ghara	Pumpkin	Cucurbitaceae	Cancer treatment or halting its progression; black bile purgative; increasing the longevity of cancer patients
Cupressus sempervirens L.	al-Sarve	Mediterranean cypress	Cupressaceae	Healing of corrosive cancerous wounds
Cuscuta epithymum Murr.	al-Afthimoon	Clover dodder	Cuscutaceae	Boosting organ's function and black bile removal
Eruca sativa Mill.	al-Jerjir	Rocket	Brassicaceae	non-ulcerative cancers
Erysimum officinale L.	Arisimun	Hedge mustard	Brassicaceae	Non-ulcerative cancer
Gundelia tournefortii L.	al-Kankarzad	Gundelia	Asteraceae	Treatment of cancerous swellings
Helleborus niger L.	Kharbagh aswad	Black hellebore	Ranunculaceae	Cleansing the body from black bile
Juglans regia L.	al-Jaws	Walnut	Juglandaceae	Ulcerative melatonic swellings
Latuca sativa L.	al-Khas	Lettuce	Asteraceae	Halting tumor progression; healing of cancerous wounds

Scientific name	Arabic common name	English common name	Family	Application
Lavandula stoechas L.	Ostokhodoos	French lavender	Lamiaceae	Cleansing the body from black bile
Lepidium sativum L.	al-Hurf	Garden cress	Brassicaceae	Indurated swellings of breasts and testicles
Linum usitatissimum L.	al-Kataan	Flax	Linaceae	Treatment of cancerous swellings
Malva rotundifolia L.	al-Khabaazi al-bostani	Dwarf mallow	Malvaceae	Healing of cancerous wounds
Matthiola incana (L.) W.T.Aiton	al-Tudari	Hoary stock	Brassicaceae	non-ulcerative cancers
Phaseolus mungo L.	Maash	Vetch	Fabaceae	Increasing the longevity of cancer patients
Physalis alkekengi L.	al-Kakenj	Bladder cherry	Solanaceae	Cleansing the body from black bile
Plantago ispaghula Roxb.	Isphaghul	Ispaghula	Plantaginaceae	Prevention of the progression and injury of the tumor
Plantago major L.	Lesaan al-hamal	Common plantain	Plantaginaceae	treatment of cancer
Plantago psyllium L.	Bazr ghatunaa	Psyllium	Plantaginaceae	Halting tumor progression; healing of cancerous wounds
Platanus orientalis L.	al-Dolab	Oriental plane tree	Plantanaceae	Healing of cancerous wounds
Polypodium vulgare L.	Basfaayaj	Common polypody	Polypodiaceae	Cleansing the body from black bile
Polyporus officinalis Fries	al-Ghaarighoon	White agaric	Polyporaceae	Black bile purgative
Portulaca oleracea L.	al-Baghlah al-hamghaa	Purslane	Portulaceae	Treatment of corrosive cancers; healing of cancerous wounds
Rhus coriaria L.	al-Sumaagh	Sumac	Anacardiaceae	Treatment of corrosive cancers; healing of cancerous wounds
Salix caprea L.	al-Khalaf	Goat willow	Salicaceae	Healing of cancerous wounds
Sempervivum tectorum L.	Hay al-aalam	Common houseleek	Crassulaceae	Halting tumor progression; healing of cancerous wounds
Solanum nigrum L.	Enab al-thaalab	Black nightshade	Solanaceae	Healing of cancerous wounds; cleansing the body from black bile; healing of tumor injury
Spinacia oleracea L.	Isphanakh	Spinach	Chenopodiaceae	Increasing the longevity of cancer patients
Terminalia chebula Retz.	Halilaj aswad	Black myrobalan	Combretaceae	Cleansing the body from black bile
Urtica dioica L.	al-Anjarah	Nettle	Urticaceae	Corrosive cancers

Table 1. List of medicinal plants mentioned in the current review for the treatment of cancer and its complications.

http://dx.doi.org/10.5772/55249

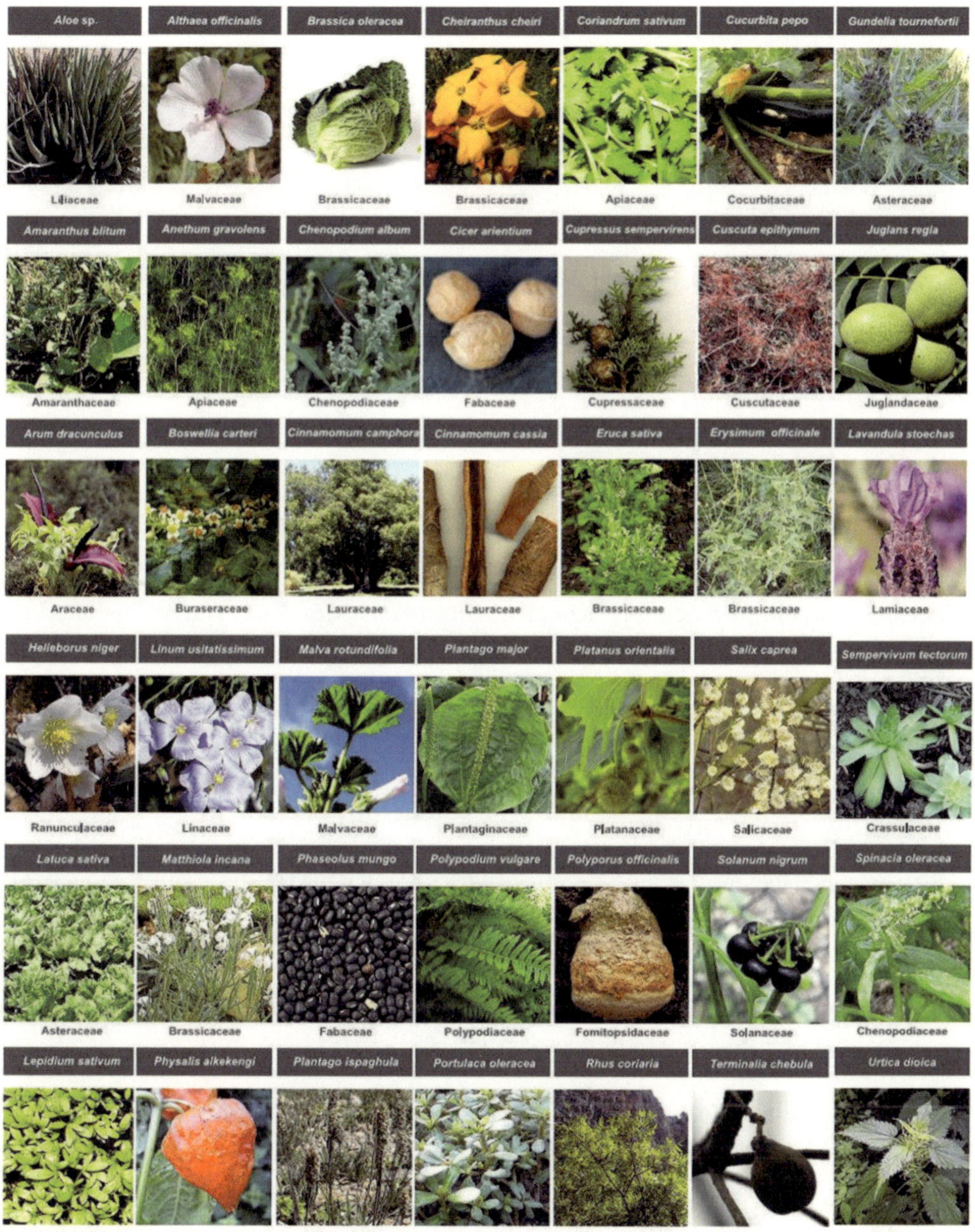

Figure 2. Figurative list of medicinal plants mentioned in this chapter. Reproduced from Wikipedia

Acknowledgements

The authors are thankful to Mr. Mohammad Naseri for his kind assistance in the preparation of pictures used in this chapter.

Author details

Amirhossein Sahebkar[1], Nilufar Tayarani-Najaran[2], Zahra Tayarani-Najaran[3] and Seyed Ahmad Emami[4*]

*Address all correspondence to: emamia@mums.ac.ir or saemami@gmail.com

1 Biotechnology Research Center and School of Pharmacy, Mashhad University of Medical Sciences, Mashhad, Iran

2 Department of Dental Prosthesis, School of Dentistry, Mashhad, University of Medical Sciences, Mashhad, Iran

3 Department of Pharmacodynamics and Toxicology, School of Pharmacy, Mashhad University of Medical Sciences, Mashhad, Iran

4 Department of Pharmacognosy, School of Pharmacy, Mashhad, University of Medical Sciences, Mashhad, Iran

References

[1] Mosaddegh M, Naghibi F. Iran's traditional medicine, past and present. In: Traditional medicine and material medica. Mosaddegh M, Naghibi F (eds). Sara Publication, Tehran, Iran, 2002; p. 19.

[2] Ibn Abi OSsaybiah AQ. Oyun al-Anba fi Tabaqat al-Atebba (The Sources of News on the Classification of the Physicians) (in Arabic). Oyun al-Soud MB, ed. Dar al-Kotob al-Ilmiyah, 1998; pp.294–295, 379–392, 401–421.

[3] Nadjmabadi M. Mohammad ibn Zakarya Razi, Iranian Physician, Chemist and Philosopher (in Persian). Razi University Publications, 1992.

[4] Nadjmabadi M. History of Medicine in Iran During the lslamic Era (in Persian). Tehran University Publications, 1995; pp. 324–640, 719–742.

[5] Safa Z. History of Rational Sciences in lslamic Civilization (in Persian). Vol. 1. Tehran University Publications, 1997; pp.165–179, 206–271.

[6] Tadjbakhsh H. History of Veterinary Medicine and Medicine of Iran (in Persian). Vol. 2. Tehran University Publications, 2001; pp. 284 –295, 301–312, 317–332.

[7] Tadjbakhsh H. History of Human and Veterinary Medicine in Iran.Fondation Merieux, 2003; pp. 127–135, 139, 145–156, 162–174.

[8] Razi MZ. Al-Hawi fi al-Tibb (Continens) (in Arabic). Abdul Muid Khan, ed. Vol. 12. Osmania Oriental Publications Bureau, 1962; pp. 1–25.

[9] Akhaweyni Bukhaari RA. Hidayat-al-Muta'allimin fi al-Tibbe (An Educational Guide for Medical Students) (in Persian). Matini J, ed., 2nd ed. Ferdowsi University press, 1992; pp. 606–607.

[10] Ahwazi Arjani AA. Kamel al-Sina'ah al-Tibbiyah (The Perfect Art of the Medicine) (in Arabic). Al-Dassuqi, I, ed. Vol. 2.,, Saadat Press, 1877; pp. 190–191.

[11] Ibn Sina HA. Al-Qanun fi al-Tibb (The Canon of Medicine) (in Arabic). Vol. 4. Jamia Hamdard, 1998; pp.195–197.

[12] Jorjani SI. Zakhireh Khaarazmshahi (Treasure of Khaarazmshah) (in Persian). edited by A.A. Saeedi Sirjani,, The lranian Culture Foundation, Tehran, 1977 (photoprint of the manuscript dated 1206 A.D.); pp. 585–586..

Chapter 2

The Cultural Perceptions, Folk Taxonomies and the Relationship with Alternative Medicine Practices Among Hong Kong People

Judy Yuen-man Siu

Additional information is available at the end of the chapter

http://dx.doi.org/10.5772/53281

1. Introduction

Alternative medicine is often embedded in a society's social and cultural beliefs. Every society has its unique social and cultural belief system in health and diseases, and this can influence how people understand and classify diseases. Such classification system embedded in local social and cultural system is referred as folk taxonomy in anthropological terms as suggested by Emile Durkheim in 1912, and this classification is often based on people's own cultural belief system rather than scientific knowledge. Folk taxonomy is noted as a form of ethnoscience, which "refers to system of classification that people construct to organize knowledge of their universe... Such systems are based on taxonomic hierarchies in which some entities are ordered hierarchically…and other entities are contrasted taxonomically" [1]. Understanding the folk taxonomies of diseases will be another important approach in understanding people's therapeutic approach(es), since their cultural understandings on diseases can be crucial in influencing their choices of remedy. As Kleinman (1980) stated,

> Since beliefs about illness are always closely linked to specific therapeutic interventions and thus are systems of knowledge and action, they cannot be understood apart from their use.

> Beliefs about illness, the central cognitive structure of every health care system, are closely tied to beliefs about treatment. Thus, ideas about the cause of illness (as well as its pathophysiology and course) are linked to ideas about practical treatment interventions. Part of medicine's therapeutic mandate is that sickness beliefs organize health care seeking choices and treatment interventions [2].

The motivations for seeking alternative medicine for therapy are many, and they are never simple. As treatment decision is closely related to the cultural beliefs about illnesses and diseases, hence Kleinman (1980) argued that a structural analysis of the cultural understandings and classification of diseases, ie. folk taxonomy of diseases, can enable the understanding of people's motivations in practicing alternative medicine. "Medical anthropologists have shown that the application of values to types of illness has an important influence upon the decisions people make in responding to particular episodes of sickness" [2].

Hong Kong is a medical pluralistic society. Alongside the mainstream medical system of biomedicine, other alternative medical systems such as traditional Chinese medicine, *qigong* (氣功) and *tai chi* (太極) co-exist. Many personal, social, and cultural forces intertwine together in influencing people's choice of remedy. Besides the perceptions on different medical systems and the illness experiences during the therapeutic process [3], the underlying cultural perceptions on diseases also explain why people turn to alternative medicine such as *qigong* and *tai chi* for remedy in Hong Kong. In other words, people's *qigong* and *tai chi* practice can be influenced by their underlying cultural health and disease beliefs, which are reflected in their folk classification of diseases. In this chapter, I therefore sought to construct a folk taxonomy of diseases of my research participants in order to understand their underlying motivation in *qigong* and *tai chi* practice.

1.2. *Qigong* and *tai chi* in Hong Kong

Qigong and *tai chi* are common alternative medicine practice in Hong Kong. According to Hong Kong Tai Chi Association, more than 300,000 people were practicing in morning *tai chi* classes in 2001 [4]. Presumably there are more than 300,000 *qigong* followers in Hong Kong after a decade now as many other followers practice outside these morning classes. Not only do *qigong* practitioners aim at reaching the balance of *qi*, the maintenance of health, and life prolongation through the practice, but *qigong* practice itself has also become a popular remedy among patients who receive biomedical treatment. Some patients' resource centres in biomedical hospitals also provide *qigong* classes for their patients.

Little literature has provided a clear definition of *qigong*. As Dong (1990) stated, "[*q*]*igong* is an ancient Chinese system of 'breathing' or 'vital energy' mind control exercises" [5]. Generally, most people would describe *qigong* as a form of "breathing exercise".

Two categories of *qigong*, hard *qigong* and soft *qigong*, can be identified according to literature. Hard *qigong* is considered as a kind of martial arts. Breaking steel rods, splitting bricks by hand, and resisting attacks by assailants with weapons are common representations of hard *qigong*. Soft *qigong* is mainly for health maintenance purpose [5]. As this chapter concerns the role of *qigong* as alternative medicine and its relation with cultural beliefs, soft *qigong* is the focus of this chapter.

Four major traditions are noted within the category of soft *qigong* according to literature. The first tradition is Taoist *qigong*, which emphasizes the training of body and mind and focuses on the relationship between the individual and the cosmic environment. Prolongation of life expectancy is a key focus of this tradition. The second tradition is Buddhist *qigong*,

http://dx.doi.org/10.5772/53281

emphasizing the cultivation of mind and moral will and aiming at escaping from "hard life". The third follows the Confucian tradition, emphasizing on the setting of the conceptual mind, righteousness, honesty of higher thought, and altruism, and the obtaining of rest, steadiness, and tranquility. The fourth tradition is medical *qigong*, which aims at the prevention and treatment of diseases, with the primary goal of health maintenance [5]. Although theoretically there are four traditions, the boundary of these traditions is not clear-cut in practice.

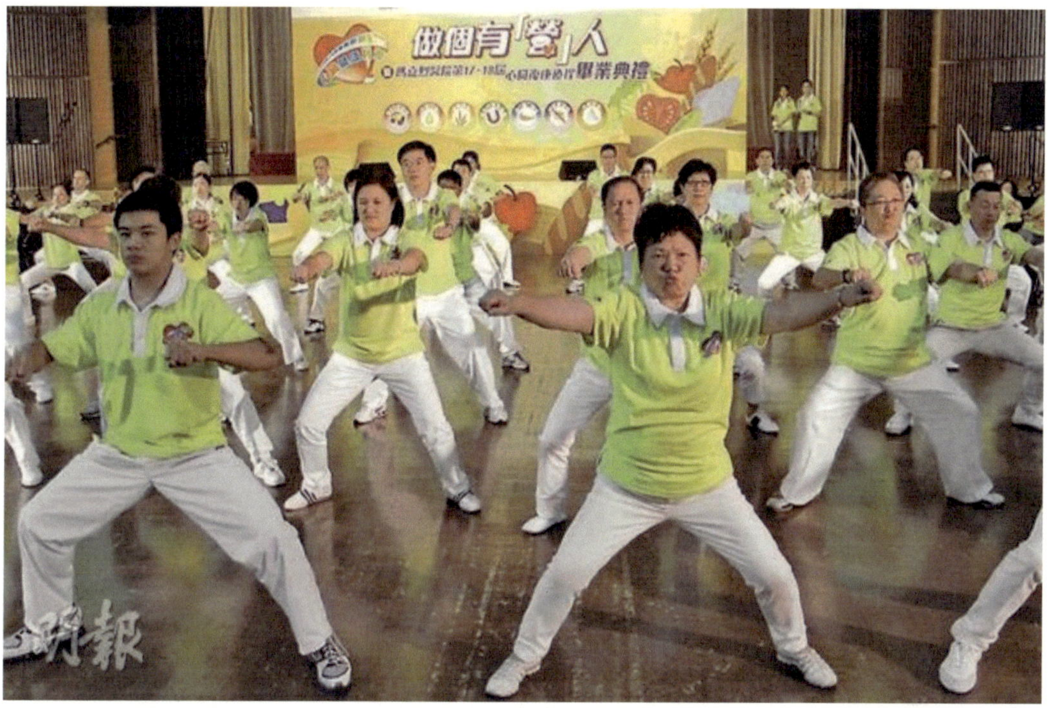

Figure 1. Heart disease patients practicing *tai chi* in a function of biomedical setting. (Photo courtesy by *Mingpao*)

Tai chi is another form of breathing exercise which falls into the category of soft *qigong*. Some people would refer it as a form of "active gong" (動功), since the practice of *tai chi* requires body movement; whereas *qigong* is often referred as "quiet gong" (靜功), since its practice mainly involves breathing and mind control as well as meditation. As Miura (1989) stated,

> Contrary to popular perception, *Qigong* is not a type of *Taiji quan*, but rather the other way around. *Taiji quan* seems to have developed through combinations of various *Qigong* styles with martial and longevity practices... They have certain basic features in common: martially inspired exercises, abdominal respiration, relaxation, and the collection of energy in the lower cinnabar field [6].

As there are different traditions of *qigong* practice, therefore the way of practice is varied. There is no single method of practice. However, health maintenance is the ultimate goal for all *qigong* traditions. Its practice emphasizes on the balance of *qi*, or the cosmic force within body, to achieve health. In traditional Chinese medicine concept, the balance of *qi* within human body is important for good health. *Qigong* practice emphasizes the attention on breathing and a relaxation of mind. Through attaining a peaceful mind in the practice, a balance of *qi*, and thus health, can be restored.

1.3. History of *qigong* development as alternative medicine in Hong Kong

In Hong Kong, the practice of "active gong" – *tai chi* – is more easily visible than the practice of "quiet gong" – *qigong*. However, this does not necessarily indicate there are more *tai chi* followers than *qigong* followers. As the practice of *tai chi* requires more space than the practice of *qigong*, the practice of *tai chi* often takes place in outdoor areas such as parks. On the other hand, as the practice of "quiet gong" – *qigong* – requires a high state of calmness and tranquility, it often takes place indoors. Hence, people are more aware of the practice of *tai chi* than the practice of *qigong* in Hong Kong.

The term *qigong* first emerged in 1949 in Mainland China,

> it was only after 1949 that *qigong* became a generally-used term in Chinese medical, scientific and popular discourse, including in a single category all Chinese gymnastic, meditation, visualization and breathing techniques, to which, over the years, were added martial, performance, trance, divination, charismatic healing, and talismanic techniques, as well as the study of paranormal phenomena… [7].

In accordance with the four traditions, *tai chi* comes from the Taoist tradition of *qigong* practice. The emergence of *tai chi* is closely related to Taoist priests. As they lived in remote hilly areas with poor transportation and medical facilities, they developed the practice of martial arts in order to strengthen their health and resist against potential attacks of wild animals. These Taoist priests pioneered the practice of *tai chi* [8].

The founder of *tai chi* is Zhang San-feng (張三豐), who was born after the Tang Dynasty China. The practice was then spread by Taoist priests. Master Cheng Tin-hung, who is the founder of the Hong Kong Tai Chi Association in 1972, is recorded as one of the pioneers who introduced *tai chi* in Hong Kong [8].

When *tai chi* first came to Hong Kong, it was more a martial arts tradition rather than for potential use of health in the period between the 1940s and the 1970s. Only until late 1975 and early 1976 that *tai chi* came to a watershed for its development in Hong Kong. Due to the introduction of the official morning *tai chi* classes by the Leisure and Physical Education

http://dx.doi.org/10.5772/53281

Division of the Department of Education of the Hong Kong Government, *tai chi* started to become a health-oriented exercise. The morning *tai chi* classes provided an opportunity for the Hong Kong people to learn about *tai chi* as an alternative means for them to enhance their health.

In Mainland China, the transition from martial arts tradition to health orientation of *qigong* practice also occurred around the same time by the end of the 1970s. One of the most famous *qigong* practitioners in this orientation is Guo Lin (郭林), who was a self-healed cancer victim teaching *qigong* in Beijing since the early 1970s. Guo Lin's "New *Qigong* Therapy", hailed as a cure for cancer, quickly spread to all parts of China [7].

The health orientation of *qigong* and *tai chi* practice was further emphasized in 2003 Hong Kong, where the Severe Acute Respiratory Syndrome (SARS) outbreak hit Hong Kong from March to May 2003. The *tai chi* athlete Li Hui, for example, introduced a new *tai chi* style called "*qi* enhancing and lung nurturing gong" (益氣養肺功) at that time, which claimed to have particular benefits to the lungs. The outbreak of the SARS epidemic led to the sudden rise in the attendance rate and the number of new *qigong* and *tai chi* learners. The health orientation of *qigong* and *tai chi*, thus, has been fully demonstrated and established in Hong Kong.

2. Methods

To understand how the cultural perceptions of *qigong* followers influence their understanding and organization of knowledge on diseases and so their therapeutic choices, free listing and pile sort [9] were conducted in Hong Kong with 57 participants. Among these 57 participants, 4 *qigong* masters and 53 *qigong* followers were asked to do two parts of qualitative study. The first part was the free listing of diseases, and the second part was the pile sort on the seventy-two diseases in which they had free listed. These 57 participants, who had the experiences in *qigong* and/or *tai chi* practice, were sampled purposively to join this qualitative exercise. The study revealed the relationship between the folk taxonomy of diseases and their alternative medicine practice. These 57 participants age ranged from 32 to 60, and were engaging in *qigong* and/or *tai chi* practice at the time of study.

2.1. Free listing

The 57 participants were asked to free list all the diseases that they knew and/or have heard at the time of study. This was to ensure the selected seventy-two diseases could represent the range of diseases that the participants, and so the public to some extent, were familiar with. The seventy-two diseases mentioned by the participants and used in the pile sort were shown in Table 1.

Diseases free listed	Codes	Chinese Terms of Diseases (Names in brackets are layman usage in Cantonese Chinese)	Best Treatment Approach(es) as suggested by 57 participants		
			Biomedicine	Chinese medicine	*Qigong / tai chi*
AIDS	AIDS	愛滋病	57	57	57
Allergic Rhinitis	ALR	過敏性鼻炎 (鼻敏感)	32	30	49
Alzheimer's Disease	ALS	腦退化症（老人痴呆症）	57	0	18
Anaemia	ANA	貧血	40	57	57
Stroke	APO	中風	57	21	53
Appendicitis	APP	闌尾炎 (盲腸炎)	57	34	35
Arthritis	ART	關節炎	15	40	57
Asthma	AST	哮喘	50	48	54
Bone Cancer	BOC	骨癌	57	57	57
Brain Cancer	BRC	腦癌	57	57	57
Bronchitis	BRO	氣管炎	51	29	42
Cataract	CAT	白障	57	3	3
Cholera	CHO	霍亂	57	18	1
Chicken-Pox	CHP	水痘	40	42	11
Cirrhosis	CIR	肝硬化	57	53	43
Cold	COL	傷風	42	48	40
Constipation	CON	便秘	23	46	36
Cough	COU	咳嗽	34	45	31
Colon and Rectal Cancer	CRC	大腸癌	57	57	57
Cystitis	CYS	膀胱炎	48	39	22
Diabetes	DBT	糖尿病	57	48	48
Dengue Fever	DEF	登革熱	57	10	4
Diarrhea	DIR	腹瀉	38	31	12
Dizziness	DIZ	頭暈	24	41	40
Down's Syndrome	DOS	唐氏綜合症	57	0	5
Eczema	ECZ	濕疹	50	45	6
Emphysema	EMP	肺氣腫	52	32	48
Epilepsy	EPI	腦癇 (癲癇)	57	20	36
Fever	FEV	發燒	45	40	2
Gastric Bleeding	GAB	胃出血	57	24	12

Diseases free listed	Codes	Chinese Terms of Diseases (Names in brackets are layman usage in Cantonese Chinese)	Best Treatment Approach(es) as suggested by 57 participants		
			Biomedicine	Chinese medicine	*Qigong / tai chi*
Gastric Cancer	GAC	胃癌	57	57	57
Gastroenteritis	GAE	腸胃炎	51	46	12
Gastric Ulcer	GAU	胃潰瘍	57	31	32
German Measles	GEM	德國痲疹	57	30	1
Glaucoma	GLA	青光眼	57	2	1
Gout	GOU	痛風	41	48	52
Headache	HEA	頭痛	32	38	40
Liver Cancer	HEC	肝癌	57	57	57
Heart Disease	HED	心臟病	57	24	45
Hemorrhoid	HEM	痔瘡	48	38	21
Hepatitis	HEP	肝炎	51	43	34
Herpes	HER	疱疹	57	28	4
Hand, Foot, and Mouth Disease	HFM	手足口病	57	11	1
Hypertension	HYP	高血壓	57	34	57
Influenza	INF	流行性感冒	43	43	2
Renal Disease	KID	腎病	57	5	40
Leukemia	LEU	白血病 (血癌)	57	57	57
Lung Cancer	LUC	肺癌	57	57	57
Malaria	MAL	瘧疾	57	3	2
Measles	MEA	痲疹	31	49	21
Mental Illness	MEI	精神病	42	23	57
Meningitis	MEN	腦膜炎	57	1	0
Nasopharyngeal Cancer	NPC	鼻咽癌	57	57	57
Osteoporosis	OST	骨質疏鬆症	32	25	57
Otitis Media	OTI	中耳炎	57	30	1
Parkinson's Disease	PAS	柏金遜症	57	2	38
Pharyngitis	PHA	喉嚨發炎	41	40	13
Pneumonia	PNE	肺炎	57	13	34
Psoriasis	PSO	牛皮癬	48	42	20

Diseases free listed	Codes	Chinese Terms of Diseases (Names in brackets are layman usage in Cantonese Chinese)	Best Treatment Approach(es) as suggested by 57 participants		
			Biomedicine	Chinese medicine	*Qigong / tai chi*
Kidney Stones	REC	腎石	57	24	19
Rheumatism	RHE	風濕	49	52	57
Sinusitis	SIN	鼻竇炎	48	32	28
Systemic Lupus Erythematosus	SLE	紅斑狼瘡	57	41	43
Sore Throat	SOT	喉嚨痛	24	38	24
Bone Spurs	SPU	骨刺	35	51	57
Stomachache	STA	胃痛	48	40	35
Syphilis	SYP	梅毒	57	2	6
Tuberculosis	TB	肺結核 (肺癆)	57	30	35
Athlete's Foot	TIP	足蘚(香港)	57	38	2
Tonsillitis	TON	扁桃腺發炎	57	24	15
Urethritis	URE	尿道炎	44	37	8
Urticaria	URT	蕁痲疹 (風癩)	34	47	3

Table 1. The 72 Diseases free listed for the Pile Sort

2.2. Pile sort

After the free listing, the names of the mentioned seventy-two diseases were printed on a set of cards. The same set of 57 participants was asked to classify these seventy-two diseases into groups according to their own knowledge and classification criteria. They were asked to put those diseases which they thought to be similar together in the same pile. The therapeutic choices on these seventy-two diseases were also asked (Table 1). By doing this, it demonstrated not only the folk taxonomy of diseases of each participant, but also the relationship between the folk taxonomy of diseases and the therapeutic choices, as well as the practice of alternative medicine, among the participants in Hong Kong context. As the folk taxonomy of diseases reflects the underlying cultural perception of health and diseases, this experiment enabled the exploration of how close the relationship between the underlying cultural health and disease belief and the practice of *qigong* and *tai chi* is. The folk taxonomy of diseases and the therapeutic choices for these seventy-two diseases could provide part of the reasons why the participants attempted *qigong* and *tai chi* for certain diseases, but not others.

http://dx.doi.org/10.5772/53281

3. Results

3.1. What was shown from the free listing?

The free listing of diseases from the participants showed that the concept of "disease" could be varied. Some of the items listed by the participants were "symptoms" rather than "diseases" from the biomedical point of view. The participants perceived uncomfortable and abnormal feelings, or "symptoms" in the biomedical sense, as diseases, and their descriptions could be different from the biomedical explanations. The fact that some of the participants perceived "symptoms" and "discomforts" as diseases introduced a conceptual distinction between "illness" and "disease". Kleinman indicated that illness could include people's responses to symptoms, and they could perceive "symptoms" as "diseases" in this sense,

---

illness…means to conjure up the innately human experience of symptoms and suffering. Illness refers to how the sick person and the members of the family or wider social network perceive, live with, and respond to symptoms and disability…

Disease is the problem from the practitioner's perspective. In the narrow biological terms of the biomedical model, this means that disease is reconfigured *only* as an alteration in biological structure or functioning [10].

In many cases, the participants had already classified the diseases into groups in their free listing. They would free list the diseases together if they perceived them as having similar elements and nature.

The participants also tended to free list those diseases that caught their attention most and that they were most familiar with in the first instance. They started with the more serious and life-threatening diseases, such as cancers and heart disease. They then proceeded to free list those diseases that occur commonly and which they often experienced, such as cold and flu.

The free listing also features common diseases in a society, those which have been present for a long time as well as those which have recently emerged. Hand, foot, and mouth disease, for example, was a new disease common in kindergartens and widely reported in the media at the time of the study, hence it was mentioned frequently by the participants.

In addition, the free listing of diseases could be time- and/or environment-bound. As the free listing was conducted in summer, therefore those diseases that mainly occur in summer, such as cholera, were often mentioned. Presumably the results of the free listing would vary depending on time and context. The free listing could thus reflect the social and cultural environment of a society.

The diseases free listed by the participants not only reflected a culture's focus on disease, but also portrayed the institutional and social forces shaping the social beliefs and ideology on health and diseases of people. Female participants tended to free list more diseases than male participants. This could be related to their higher ratio in engaging domestic role in which they could have more time to learn about diseases from various media. The "women's television programmes" in the afternoon, in particular, could be a popular medium for housewives to learn about diseases that were of current concern. On the other hand, male participants were more reluctant to free list sexually-transmitted diseases and those diseases that were suffered by females exclusively.

The free listing gives a general picture of how people of a culture view diseases, and how the social, environmental, and institutional forces influence people's views on diseases. The free listing shows how people organize the knowledge of diseases, and the diseases in which a society is familiar with and concerns about. Therefore, free listing of diseases can reveal the difference between cultural belief system of "diseases" and biomedical point of view.

3.2. Folk taxonomies of diseases as mentioned by the participants

After the disease free listing, the participants were asked to do pile sort in which they were asked to classify the free listed diseases into groups. They were asked to put those diseases which they thought to be similar together in the same pile according to their own knowledge and understanding. The 57 pile sorts were analyzed by ANTHROPAC. A multidimensional scaling diagram of the 72 diseases was generated and constructed by ANTHROPAC according to the classification of the 57 participants (Figure 2). This showed how the participants classified diseases according to their own knowledge. Those diseases that were located closely together were perceived as similar by the participants.

Several clusters, ie. folk taxonomies, of diseases in Hong Kong context were illustrated from the multidimensional scaling diagram (Table 2). The folk taxonomies illustrated how the participants perceived and organized the knowledge of the free listed diseases. Those diseases in the same taxonomy were sharing similar nature and characteristics according to the participants.

Eight clusters were noted in participants' folk taxonomy of diseases.

Cluster	Diseases
1	Bone cancer, brain cancer, nasopharyngeal cancer, leukemia, colorectal cancer, gastric cancer, lung cancer, liver cancer, cirrhosis, renal disease, kidney stone, gallstone, hepatitis.
2	Cholera, malaria, Dengue Fever, Hand foot and mouth disease, German measles, measles, urticaria, psoriasis, eczema, chicken-pox, athlete's foot, syphilis, herpes.
3	Fever, cold, asthma, tuberculosis, allergic rhinitis, cough, influenza, sore throat, pharyngitis, otitis media, bronchitis, sinusitis, tonsillitis.
4	Appendicitis, hemorrhoid, cystitis, urethritis, gastric ulcer, gastric bleeding, pneumonia, emphysema.

http://dx.doi.org/10.5772/53281

Cluster	Diseases
5	Osteoporosis, spurs, rheumatism, gout, stroke, arthritis.
6	Glaucoma, cataract.
7	Parkinson's Disease, Alzheimer's Disease, Down's Syndrome, epilepsy, mental illness.
8	Systemic Lupus Erythematosus, meningitis, dizziness, headache.

Table 2. The folk taxonomies of diseases that are suggested by the participants

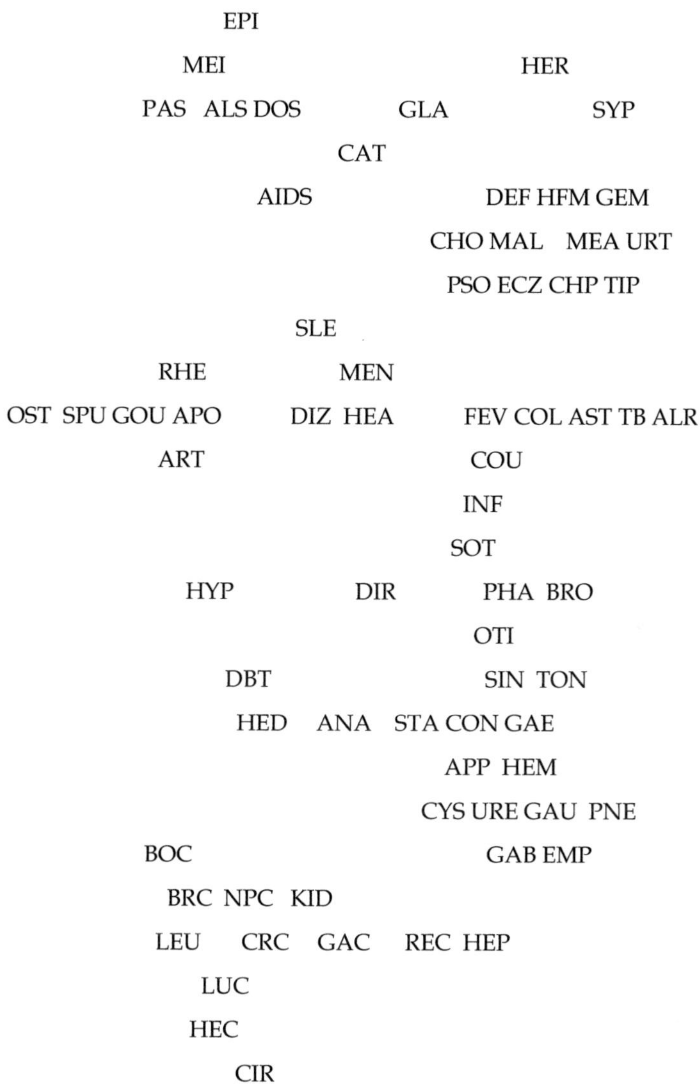

Figure 2. The Multidimensional Scaling Diagram of Diseases as classified by the participants

Cluster 1

This cluster consisted those diseases that were serious and life-threatening from the participants' point of view and those diseases that often required surgical treatment, such as cancers, kidney stones, and gallstones. On the other hand, the language of a culture also influenced the perceptions and cultural beliefs of people and the ways in which they classified diseases. Hepatitis was situated next to the gallstone in this cluster because, according to some participants, there was a Chinese slang expression which literally means "liver and gall bladder help and complement with each other" (肝膽相照). See the Sapir-Whorf Hypothesis, as recounted in Bonvillain (2000),

---

Some elements of language, for example, in vocabulary or grammatical systems, influence speakers' perceptions and can affect their attitudes and behavior… In fact, both Sapir and Whorf wavered in their statements on the issue of causal or directional relationship between language and thought [1].

Cluster 2

This cluster consisted infectious and contagious diseases from the participants' point of view. This mainly included dermatological diseases. All dermatological diseases were included in this cluster. Other infectious diseases that are not dermatological but with skin symptoms were also classified in this category. Some other infectious diseases such as cholera, malaria, and Dengue Fever were in this cluster as well. Such lay classification revealed the underlying perceptions of the participants on dermatological diseases as contagious (though not all of them were contagious), which were perceived as similar to those infectious diseases such as cholera, malaria, and Dengue Fever. On the other hand, the participants perceived some infectious diseases as dermatological, even though they are infectious in nature. For example, German measles, measles, and hand, foot and mouth disease are infectious in nature. However, because the symptoms of these diseases often appear on skin, this led the participants to have an impression that infectious diseases were similar to dermatological diseases.

The sexually-transmitted diseases, such as syphilis and herpes, were located closely to this cluster of infectious and dermatological diseases. Besides the contagious nature and the skin symptoms, the specialty classification in Hong Kong's biomedicine also played a role in influencing participants' perceptions, since both the sexually-transmitted diseases and dermatological diseases were under the same specialty – Dermatology and Venereology [11]. The biomedical institution thus constructed the disease perceptions of the participants. From the participants' viewpoints, the diseases in this cluster were infectious and contagious.

Cluster 3

This cluster consisted the diseases and symptoms of the upper and lower respiratory system, which were perceived as common for anyone to suffer. Again, the specialty classifica-

http://dx.doi.org/10.5772/53281

tion in Hong Kong's biomedicine played a role in influencing participants' perceptions in this group of diseases, as some participants indicated that most of the diseases in this cluster were under the specialty of otorhinolaryngology [11].

Cluster 4

This cluster mainly contained the diseases in relation to gastrointestinal and urological system. However, two diseases in relation to breathing system were also grouped in this category. In participants' terms, the diseases in this cluster were related to "internal organs".

Cluster 5

This cluster was made up of those diseases that were perceived as having a long-term impact on patients, or chronic diseases. This cluster mainly consisted bone and joint diseases. Some participants used age as a criterion in grouping these diseases together in the same category, having the impression that these diseases were mainly suffered by the elderly.

Cluster 6

This cluster consisted of ophthalmological diseases in participants' understanding. The diseases of glaucoma and cataract were usually straightforward to participants, since they often grouped these two diseases together in the same pile quickly.

Cluster 7

This cluster contained those diseases that were related to mind, nerve, and brain function, and the participants often had the impression that these diseases were chronic and incurable. Another feature noted in this cluster was that the participants often did not have much knowledge on these diseases, since many of these names were new and "foreign" to them.

Cluster 8

This cluster contained diseases in relation to head, though Systemic Lupus Erythematosus was located in this cluster as well. Some participants commented as Systemic Lupus Erythematosus has skin symptoms, especially in the area of face. Therefore, they grouped this disease under the category of "head".

The folk taxonomies of the seventy-two diseases showed how the participants organized and understood diseases by using their own cultural beliefs. From the multidimensional scaling diagram as shown in Figure 2, there were at least two scales at work regarding the nature of the diseases. On the first scale, the diseases perceived as life-threatening were located at one end, while the diseases perceived as infectious and contagious, and as chronic and incurable, were located at the other. In the second scale, the diseases perceived as chronic and long term were located at one end, and the diseases perceived as acute and short term were located at the other. Such scaling demonstrated when the participants made classifications, whether the diseases are life-threatening or not and whether they are acute or chronic were the subconscious force at work in their perceptions.

3.3. The interrelationship between the folk taxonomy of diseases and the choices of remedy

Cultural belief system affects how people organize their knowledge on diseases. In addition, common sense, lay perceptions, and illness and treatment experiences also influence people's decisions in choosing remedy. This section will examine the interrelationship between the folk taxonomy of diseases and the choice of therapies, and whether the same choice of therapies were to be used on the same clusters of diseases among the participants. The participants' choices on the therapeutic approaches provide a framework of the underlying reasons for their *qigong* and *tai chi* practice.

After the pile sorts, the participants were asked about their choice of therapies in dealing with those seventy-two diseases. They were asked to rank their choice of therapeutic approaches for suitability (Table 1). Their treatment decisions were to be compared with their folk taxonomy of diseases. Treatment choices are to be influenced by one's cultural beliefs. As Kleinman (1988) stated:

> local cultural orientations (the patterned ways that we have learned to think about and act in our life worlds and that replicate the social structure of those worlds) organize our conventional common sense about how to understand and treat illness; thus we can say of illness experience that it is always culturally shaped... Expectations about how to behave when ill also differ owing to our unique individual biographies [10].

An obvious interrelationship between the folk taxonomy and treatment choices was noted for cluster 1 diseases, which were perceived as life threatening and serious. As most of the diseases in this cluster were cancers that were life-threatening, all 57 participants had no hesitation in asserting that they would try all forms of remedies, including biomedicine, traditional Chinese medicine, *qigong, tai chi,* and even other folk remedies. All the participants except two would choose biomedicine first, and then traditional Chinese medicine and *qigong* as the complement. The participants had more confidence and trust in biomedicine to cope with the life-threatening diseases. They believed they would need biomedical investigation and treatment at the beginning stage. Once the diagnosis was confirmed, then they would seek traditional Chinese medicine and *qigong* afterwards as a complement.

Although the participants would use all the remedies they knew for life-threatening diseases, the acceptability of alternative medicine was much higher for cancers than for renal disease, kidney stones, and gallstones. Some participants even would try all sorts of alternative medicine for the treatment of cancers, no matter how "strange" the remedies were. However, participants tended not to search alternative remedies for renal disease, though a few would search for *qigong,* and then traditional Chinese medicine for treatment. As most participants recognized the necessity of adopting biomedical therapy such as dialysis (for renal disease) and surgery (for kidney stones and gallstones), they would only seek traditional Chinese medicine and *qigong* afterwards as a supplementary remedy. As participants per-

http://dx.doi.org/10.5772/53281

ceived cancers as more life-threatening and dangerous than renal disease, hence they were more motivated to search for other alternative medicine for remedy in cancers. Also, the known and established remedies of biomedicine in renal disease, kidney stones and gallstones explain why the participants tended to only attempt biomedicine for treatment.

Another cluster of disease which showed clear corelation between folk taxonomy and treatment choices was dermatological, sexually-transmitted, and infectious diseases. Most participants would first seek biomedicine for therapy for this cluster of diseases, and then some of them, especially those older ones, would use traditional Chinese medicine afterwards. The underlying Chinese cultural belief in health motivated these participants considering traditional Chinese medicine for remedy. In that case they would perceive their body suffered from "wet toxin" (濕毒). As this concept is embedded in traditional Chinese medicinal belief, therefore adopting the remedy with the same cultural medicinal belief would be perceived as a "sensible" solution for the participants. On the other hand, the participants believed biomedicine was the best remedy for contagious diseases. As contagious diseases were more "polluting" in both physical and cultural sense, participants would prefer the remedy that they were most confident. Also, biomedicine often gave an impression "quick" to the participants, therefore biomedicine was often attempted in order to get rid of such social labeling as soon as possible.

Social and cultural environment and gaze on certain groups of diseases also influenced participants' decision in remedies. As shown from the folk taxonomies in the multidimensional scaling diagram, dermatological diseases located closely to sexually-transmitted diseases. Sexually-transmitted diseases receive much stigmatization in Chinese culture. As dermatological diseases located closely to the cluster of sexually-transmitted diseases, which indicated these two types of diseases were similar from participants' viewpoint, presumably the participants would want to get rid of dermatological diseases in order to avoid being stigmatized. As biomedicine was perceived as giving a quick treatment, the participants were thus motivated to choose biomedicine in the first instance.

Age was another influential element in predicting how participants choose treatment approach. Same disease could be perceived differently by different age groups. Take inflammatory disease as an example, the treatment choices can be varied for different age groups. Younger participants were more under western cultural exposure so they were more motivated and ready in choosing biomedicine. Antibiotics were widely known by these young participants. In contrast, middle-aged and the elderly participants would prefer traditional Chinese medicine more as they were under more influence of Chinese culture. They believed many inflammatory diseases, and dermatological diseases, were induced by the "wet hot" (濕熱) and the toxins of the body, and the best way to deal with these bad forces was the use of traditional Chinese medicine in order to "clear the root".

Whether the disease itself has a cultural medicinal explanation would be remarkable in participants' choice of alternative medicine. If the disease had a cultural medicinal explanation, participants would be more motivated in using alternative medicine. As alternative medicine is embedded in a community's cultural belief, therefore using the same cultural medicinal approach is to be perceived as the most optimal approach. Just like "wet hot" and toxins is a Chinese cultural medicinal concept, hence these problems are believed to be best overcome by the Chinese approaches.

Another cluster which demonstrated a clear relationship between folk taxonomy and treatment choices were ophthalmological diseases. There was a strong preference in biomedical treatment among the participants in this category of diseases. As the biomedical treatment of ophthalmological diseases has long been established, hence the participants believed that only biomedicine and surgery could treat these diseases. Only a few older participants would attempt traditional Chinese medicine and *qigong* as a follow up treatment, since surgery was perceived as "hurt" to human body. Traditional Chinese medicine and *qigong* would be adopted only for rebuilding the body status after biomedical surgery according to these few participants.

Language influences how people think and perceive things. As demonstrated by the participants, the names of diseases could serve as an influential factor for determining suitable remedy. The participants tended to seek biomedical remedies for the cluster of brain, mind, and nerve diseases. As the names of the diseases, ie. Parkinson's Disease, Alzheimer's Disease, Down's Syndrome, in this cluster are "western" and "foreign" to them, they believed biomedicine was better in treating these "western" diseases. Another example was German Measles. All the participants would choose biomedicine as treatment for German Measles, though more participants would choose traditional Chinese medicine for ordinary measles instead.

Although gastrointestinal, urological, and lung diseases were in the same cluster according to the participants, treatment choices varied for these three groups of diseases. Participants preferred adopting biomedicine as the first line of treatment for the gastrointestinal and lung diseases, whereas they preferred traditional Chinese medicine in urological diseases such as cystitis and urethritis, and hemorrhoid, though younger participants would prefer biomedicine for urological diseases. For lung diseases, the acceptability of alternative medicine such as traditional Chinese medicine and *qigong* was higher for emphysema than for pneumonia. Since emphysema is a chronic lung disease, therefore the participants would search for alternative medicine as a complement. Pneumonia, on the other hand, is an acute disease, therefore biomedicine was still the first option for them.

Alternative medicine was shown to be popular in dealing chronic and long-term diseases, and the findings from the participants demonstrated the same picture. Traditional Chinese medicine and *qigong* were regarded as in a higher priority as treatment choice among the participants in managing chronic diseases.

Bone and joint diseases was another cluster which showed the strongest correlation between the folk taxonomy and alternative medicine practice as suggested by the participants. Most participants would choose *tai chi* in the first instance for this cluster of bone and joint diseases, since they recognized the weaknesses and experienced the limitations of biomedicine in managing bone and joint problems from their personal experiences. Besides practicing *tai chi*, acupuncture in traditional Chinese medicine was another popular treatment option as suggested by the participants, since acupuncture has a long history in dealing bone and joint diseases in Chinese society.

http://dx.doi.org/10.5772/53281

For the cluster of diseases that were more common and less serious, such as those in relation to upper respiratory tract infections, the acceptability of traditional Chinese medicine as a remedy was high among the participants. However, the interrelationship between the diseases in this cluster and the choice of remedy was rather weak. Some participants would choose biomedicine as first line for remedy on account of its fast relief and efficacy, while others would choose traditional Chinese medicine as first line treatment. But in general older participants tended to choose traditional Chinese medicine as the first option for these diseases. Only when they failed to experience the efficacy that they would then turn to biomedicine for treatment.

The above findings illustrate that the folk taxonomies of diseases are closely related to people's organization of disease knowledge and perceptions, which is often based on their cultural belief system. This influence their treatment choices and decisions to a certain extent. From the participants' choices of therapies and their explanations on their treatment decisions, they usually had their own interpretations on the best treatment for those diseases. These revealed how they perceived the strengths and weaknesses of biomedicine, traditional Chinese medicine, and *qigong* to a certain extent. These underlying perceptions served as the underlying motivations for the participants' practice of alternative medicine such as traditional Chinese medicine and *qigong*. The folk taxonomies of diseases and the treatment decisions showed that their alternative medicine practice was to be related to the perceived weaknesses of biomedicine and the perceived strengths of traditional Chinese medicine and *qigong* on managing different diseases.

From the participants, the folk taxonomy consisting the relatively more serious diseases such as the life threatening diseases, the contagious and dermatological diseases, and ophthalmological diseases, a remarkable correlation with biomedicine was observed. In contrast, for the folk taxonomy that consisted of the less serious diseases such as the non-life threatening chronic diseases and the bone and joint problems, a strong correlation with alternative medicine practice such as traditional Chinese medicine and *qigong* was noted. As Lupton (2000) stated, "[t]he more common and the less serious the illness, the more likely it is that lay theories of causation and treatment draw upon traditional folk-models of illness" [12]. Although apparent correlation was observed between some taxonomies of diseases and remedy preferences, such correlation was not applicable to all taxonomies. The cultural perceptions of a disease were still a more decisive factor in influencing the treatment choices of the participants. On the other hand, another point to be noted is the common belief among the participants that they could still practice alternative medicine, in particular *qigong*, in almost all kinds of health problems, since it could strengthen their health and alleviate the suffering without conflicting with other remedies and exerting any harm to the body.

4. *Qigong* practice and the Chinese philosophical teaching

As alternative medicine practice is embedded in a community's cultural belief system, therefore, the cultural values and ideal will be transmitted and reinforced through people's practice. Alternative medicine practice also conveys other symbolic meanings as discussed by Lupton (2000), particularly the aspects of virtue and goodness within the Chinese culture.

Other than traditional Chinese medicine, *qigong* is another popular alternative medicine in Hong Kong. The operating logic of *qigong* reaffirms Chinese philosophical ideas and teachings. As its followers are more concerned with the pragmatic and therapeutic value of *qigong*, its connections with Chinese philosophical teachings are under-emphasized in contemporary practice. Although these philosophical ideas and teachings are not the focus of the practice, they still feature in the lectures in some traditions of *qigong* practice. These lectures are closely tied to the Chinese cultural medical belief system, as well as the Chinese cultural beliefs and values.

In the lectures of a *qigong* class during fieldwork, the master often emphasized the importance of reaching a highly relaxed and tranquil state in order to achieve the "highest" state of the practice, ie. trance. In order to reach such a state, the followers ought to control their emotions and feelings by forgetting all happiness and unhappiness, and their social roles in the real world. They ought to imagine that they are relaxing in a quiet and beautiful environment.

The importance of reaching a highly tranquil state recalls the importance of the ancient Chinese teaching about controlling the "seven emotions" (七情) properly, linking this with health. The ancient Chinese teachings, particularly the Confucian ideas, emphasize that one should not expose one's emotions in a vigorous manner. The "seven emotions" include: happiness (喜), anger (怒), worry (憂), puzzle (思), sadness (愁), fright (驚), and fear (恐). If one expresses these emotions in a vigorous manner, one will fall short of the model of an ideal human. In the practice of *qigong*, it is believed that failure to control emotions or to express them in an inappropriate manner can be harmful to one's health. As one female informant who has recovered from cancer stated:

> In the past, I often felt unhappy and got angry easily. I was often annoyed with the staff. As I could not scold them, so I lost my temper to my family instead… Perhaps I expected too much on the job, so it exerted a lot of pressure on myself… I think these negative emotions accumulated to cause the disease. If I had known how to control my emotions and express them properly in the past, I would not need to suffer [from cancer]. The practice [of *qigong*] can let me learn how to control my emotions and attain calmness. I feel like I am having a rebirth in personality now.

Hence, not only does *qigong* practice affirm Chinese ideas of morality, virtue and goodness, but it also provides a sense of renewal for some participants. Such sense of renewal not only confines to the restoration of health, but which also includes a renewal in the psychological state of some participants.

Some *qigong* masters, thus, insisted that controlling emotions is the key in maintaining health, since a follower has to control emotion and keep calm so that he or she can achieve the "trance" state. Through the practice of *qigong*, not only can health be maintained or improved by emotional control, but the Chinese teachings of the ideal emotional expression – neutral expression of emotion – can also be reaffirmed.

The *qigong* practice, in addition, tries to reaffirm the importance of morality. As some masters indicated during lectures, since the practice requires appropriate control of emotional expression, there is a close relationship between the practice and the enhancement of morality. One *qigong* master indicated in his lecture:

Morality in contemporary society is a result of the control of laws, which aim at controlling one's behavior. It is very similar to *qigong*, since it emphasizes that a follower has to control himself or herself in a highly relaxed and tranquil state, so as to reach the "highest" [trance] state of the practice.

Some traditions of *qigong* also reaffirm the Chinese perception of the world and the cosmic order. The "five elements" (五行) – gold (金), wood (木), water (水), fire (火), and earth (土) – are the keys to achieving order and disorder. "Five element" should be in an appropriate order; otherwise, bad consequences can occur. Some traditions of *qigong* claim they can restore the order of the "five elements" within the human body in order to achieve health. The imbalance of the "five elements" within the human body can lead to diseases.

The practice of *qigong*, therefore, reaffirms the traditional Chinese moral teachings, the idea of cosmic order, and worldview. However, as the contemporary practice in Hong Kong focuses on its pragmatic usage to treat diseases and maintain health, its close relationship with the Chinese philosophical ideas is not emphasized. Anyway, the folk taxonomies of diseases among the participants are discussed, and the interrelationship between the folk taxonomies of diseases and the treatment options in Hong Kong context are examined in this chapter. All these have to do with the cultural belief system of a community, and the cultural backgrounds, traditions, and the personal experiences of people. The cultural understanding of diseases can thus provide another perspective on understanding alternative medicine practice.

5. Conclusion

As demonstrated in this chapter, a community's social and cultural belief system is remarkable in influencing people's understandings on diseases. This affects how they perceive and classify diseases, which can be reflected from the folk taxonomy of diseases. As folk taxonomy is a classification system embedded in a community's social and cultural beliefs, therefore each society has its own folk taxonomy of diseases. People's cultural perceptions on diseases can also influence how they choose remedy, whether biomedicine and/or alternative medicine should be adopted. Alternative medicine is mostly embedded in the cultural beliefs of a community, hence it is mostly used on those diseases which can fit with their cultural understandings. Also, biomedicine has its own weaknesses and limitations, therefore, alternative medicine is often used on those diseases which cannot be handled by biomedicine. This chapter demonstrates how people's cultural understandings on diseases can influence treatment approaches, and thus the practice of alternative medicine in Hong Kong.

Although cultural belief system can influence how people perceive and classify diseases and thus the disease folk taxonomy as well as their treatment choices, the interrelationship between folk taxonomy of diseases and treatment choices is not always absolute. As demonstrated by the participants, only some taxonomies of diseases, such as those that are life-threatening, serious, ophthalmological, and chronic bone and joint diseases show apparent relationship in the treatment choices. Treatment choices, however, are still more embedded in people's cultural perceptions on individual diseases.

The use of alternative medicine was widely welcome by the participants, since they would attempt alternative medicine (traditional Chinese medicine and/or *qigong/ tai chi*) for most common diseases. The key message is although alternative medicine may not treat all diseases efficaciously, still it is effective in maintaining and enhancing health, which is required for all kinds of diseases. From the participants' point of view, qigong and tai chi practice can be used on most diseases, since the balance of qi inside human body will be important for maintaining health and helping to fight against diseases. It is particularly common in the use of health restoration after biomedicine treatment.

Author details

Judy Yuen-man Siu

Address all correspondence to: judysiu@hkbu.edu.hk

David C. Lam Institute for East-West Studies, Hong Kong Baptist University, Hong Kong, China

References

[1] Bonvillain N. Language, Culture and Communication: The Meaning of Messages. NJ: Prentice-Hall Inc; 2000.

[2] Kleinman A. Patients and Healers in the Context of Culture: An Exploration of the Borderland between Anthropology, Medicine, and Psychiatry. Berkeley, CA: University of California Press; 1980.

[3] Siu J.Y.M. The Use of Qigong and Tai Chi as Complementary and Alternative Medicine (CAM) among Chronically Ill Patients in Hong Kong. In: Bhattacharya A. (ed). A Compendium of Essays on Alternative Therapy. Rijeka: InTech; 2012. p.175-192.

http://dx.doi.org/10.5772/53281

[4] Hong Kong Tai Chi Association.《太極拳功三百問》Tai Chi Quan Gong Shan Bai Wen. [Three Hundred Questions in Tai Chi Quan]. Hong Kong: Hong Kong Tai Chi Association; 2001.

[5] Dong P., Aristide H.E. Chi Gong: The Ancient Chinese Way to Health. New York: Marlowe and Company; 1990.

[6] Miura K. The Revival of Qi: Qigong in Contemporary China. In: Kohn L., Sakade Y. (eds.). Taoist Meditation and Longevity Techniques. Ann Arbor: Center for Chinese Studies, University of Michigan; 1989. p. 331 – 358.

[7] Palmer D.A. Modernity and Millenialism in China: Qigong and the Birth of Falun Gong. Asian Anthropology 2003; 2(3): 79 – 109.

[8] Cheng T.H., Tsui W.K, editors.《鄭天熊太極武功》。Zheng Tian Xiong Tai Chi Wu Gong Lu. [Cheng Tin-hung's style in tai chi and martial arts]. Hong Kong: Hong Kong Tai Chi Association; 1996.

[9] Bernard H.R. Research Methods in Anthropology: Qualitative and Quantitative Approaches, 3rd ed. Walnut Creek, CA: AltaMira Press; 2002.

[10] Kleinman A. The Illness Narratives: Suffering, Healing, and the Human Condition. NY: Basic Books; 1988.

[11] The Medical Council of Hong Kong. List of Registered Doctors: Specialist Registration. http://www.mchk.org.hk/doctor/spec/index.htm. (accessed on 6 July 2012).

[12] Lupton D. Medicine as Culture: Illness, Disease and the Body in Western Societies. London: Sage Publications Ltd; 2000.

Section 2

Compositional Analysis

Chapter 3

Herbal Drugs in Traditional Japanese Medicine

Tsutomu Hatano

Additional information is available at the end of the chapter

http://dx.doi.org/10.5772/53126

1. Introduction

Medicinal herbs are used in the context of ethnic traditions in various regions of the world. Although modern medicine, based on Western medicine, is practiced in developed countries, traditional medicine is also an important part of treatment in Asian countries.

Traditional Chinese medicine (TCM) influences traditional medicine in Asian countries as a function of the cultural and historical relationships between each country and China. That is, traditional medicine has developed in each country under the influence of TCM in the context of its own cultural background.

This chapter examines traditional Japanese medicine (TJM), an alternative form of medicine used in Japan. Although acupuncture, moxibustion, and several related medical practices also play important roles in TJM, herbal medicine, as the most characteristic treatment within TJM, is the focus of this chapter.

2. Relationship between TJM and TCM

Western medicine often regards patients as sets of individual organs, and illnesses are often attributed to pathogens or morbid organs that should be removed. However, Asian traditional medicine, including TJM and TCM, understand patients from a holistic perspective that emphasizes the importance of balancing and harmonizing the entire patient, including her or his mind and body. Asian forms of medicine explain changes in symptoms in terms of causes, and treatments are prescribed based on a view of diseases as dynamic processes [1,2].

Basic medical concepts are common to both TJM and TCM, and practitioners of these disciplines arrive at diagnoses via four basic approaches.

1. Visual examination: Observation of the status of the face, tongue, skin, and behavior of the patient.
2. Auditory examination: Auscultation of the patient speaking, sighing and wheezing and examination of the patient's olfaction.
3. Interview: Questions posed to the patient about the history of the illness.
4. Tactile examination: Evaluation of the pulse and determination of abdominal status.

However, differences between TCM and TJM exist with regard to how each makes diagnoses and prescribes treatment.

Diagnosis in the TCM treatment involves the following steps:

1. Gathering data about symptoms to determine a diagnosis. Ba-bang-bian-zheng (in Chinese, assignment of body conditions to one of the eight principal states) is an important step in the diagnostic process of TCM and is based on discriminating between members of pairs: ying (negativity/hypo-functioning) and yang (positivity/hyper-functioning), xu (deficiency) and shi (excessiveness), han (cold/chills) and re (heat/fever), and biao (exterior) and li (interior).
2. Identifying the cause of the illness based on the theory underpinning TCM, including the five-element theory described later.
3. Determining the appropriate prescription based on the theory underpinning TCM. According to TCM, herbal prescriptions are based on imbalances in the viscera and bowels.

In contrast, TJM diagnoses, particularly those based on the Koho school, involve selecting an appropriate prescription; each prescription corresponds to specific symptoms associated with the constituents of herbal drugs. The most characteristic feature of TJM is that diagnosis is directly linked to selection of a prescription. The differences between TJM and TCM became especially pronounced during the Edo era in the 17th–19th centuries. Indeed, important diagnostic concepts often have different meanings in TJM and TCM. Thus, different uses of the concepts result in confusion, even among apprentices in TJM.

3. Short history of TJM

Drug use has long been part of the ethnic traditions in Japan, and various folk medicines have been applied in these contexts. The Geranium herb (over-ground part of *Geranium thunbergii* Sieb. et Zucc.), which is used as an anti-diarrheic, and Mallotus bark (bark of *Mallotus japonicus* Muell.-Arg.), which is used for stomach disorders, are examples of herbal drugs introduced into the Japanese Pharmacopeia (Fig. 1). The leaf of *Quercus stenophylla* (Urajiro-gashi in Japanese) is used for urinary tract calculi.

Historical books, such as Koji-ki (Records of Ancient Matters) (712), include descriptions of the use of reed mace (*Typha* spp., Fig. 2) for injury. Koji-ki records historical matters or folklores of the prehistoric ages in Japan.

Cultural exchanges, including those involving envoys to the Tang Dynasty (7th–9th centuries), and trade with China brought various crude drugs to Japan. Some of these drugs are the "Shosoin drugs" of today.TJM was practiced by Buddhism priests during those eras.

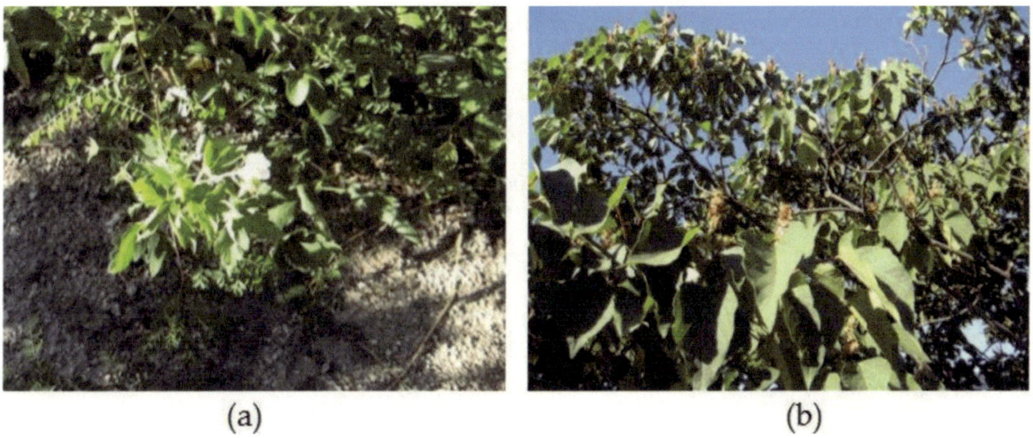

Figure 1. Examples of plants used as Japanese folk medicines. (a) *Geranium thunbergii* Sieb. et Zucc. (family Geraniaceae), and (b) *Mallotus japonicas* Muell.-Arg. (family Euphorbiaceae)

Chinese medicine changed based on historical changes in the dynasties, and the Chinese medicine of each era, until the present one, has influenced Japanese medicine. Chinese medicine was introduced during the Yuan dynasty in Japan and was practiced by Sanki Tashiro (1465–1537) and his successors, including Dosan Manase (1507–1594), who developed the medicines. They were known as the Gosei-ho-ha (the Latter-day Medicine School). The medicine taught by this school was based on two principles [Yin (active/positive) and Yang (inactive/negative)] combined with five elements (wood, fire, earth, metal, and water). The pharmacological characteristics of the herbal/crude drugs were separated into five tastes (pungent, sweet, sour, bitter, and salty) based on the five-element theory. Other characteristics, such as emotions, which may affect illnesses, are also attributed to the five elements (Table 1) [2, 3].

A trend toward a return to the fundamentalism of Confucianism appeared in China during the Ming Dynasty (14th–17th centuries), and an analogous fundamentalism was also seen in Chinese medicine. Some leaders in this field advocated reliance on the ideas or spiritual content related to medicine in the Shokan-zatsubyo-ron (*Shang-Han-Za-Bing-Lun* in Chinese, "Treatise on Cold Damage Disorders and Accompanied Various Diseases") edited by Zhong-Jing Zhang during the Han Dynasty (BC200–AD200).

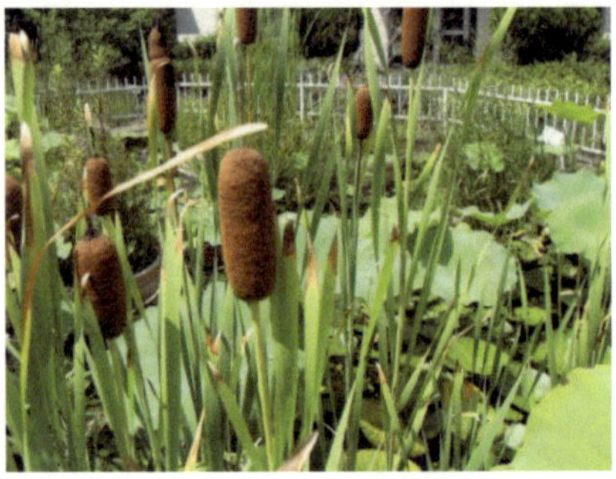

Figure 2. *Typha latifolia* L. (Typhaceae)

Element	*Mu (Wood)*	*Huo (Fire)*	*Tu (Earth)*	*Jin (Metal)*	*Shui (Water)*
Viscera	Heart	Liver	Spleen	Lung	Kidney
Bowel	Gallbladder	Small intestine	Stomach	Large intestine	Urinary bladder
Taste	Sour	Bitter	Sweet	Pungent	Salty
Emotion	Joy	Anger	Anxiety	Sorrow	Fear

Table 1. Five-element theory based on traditional Chinese medicine (TCM) and Gosei-ho-ha medicine in traditional Japanese medicine (TJM)

These ideas affected the leading physicians in Japan, who stressed that medicine in Japan should be based on Shokan-zatsubyo-ron, which was established in the Han Dynasty. Gonzan Goto (1659–1733) was such a physician, and he insisted on considering diseases to be based on ki (*qi* in Chinese) stagnation. Goto mentored many younger physicians, who were known as Koho-ha (fundamentalists). Toyo Yamawaki, one such physician, guided dissections and prepared a book entitled Zo-shi ("Records of Human Organs"), in which he clarified the differences between the actual structure of the human body and the structure depicted by TCM. Followers of this school insisted on practical evidence or actual results from medical trials. Todo Yoshimasu established a new approach to medicine based on this foundation.

4. Yoshimasu's TJM

Todo Yoshimasu established a new approach to medicine based on the notions described above. He was regarded as a highly skilled physician and contributed to new developments in the area of medical diagnosis. He stressed the importance of the abdomen, in addition to that of the radial artery pulse, in diagnosis. He actually simplified the causes of various diseases based on his unique "one-poison theory" and thereby eliminated conceptual confusion [1, 3-5].

http://dx.doi.org/10.5772/53126

However, Yoshimasu's most important contribution concerned the use of herbal prescriptions. During the Edo era, Honzo-komoku (*Ban-Cao-Gang-Mu* in Chinese, "Compendium of Materia Medica") (1590, Ming Dynasty), written by Shi-Zhen Li (1518–1593), was the most authoritative book in Asia, including Japan, to describe the efficacy of herbal drugs. However, Yoshimasu decided to revise sections on the effects of herbal drugs as he thought that the descriptions in the book were useless in terms of practical clinical applications. Yoshimasu thought that the descriptions were written under the influence of delusions/superstitions based on ethnic religion.

Thus, he first addressed cases in which major prescriptions are used for Shokan-zatsubyo-ron. Shokan-zatsubyo-ron is composed of two parts, which were identified separately. Shokan-ron (*Shang-Han-Lun* in Chinese, "Treatise of Cold Damage Disorders"), which addresses acute feverish diseases and Kinki-yoryaku (*Jin-Gui-Yao-Lue* in Chinese, "Essential Prescriptions as A Treasure Box"), which addresses sub-acute and chronic diseases.

He also added discussion based on his clinical experience concerning the uses of each prescription. These were gathered in Ruiju-ho ("a classified collection of prescriptions"). In Shokan-zatsubyo-ron, the author indicated the uses of each prescription during the course of an illness. However, the author did not explain the reasons for using each prescription, but instead stated that the physician should "just use it in exemplar cases." In this way, Todo Yoshimasu clarified the actions of the prescriptions by analyzing the kind of case in which it should be used.

Yoshimasu then began to collect the herbal drugs to be used in prescriptions. He gathered descriptions of the prescriptions containing each herbal drug from Shokan-zatsubyo-ron and discussed the effects of each herbal drug based on commonalities in the properties of prescriptions containing the drug. In other words, common symptoms referenced in the descriptions of the prescriptions were regarded as related to the herbal drug that was common to the prescriptions. He learned about the efficacy of each of the herbal drugs from Shokan-zatsubyo-ron by comparing it with his clinical experience. Such knowledge was collected in Yaku-cho ("Properties of Herbal Drugs").

For example, the action of the herbal drug licorice is discussed as follows: Although licorice (root with stolon of *Glycyrrhiza uralensis* Fisch. or *G. glabra* L.) is included in many prescriptions, prescriptions containing a particularly large quantity of licorice are shakuyaku-kanzo-to ("peony and licorice combination"), kanzo-kankyo-to ("licorice and ginger combination"), kanzo-shashin-to ("pinellia and licorice combination"), and kan-baku-taiso-to ("licorice and jujube combination"). Based on the cases described in the literature that involved use of these prescriptions and on comparisons with his own clinical experience, he concluded that licorice suppressed various otherwise imminent symptoms.

He next listed the effects of each prescription based on the actions of the constituent crude drugs he had examined. These findings are summarized in the book Ho-kyoku ("The Ultimate Properties of the Prescriptions").

For example, the keishi-to ("cinnamon combination") prescription, which is composed of cinnamon (bark of *Cinnamomum cassia* Blume), peony (root of *Paeonia lactiflora* Pall.), licorice, jujube (fruit of *Zizyphus jujuba* Mill. var. *inermis* Rehd.), and ginger (rhizome of *Zingiber officinalis* Rosc.), is used for patients with some upward streams such as hot flashes, headaches, fevers, sweats, and dislike of wind (feeling sick when exposed to wind). According to Yoshimasu, keishi-ka-kakkon-to ("cinnamon and pueraria combination"), formed by adding pueraria (root of *Pueraria lobata* Ohwi), should be used for patients with keishi-to symptoms in combination with "tension from the nape to the back," which indicated that pueraria should be added.

Another example is seen in the addition of peony (i.e., an increase in the amount of peony in keishi-to) to form keishi-ka-shakuyaku-to ("cinnamon and peony combination"). If the patient exhibited intense convulsions of the rectus abdominis in addition to the symptoms of keishi-to, a prescription with an excess amount of peony was used, as per Ho-kyoku.

In summary, Yoshimasu reorganized descriptions of the efficacy of prescriptions using the following analytical procedures:

1. Collecting information on the uses of prescriptions from Shokan-zatsubyo-ron.
2. Clarifying the efficacy of the respective herbal drugs based on the uses of the prescriptions containing those herbal drugs.
3. Identifying the effectiveness of prescriptions based on the efficacy of the constituent herbal drugs.

This simplification by Yoshimasu was quite useful for understanding the uses of herbal prescriptions in TJM today and also for clarifying the pharmacological properties of the herbal drugs constituting the prescriptions. Based on this simplification, herbal drugs can be linked to modern analyses of Oriental medicine to understand drug actions in ways that are analogous to those that enable understanding of Western medicine.

However, such a simplification ignores the notion that an illness should be understood in terms of sequential stages or states of the patient. Considering that, physicians of the Secchu (compromising) School, including Sohaku Asada (1815–1894), avoided extreme simplification and proposed that the good points of the theories underpinning both the Koho and the Gosei-ho should be used. The current major trend in TJM is based on his efforts.

5. Differences in herbal drugs used in TJM and TCM

The two forms of herbal medicine differ with respect to prescriptions and crude drugs. Many herbal drugs used in TCM are also used in TJM. However, it had been difficult to import herbal products from China to Japan during the Edo era because of the Japanese national policy of isolation. During this era, Japanese herbalists searched for plant materials that could act as alternatives to Chinese materials. Thus, the following are examples of differences between the plant materials used in TCM and TJM [6].

1. (Fig. 3a and b) Nin-jin: Japanese ginseng (chiku-setsu-nin-jin in Japanese, rhizome of *Panax japonicus* C. A. Meyer, family Araliaceae) used in TJM is much more effective

than is Korean ginseng (ninjin in Japanese, root of *P. ginseng* C. A. Meyer, *ren-shen* in Chinese) for stomach diseases accompanied by an epigastric obstruction (shin-ka-hi, *Xin-xia-pi* in Chinese). Thus, TJM and TCM both use *P. ginseng* root as a nourishing tonic.

2. (Fig. 3c) To-ki: Root of *Angelica acutiloba* Kitagawa (or *A. acutiloba* Kitagawa var. *sugiyamae*, family Umbelliferae) is used as To-ki (for soothing pain, corresponding to dong-gui in Chinese) in TJM, whereas the root of *A. sinensis* Diels is used in TCM.

3. (Fig. 3d) Sen-kyu (Kyu-kyu): Rhizome of *Cnidium officinale* Makino (family Umbelliferae) is used as sen-kyu (Cnidium rhizome) in Japan (corresponding to *chuan-xiong* in Chinese) for soothing pain and is often used in combination with to-ki. The use of *Ligusticum chuangxiong* (family Umbelliferae) originated in TCM.

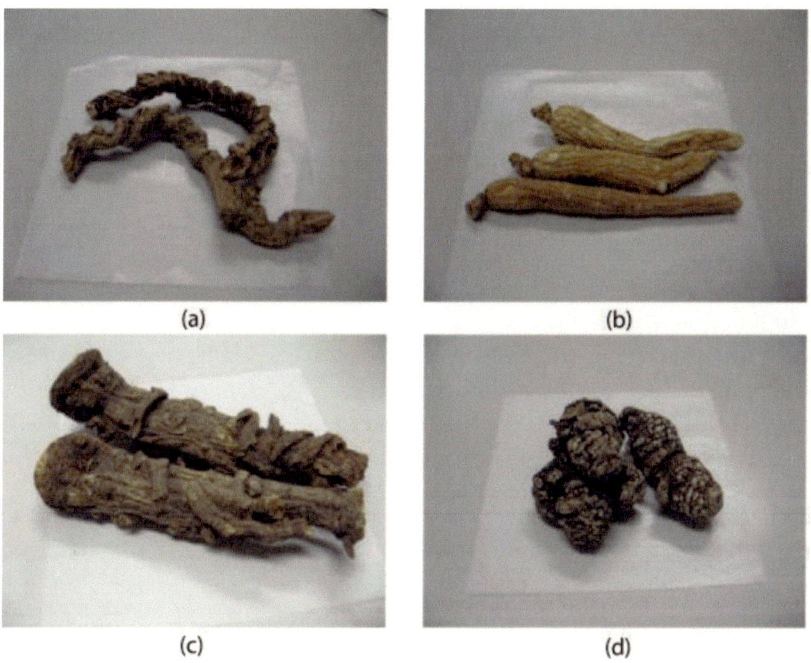

Figure 3. Examples of herbal drugs used in traditional Japanese medicine (TJM). (a) chiku-setu-nin-jin (rhizome of *Panax japonicus* C. A. Meyer), (b) nin-jin (root of *P. ginseng* C. A. Meyer), (c) to-ki (root of *Angelica acutiloba* Kitagawa), and (d) sen-kyu (rhizome of *Cnidium officinale* Makino)

4. Sai-ko: Root of *Bupleurum falcatum* L. (family Umbelliferae) is used as sai-ko (Bupleurum root), an antifebrile agent and to regulate liver functions in TJM, whereas *chai-hu*, the root of *B. chinense* DC (and *B. scorzonerifolium* Willd.) is considered a diaphoretic in TCM.

5. Ko-boku: Magnolia bark is used in both TJM and TCM for distension from the chest to the stomach that is due to a digestive organ disorder, which is often accompanied by

pain, and also for relief of bronchitis. The bark of *Magnolia obovata* Thunb. (family Magnoliaceae), regarded as wa-ko-boku (Japanese Magonolia bark), is different from the Chinese preparation (*hou-po* in Chinese) from *M. officinalis* Rehd. et Wils. and *M. officinalis* var. *biloba* Rehd. et Wills. In this case, Yoshimasu preferred the Chinese version.

6. Byaku-jutsu: Rhizomes from the following *Atractylodes* species are used for dyspepsia. That derived from *Atractylodes japonica* Koidz. ex Kitam. (family Compositae) is regarded as wa-byaku-jutsu (Japanese Atractylodes rhizome). In contrast, kara-byaku-jutsu (Chinese Atractylodes rhizome, *bai-zhu* in Chinese) is derived from *A. macrocephala* Koidz. (=*A. ovata* DC.). The latter is used in both China and Japan.

7. O-ren: Rhizome derived from the following *Coptis* species is used to eliminate fever of the upper body, particularly in the heart. *Coptis japonica* Makino (family Ranunculaceae) is cultivated in Japan, and its rhizome, particularly that from Ishikawa Prefecture has been used since the Edo era. In contrast, Chinese products, used in both in China (*huang-lian* in Cinese) and Japan, are derived from *C. chinensis* Franchet, *C. deltoidea* C. Y. Cheng, and *C. teeta* Wallich.

8. San-sho: Fruit of *Zanthoxylum piperitum* DC. (family Rutaceae) is known as "Japanese pepper," and its peel is used for dyspepsia in TJM. *Z. bugeanum* Maxim. or *Z. simulans* Hance are the source plants of Sichuan pepper (*hua-jiao* or *chuan-jiao* in Chinese), and they are used in analogous ways in TCM. However, they are not used for medicinal purpose in Japan.

9. Bo-fu: Root (including rhizome) of *Saposhnikovia divaricata* Schischk. (family Umbelliferae) is used for fever, pain, and spasms in TJM and TCM (*fang-feng* in Chinese). The root (with rhizome) of *Glehnia littoralis* Fr. Scmidt ex Miq. (family Umbelliferae) was developed as a subsitute for bo-fu in Japan and is called hama-bo-fu in Japanese. In contrast, *G. littoralis* is regarded as *bei-sha-shen* in China, and the root is used for coughs.

10. In-chin-ko: Spike composed of many minor flowers of *Artemisia capillaris* Thunb. (family Compositae) is used for thirst and jaundice in TJM, whereas young shoots of this plant are used for the same purpose under the name of *yin-chen* in China.

These differences should be understood when these herbal drugs are used clinically and studied in research settings.

6. Constituents of herbal drugs used in TJM

This section discusses studies on the constituents of the herbal drugs that are used in TJM and in our laboratory. Yoshimasu's work on the practical aspects of herbal drugs is quite useful for researchers attempting to understand the uses of herbal drugs in TJM, and the researchers in our laboratory are searching for new constituents based on such materials rather than considering the implications of the complex theories underlying TCM.

http://dx.doi.org/10.5772/53126

6.1. Tannins and related compounds: Major constituents of Japanese folk medicines or TJM

6.1.1. Hydrolyzable tannins of Geranium thunbergii

Hydrolyzable tannins are esters of galloyl and related polyphenolic acyl groups with glucose or some other sugars/polyalcohols. Although various types of hydrolyzable tannins have been found in plants, geraniin (**1**) is a representative one among them [7]. One of the most important herbal drugs in Japan is the geranium herb, the overground parts of *G. thunbergii*. The main constituent is crystalline tannin geraniin (**1**), and the structure containing a dehydrohexahydroxydiphenoyl group (**1'**) was reported in 1977 [8]. Although this compound equilibrates in a mixture, the structural factor forming the mixture was not clarified at that time. Detailed analysis with ^{1}H and ^{13}C nuclear magnetic resonance spectra revealed that it forms a mixture of six-membered (**1a**) and five-membered hemi-ketal structures (**1b**) (Fig. 4) [9]. An X-ray analysis of crystalline geraniin revealed the **1a** form with seven molecules of water [10].

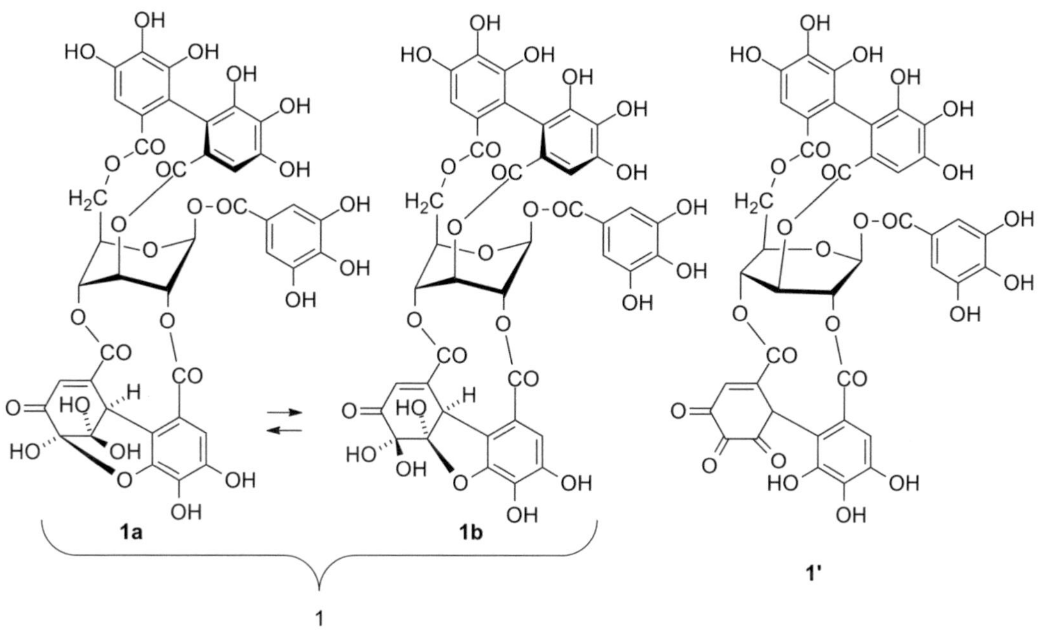

Figure 4. Structure of geraniin (**1**) forming an equilibrium mixture of six-membered hemi-ketal (**1a**) and five-membered hemi-ketal (**1b**) forms. Structure **1** was assigned to geraniin, firstly.

Further examination of this source plant revealed the presence of the co-existing hydrolyzable tannins furosin; didehydrogeraniin; furosinin [11]; geraniinic acids B and C; phyllunthusiins B, C, E, and F [12]; and acalyphidin M1 [13]. However, several compounds are formed after linking with ascorbic acid in the plant; these include ascorgeraniin (= elaeocarpusin) (**2**) [14,15] and furosonin (**3**) [13] (Fig. 5). We also found that geraniin is easily converted to corilagin (**4**) and repandusinic acid A (**5**) (Fig. 5) under near physiological conditions (pH 7.4) [13].

Because some hydrolyzable tannins show noticeable effects on β-lactam resistance of methicillin-resistant *Staphylococcus aureus* (MRSA) [16-18], we examined the effects of several available tannins, and repandusinic acid A and corilagin showed a noticeable suppressive effect on oxacillin resistance of MRSA [13].

The presence of tannins with analogous structures including mallotusinic acid (**6**) in *Mallotus japonicus* is shown in Fig. 5 [8,19].

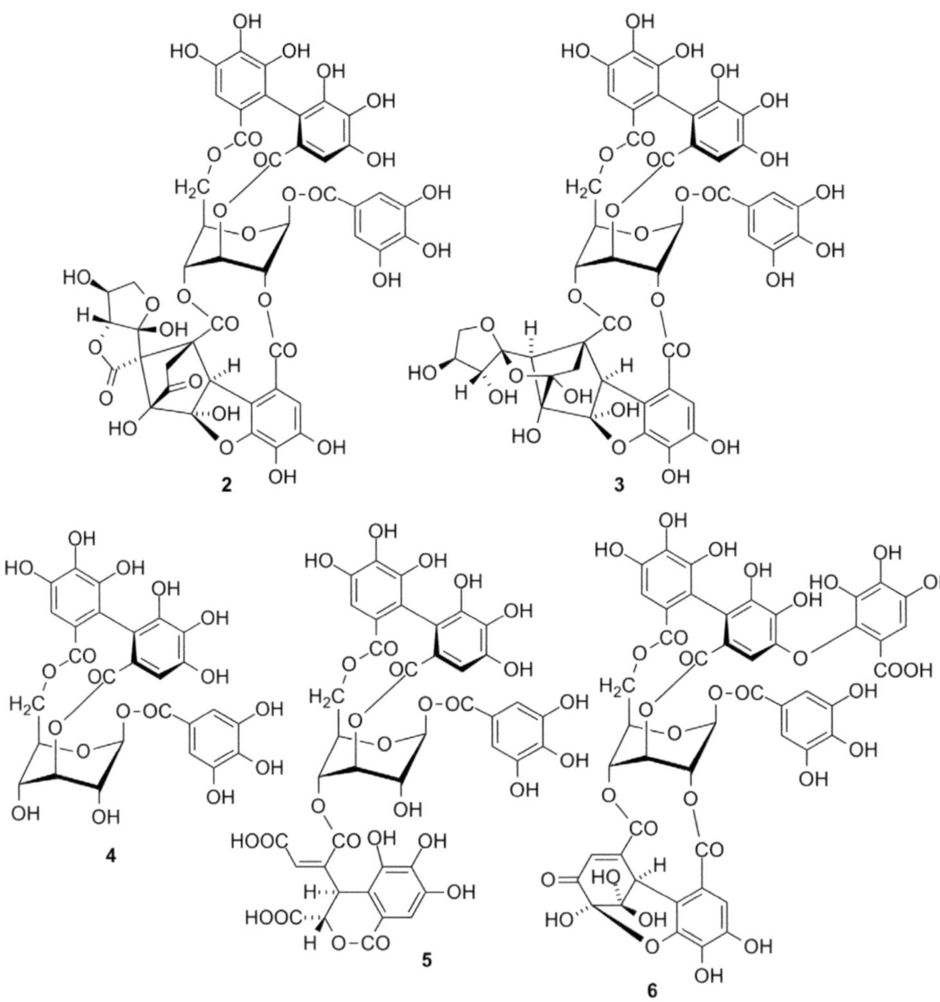

Figure 5. Tannins structurally related to geraniin. Compound 6 was isolated from *M. japonicus*.

http://dx.doi.org/10.5772/53126

6.1.2. Proanthocyanidins of Saxifraga stolonifera

Saxifraga stolonifera Curtis (family Saxifragaceae) is used as an ethnic medicine in Japan and China. A study of the constituents of this plant revealed that the major polyphenolic constituents of the overground part are proanthocyanidins, which are highly galloylated at O-3 of the respective flavan [(-)-epicatechin unit] in addition to 11-*O*-galloylbergenin (7) [20,21]. An oligomeric proanthocyanidin fraction, Ss-tannin-1 (8), with a molecular weight of 2300 shows potent antioxidant effects on lipid peroxidation in rat mitochondria induced by adenosine diphosphate (ADP) and ascorbic acid, and on that in rat microsomes induced by ADP and nicotinamide adenine dinucleotide phosphate [21]. Among the isolated constituents from this plant (Fig. 6), the administration of 3-*O*-galloylepicatechin-(4β→8)- 3-*O*-galloylepicatechin (**9**) and 3-*O*-galloylepicatechin-(4β→6)-3-*O*-galloylepicatechin (**10**) results in a noticeable increase in the life span of mice after inoculation of Sarcoma-180 [22].

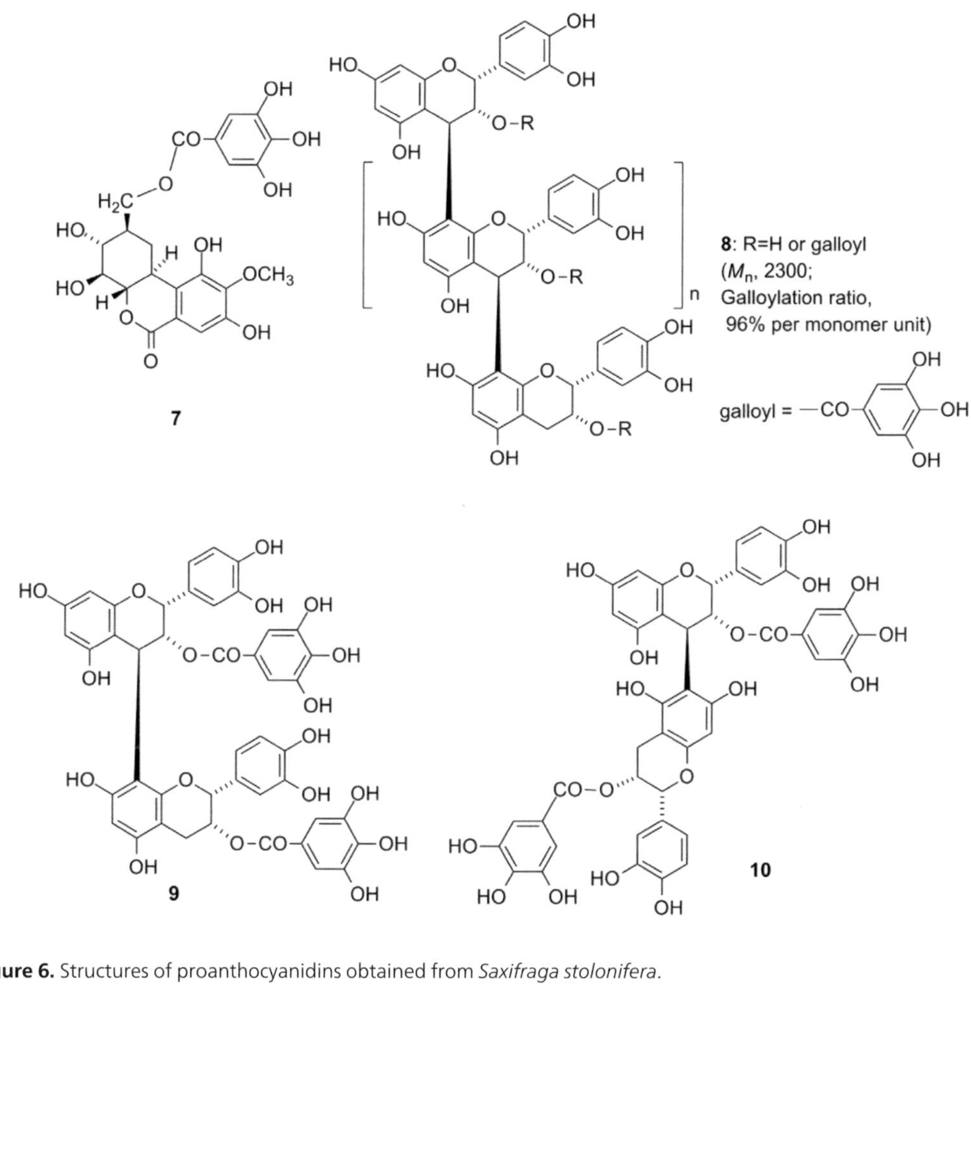

Figure 6. Structures of proanthocyanidins obtained from *Saxifraga stolonifera*.

6.2. Polyphenolics in herbal drugs used in TCM and TJM

6.2.1. Caffeic acid derivatives of Artemisia leaf and Perilla herb

The leaves of *Artemisia princeps* Pamp. or *A. montana* Pamp. (family Compositae) are used as gai-yo to stop bleeding and blood circulation difficulties in Japan, and the corresponding *A. argyi* Levl. et Vant. is used as *ai-ye* in China. Investigations of the constituents of the leaf revealed that dicaffeoylquinic acids [particularly 3,5-di-*O*-caffeoylquinic acid (**11**)] are the major constituents of *A. princeps* and *A. montana* [23] (Fig. 7).

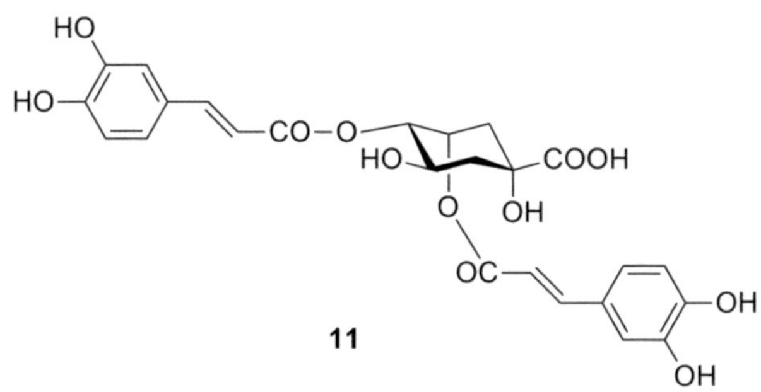

11

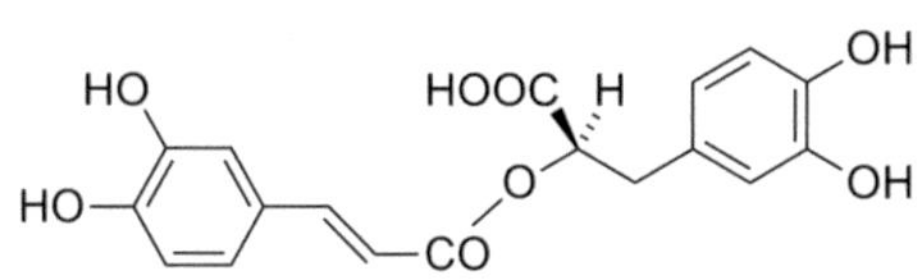

12

Figure 7. Structures of caffeic acid derivatives found in Artemisia leaf and Perilla herb

The aboveground part of *Perilla frutescens* Brit. var. *acuta* Kudo (or *P. frutescens* Brit. var. *crispa* Decne., family Labiatae) is used as so-yo or shi-so-yo for regulating energy flow or treating bronchial asthma and bronchitis in TJM and is used in analogous ways in TCM under the name *zi-su-ye*. Our study on the leaf constituents revealed that rosmarinic acid (an ester of caffeic acid with 3,4-dihydroxyphenyllactic acid, **12**) is a major constituent and showed that instability during the drying process of the leaves should be considered when using this herbal drug [24] (Fig. 7).

Caffeoylquinic acids show inhibitory effects on histamine release from rat peritoneal mast cells [25,26] and also on the formation of leukotriene B4 (LTB4) in human polymorphonuclear leukocytes (PMN-L). Rosmarinic acid shows a strong inhibitory effect on the formation of 5-hydroxy-6,8,11,14-eicosatetraenoic acid and LTB4 in PMN-L [25]. Because arachidonate metabolism is related to allergic inflammation and asthma, these results suggest that the effects of these constituents may participate in the actions of the herbal drugs containing them.

http://dx.doi.org/10.5772/53126

6.2.2. Flavonoids and 3-arylcoumarins from licorice

Licorice, the root (with stolon) of *Glycyrrhiza uralensis* and *G. glabra*, is widely applied in various TCM and TJM prescriptions. Although glychyrrhizin and related triterpene glycosides are regarded as the major constituents, Japanese researchers have reported on the importance of flavonoids and related phenolics [27].

Our investigation of licorice constituents revealed the inhibitory effects of flavonoids, including new ones, on xanthine oxidase [28] and monoamine oxidase [29]. Several also effective against the cytopathic effects of human immunodeficiency virus (HIV). The inhibitory effects of those constituents on giant cell formation induced by HIV were constituents are examined using a cell line sensitive to the cytopathic activity of HIV. Licochalcone A (**13**), isolicoflavonol (**14**), glycycoumarin (**15**), glycyrrhisoflavone (**16**), and licopyranocoumarin (**17**) inhibited at a 1:25 concentration (20 μg/ml) relative to that of glychyrrhiziin showed an analogous effect (500 μg/ml) (Fig. 8) [30]. Further investigation revealed that the HIV promoter activity induced by 12-O-tetradecanoylphorbol-13-*O*-acetate is suppressed by licorice phenolics. Those including glycycoumarin, and tetrahydroxymethocychalcone showed a specific suppressive effect on the HIV promoter; this effect was in contrast to its effects on the cytomegalovirus promoter [31].

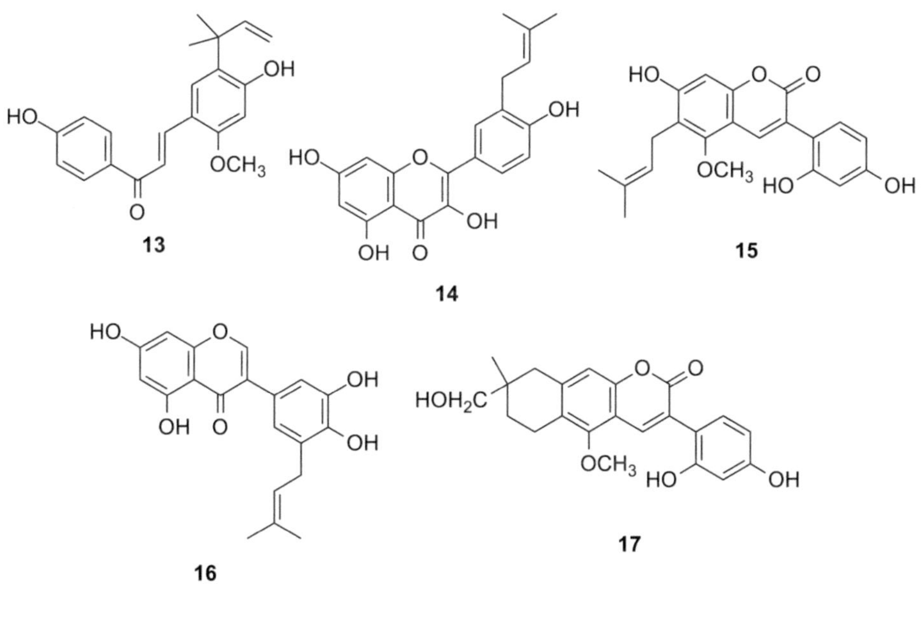

Figure 8. Structures of licorice phenolics that suppress human immunodeficiency virus (HIV) cytopathic effects.

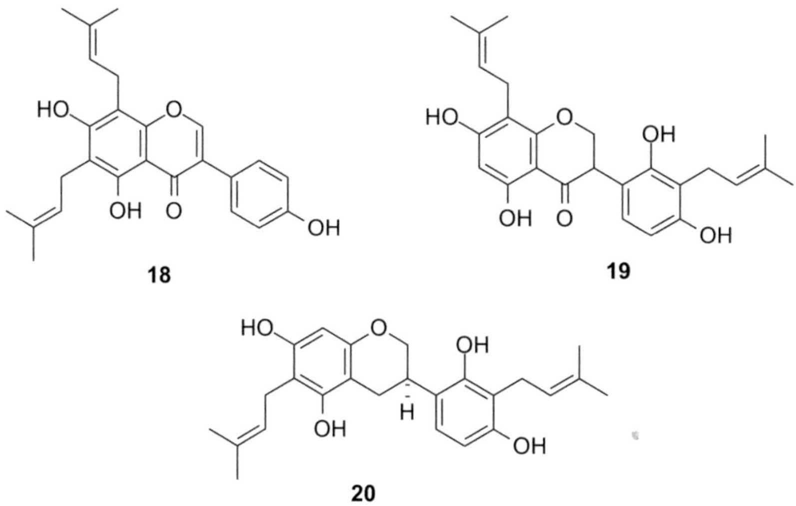

Figure 9. Licorice phenolics that show the most potent antibacterial effects on methicillin-resistant *Staphylococcus aureus* (MRSA) (compounds **18** and **19**) and noticeable suppressive effects on oxacillin resistance of MRSA.

Minimum inhibitory concentration (MIC) of oxacillin (μg/ml)					
Licoricidin	MRSA strains				MSSA
concentration	OM481	OM505	OM584	OM623	209P
None	512	64	256	512	<0.5
8 μg/ml	<0.5	<0.5	<0.5	<0.5	<0.5
4 μg/ml	16	8	16	16	<0.5

Table 2. Effect of licoricidin on the antibacterial activity of oxacillin.

The effects of licorice phenolics on MRSA were also investigated. Two flavonoids, 8-(γ,γ-dimethyally)-wighteone (**18**) and 3′-(γ,γ-dimethylallyl)-kievitone (**19**) showed their most potent antibacterial effects at a minimum inhibitory concentration (MIC) of 8 μg/ml. Furthermore, licoricidin (**20**) induced an effective decrease in oxacillin MIC (Fig. 9, Table 2) [32].

These findings suggest that licorice is a useful herbal source for the development of the primary constituents of the compounds used in modern medicine.

6.3. Ameliorating effect of extracts from Polygala root and Uncaria hook on scopolamine-induced impairment of spatial cognition

It is very important to develop new drugs for the treatment of patients with dementia as the number of individuals with this condition is now rapidly increasing due to the increase in the elderly population. The root of *Polygala enuifolia* Willd. (on-ji in Japanese and *yuan-zhi* in Chinese; family Polygalaceae) is used in TJM and TCM prescriptions for forgetfulness, neurasthenia, and insomnia. An investigation to identify the constituents of this herbal drug that are effective for impaired spatial cognition was conducted in rats using an eight-arm radial maze task. This task is useful for discriminating shshort-term memory from long-term one. The results showed that sinapic acid had the most potent effect among the cinnamic acid derivatives examined. Sinapoyl derivatives such as 3,6′di-*O*-sinapoylsucrose (21) are contained in this plant [33]. Analogous results have been obtained for phenolic constituents, including (+)-catechin of Uncaria hook (stem with hooks of *Uncaria rhynchophylla* Miq., *U. sinensis* Havil., and *U. macrophylla* Wall.; cho-to-ko in Japanese, *gou-teng* in Chinese; family Rubiaceae) [34]. Further studies of the adsorption/metabolism process and the mechanisms are required.

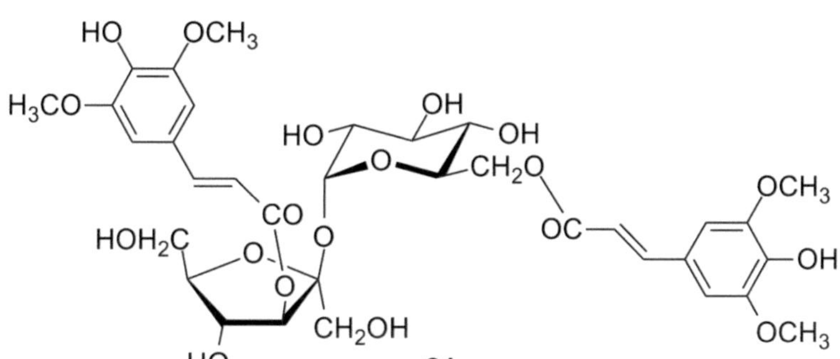

21

Figure 10. Structure of 3′,6-di-O-sinapoyl-sucrose contained in *Polygala tenuifolia* root.

7. Conclusion

Explanations of the pharmacological properties of herbal drugs based on TJM concepts have been useful for identifying new compounds with various structures. These explanations are also useful for understanding the roles of herbal prescriptions and applications in modern medicine. Modern medicine should consider some of the basic concepts of traditional medicine as they may contain wisdom.

Author details

Tsutomu Hatano

Okayama University Graduate School of Medicine, Dentistry and Pharmaceutical Sciences, Tsushima-naka, Kita-ku, Okayama, Japan

References

[1] Otsuka K. (translated by de Soriano G, Dawes N.) Kampo, a Clinical Guide to Theory and Practice. Edinburgh: Churchill Livingstone: 2010.

[2] Xie Z, Huang X. (eds.) Dictionary of Traditional Chinese Medicine. Hong Kong: Commercial Press: 1984.

[3] Deal WE. Handbook to Life in Medieval and Early Modern Japan. Oxford: Oxford Press: 2006.

[4] Kure S. (ed.) Todo Zenshu (The Complete Works of Todo). Kyoto: Shibun-kaku: 1970 (in Japanese).

[5] Hirose H, Nakayama S, Otsuka Y. (eds.) Kinsei Kagaku Shiso (Scientific Thoughts in Early Modern Japan). II. Tokyo: Iwanami Shoten: 1971 (in Japanese).

[6] Okuda T. (ed.) Kampo Yakugaku (Pharmaceutical Sciences in Kampo Medicine). Tokyo: Hirokawa Publishing Co.: 2009 (in Japanese).

[7] Haslam E. Plant Polyphenols: Vegetable Tannins Revisited. Cambridge: Cambridge University Press: 1989.

[8] Okuda T, Yoshida T, Naeshiro H. Constituents of *Geranium thunbergii* Slieb. et Zucc. IV. Ellagitannins. (2). Structure of Geraniin. Chemical and Pharmaceutical Bulletin 1977; 25 1862-1869.

[9] Okuda T, Yoshida T, Hatano T. Constituents of *Geranium thunbergii* Sieb. et Zucc. Part 12. Hydrated Stereostructure and Equilibration of Geraniin. Journal of the Chemical Society, Perkin Transactons 1 1982; 9-14.

[10] Luger P, Weber M, Kashino S, Amakura Y, Yoshida T, Okuda T, Beurskensd G, Dauter Z. Structure of the Tannin Geraniin Based on Conventional X-ray Data at 295 K and on Synchrotron Data at 293 and 120 K. Acta Crystllographica 1998; B54 687-694.

[11] Yazaki K, Hatano T, Okuda T. Constituents of *Geranium thunbergii* Sieb. et Zucc. Part 14. Structures of Didehydrogeraniin, Furosinin, and Furosin. Journal of the Chemical Society, Perkin Transactons 1 1989; 2289-2296.

[12] Ito H, Hatano T, Namba O, Shirono T, Okuda T, Yoshida T. Constituents of *Geranium thunbergii* Sieb. et Zucc. XV. Modified Dehydroellagitannins, Geraniinic Acids B and C, and Phyllanthusiin F. Chemical and Pharmaceutical Bulletin 1999; 47 1148-1151.

[13] Taniguchi S, Nogaki R, Bao LM, Kuroda T, Ito H, Hatano T. Furosonin, a Novel Hydrolyzable Tannin from *Geranium thunbergii*. Heterocycles, published on line. DOI: 10.3987/COM-12-S(N)65.

[14] Okuda T, Yoshida T, Hatano T, Ikeda Y. Biomimetic Synthesis of Elaeocarpusin. Heterocycles 1986; 24 1841-1843.

[15] Nonaka G, Morimoto S, Nishioka I. Elaeocarpusin, a Proto-type of Geraniin from *Geranium thunbergii*. Chemical and Pharmaceutical Bulletin 1986; 34 941-943.

[16] Shiota S, Shimizu M, Mizusima T, Ito H, Hatano T, Yoshida T, Tsuchiya T. Restoration of Effectiveness of beta-Lactams on Methicillin-resistant *Staphylococcus aureus* by Tellimagrandin I from Rose Red. FEMS Microbiology Letters 2000; 185 135-138.

[17] Shimizu M, Shiota S, Mizushima T, Ito H, Hatano T, Yoshida T, Tsuchiya T. Marked Potentiation of Activity of beta-Lactams against Methicillin-resistant *Staphylococcus aureus* by Corilagin. Antimicrobial Agents and Chemotherapy 2001; 45 3198-3201.

[18] Shiota S, Shimizu M, Sugiyama J, Morita Y, Mizushima T, Tsuchiya T. Mechanisms of Action of Corilagin and Tellimagrandin I That Remarkably Potentiate the Activity of beta-Lactams against Methicillin-resistant *Staphylococcus aureus*. Microbiology and Immunology 2004;48 67-73.

[19] Saijo R, Nonaka G, Nishioka I. Tannins and Related Compounds. LXXXIV. Isolation and Characterization of Five New Hydrolyzable Tannins from the Bark of *Mallotus japonicus*. Chemical and Pharmaceutical Bulletin 1989; 37 2063-2070.

[20] Okuda T, Kimura Y, Yoshida T, Hatano T, Okuda H, Archi S. Studies on the Activities of Tannins and Related Compounds from Medicinal Plants and Drugs. I. Inhibitory Effects on Lipid Peroxidation in Mitochondria and Microsomes of Liver. Chemical and Pharmaceutical Bulletin 1983; 31 1625-1631.

[21] Hatano T, Urita K, Okuda T. Tannins and Related Constituents of *Saxifraga stolonifela*. Journal of Medical and Pharmaceutical Society for Wakan-Yaku 1986; 3 434-435 (in Japanese).

[22] Miyamoto K, Kishi N, Koshiura R, Yoshida T, Hatano T, Okuda T. Relationship between the Structures and the Antitumor Activities of Tannins. Chemical and Pharmaceutical Bulletin 1987; 35 814-832.

[23] Okuda T, Hatano T, Agata I, Nishibe S, Kimura K. Tannins in *Artemisia montana*, *A. princeps* and Related Species of Plant. Yakugaku Zasshi 1986; 106 894-899 (in Japanese).

[24] Okuda T, Hatano T, Agata I, Nishibe S. The Components of Tannic Activities in Labiatae Plants. I. Rosmarinic acid from Labiatae Plants in Japan. Yakugaku Zasshi 1986; 106 1108-1111 (in Japanese).

[25] Kimura Y, Okuda H, Okuda T, Hatano T, Arichi S. Studies on the Activities of Tannins and Related Compounds, X. Effects of Caffeetannins and Related Compounds on Arachidonate Metabolism in Human Polymorphonuclear Leukocytes. Journal of Natural Products 1987; 50 392-399.

[26] Kimura Y, Okuda H, Okuda T, Hatano T, Agata I, Arichi S. Studies on the Activities of Tannins and Related Compounds from Medicinal Plants and Drugs. VI. Inhibitory Effects of Caffeoylquinic Acids on Histamine Release from Rat Peritoneal Mast Cells. Chemical and Pharmaceutical Bulletin 1985; 33 690-696.

[27] Shibata S, Saito T. Flavonoid Compounds in Licorice Root. Journal of Indian Chemical Society 1978; 11 1184-1194.

[28] Hatano T, Yasuhara T, Fukuda T, Noro T, Okuda T. Phenolic Constituents of Licorice. II. Structures of Licopyranocoumarin, Licoarylcoumarin and Glisoflavone, and Inhibitory Effects of Licorice Phenolics on Xanthine Oxidase. Chemical and Pharmaceutical Bulletin 1989; 37 3005-3009.

[29] Hatano T, Fukuda T, Miyase T, Noro T, Okuda T. Phenolic Constituents of Licorice. III. Structures of Glicoricone and Licofuranone, and Inhibitory Effects of Licorice Constituents of Monoamine Oxidase. Chemical and Pharmaceutical Bulletin 1991; 39 1238-1243.

[30] Hatano T, Yasuhata T, Miyamoto K, Okuda T. Anti-human Immunodeficiency Virus Phenolics from Licorice. Chemical and Pharmaceutical Bulletin 1988; 36 2286-2288.

[31] Uchiumi F, Hatano T, Ito H, Yoshida T, Tanuma S. Transcriptional Suppression of the HIV Promoter by Natural Compounds. Antiviral Research 2003; 58 89-98.

[32] Hatano T, Shintani Y, Aga Y, Shiota S, Tsuchiya T, Yoshida T. Phenolic Constituents of Licorice. VIII. Structures of Glicophenone and Glicoisoflavanone, and Effects of Licorice Phenolics on Methicillin-Resistant *Staphylococcus aureus*. Chemical and Pharmaceutical Bulletin 2000; 48 1286-1292.

[33] Sun XL, Ito H, Masuoka T, Kamei C, Hatano T. Effect of *Polygala tenuifolia* Root Extract on Scopolamine-Induced Impairment of Rat Spatial Cognition in an Eight-Arm Radial Maze Task. Chemical and Pharmaceutical Bulletin 2007; 30 1727-1731.

[34] Sun XL. Studies on the Ameliorating Effects of On-ji and Cho-to-ko on Spatial Cognition. PhD thesis. Okayama University; 2008 (in Japanese).

Chapter 4

Phytochemicals of the Chinese Herbal Medicine *Tacca chantrieri* Rhizomes

Akihito Yokosuka and Yoshihiro Mimaki

Additional information is available at the end of the chapter

http://dx.doi.org/10.5772/53668

1. Introduction

The family Taccaceae is composed of two genera, *Tacca* and *Schizocapsa,* and about 10 species, with most distributed in tropical regions of Asia, the Pacific Islands, and Australia [1]. *Tacca chantrieri* André is a perennial plant that occurs in the southeast region of mainland China, and its rhizomes have been used for the treatment of gastric ulcers, enteritis, and hepatitis in Chinese folk medicine. According to a Chinese herbal dictionary, *T. plantaginea* has also been used for the same purposes as *T. chantrieri* [2]. The chemical constituents of *T. plantaginea* have been extensively examined and a series of highly oxygenated pentacyclic steroids named taccalonolids, which have a γ-enol lactone, have been isolated as characteristic components of the herb [3], but there has been only one report of the secondary metabolites of *T. chantrieri,* in which a few trivial sterols such as stigmasterol and daucusterol, and a diosgenin glycoside were found [4]. Therefore, we focused our attention on the constituents of *T. chantrieri* rhizomes, and a detailed phytochemical investigation of this herbal medicine has been carried out.

In this chapter, we describe the phytochemicals isolated from *T. chantrieri* rhizomes and their biological activities with a focus on cytotoxicity against human cancer cells.

2. Isolation and structural determination

T. chantrieri specimens were collected in Yunnan Province, People's Republic of China. The rhizomes of *T. chantrieri* (fresh weight, 7.3 kg) were extracted with hot MeOH (3 L × 2). The MeOH extract was concentrated under reduced pressure, and the extract was passed through a polystyrene resin (Diaion HP-20) column eluted with MeOH/H_2O gradients,

EtOH, and EtOAc. The 50% MeOH and MeOH eluate portion was subjected to silica gel and octadecylsilanized silica gel column chromatography to afford a total of 41 compounds, classified into diarylheptanoids (**1** and **2**), diarylheptanoid glucosides (**3–9**), ergostane glucosides (**10–21**), withanolide glucosides (**22** and **23**), spirostan glycosides (**24–28**), furostan glycosides (**29–32**), pseudofurostan glycosides (**33–37**), pregnane glycosides (**38–40**), and a phenolic glucoside (**41**) (Fig.1). Their structures were determined through extensive spectroscopic studies and through chemical transformations followed by chromatographic and spectroscopic analysis.

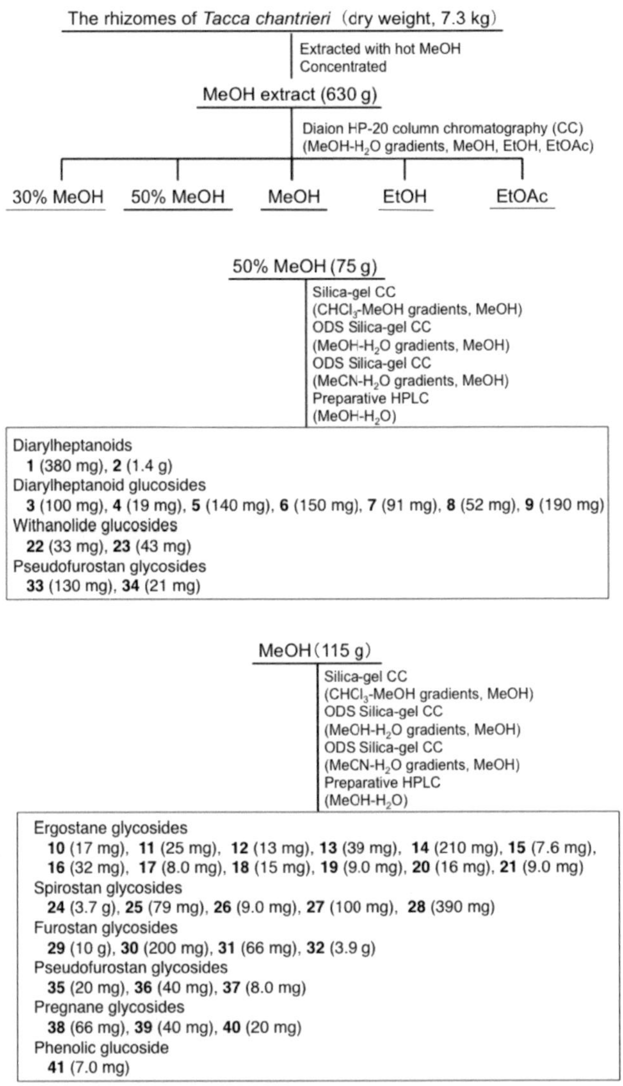

Figure 1. Extraction, partition, and purification procedures

http://dx.doi.org/10.5772/53668

3. Diarylheptanoids and diarylheptanoid glucosides

Diarylheptanoids consist of two phenyl groups linked by a linear seven-carbon aliphatic chain. Compounds **1** and **2** are diarylheptanoids and **3–9** are diarylheptanoid monoglucosides (Fig. 2) [5].

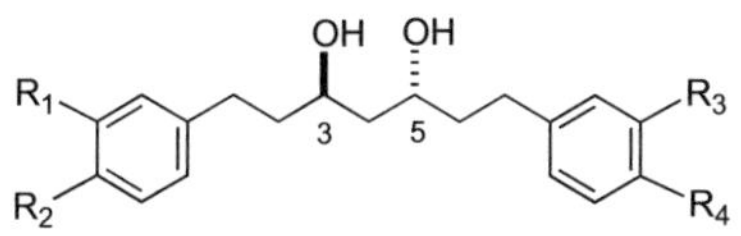

	R_1	R_2	R_3	R_4
1	OH	OH	H	OH
1a	OMe	OMe	H	OMe
2	OH	OH	OH	OH
2a	OMe	OMe	OMe	OMe
5a	OMe	OH	H	OH
7a	OMe	OH	OH	OH
8a	OMe	OH	OMe	OH
9a	H	OH	H	OH
9b	H	OMe	H	OMe

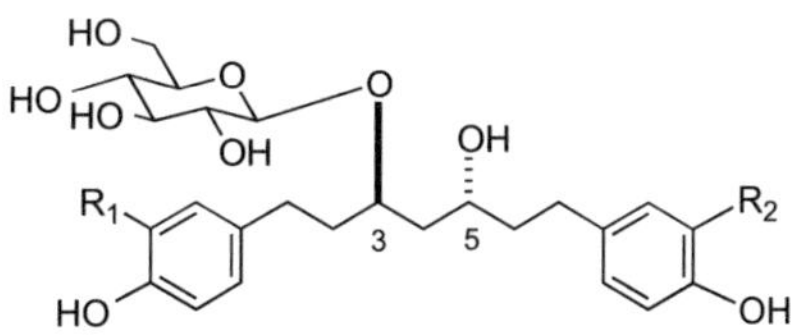

	R_1	R_2
3	OH	H
5	OMe	H
6	OH	OH
7	OMe	OH
8	OMe	OMe
9	H	H

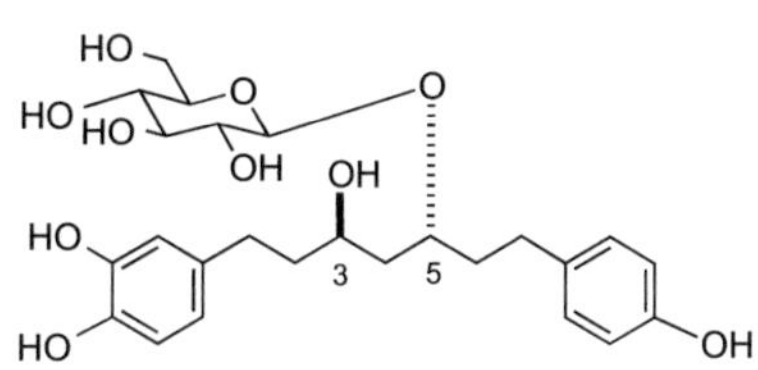

4

Figure 2. Structures of **1–9** and their derivatives

Compound **1** was isolated as a viscous syrup, $[\alpha]_D$ +1.7° (MeOH). HREIMS of **1** showed an $[M]^+$ peak at *m/z* 332.1623, corresponding the empirical molecular formula of $C_{19}H_{24}O_5$, which was also deduced by analysis of its ^{13}C NMR and DEPT spectral data. The IR spectrum suggested the presence of hydroxy groups (3347 cm^{-1}) and aromatic rings (1611 and 1515 cm^{-1}). The UV spectrum showed an absorption maximum due to substituted aromatic rings (281.4 nm). The planar structure of **1** was assigned as 3,5-dihydroxy-1-(3,4-dihydroxyphenyl)-7-(4-hydroxyphenyl)heptane by analysis of the 1D (^1H and ^{13}C) and 2D (^1H-^1H COSY, HMQC, and HMBC) spectra. The absolute configuration of the 3,5-dihydroxy moieties of the new diarylheptanoids were determined by applying the CD exciton chirality method to acyclic 1,3-dibenzoates [6]. The trimethyl derivative (**1a**) was converted to the corresponding 3,5-bis(*p*-bromobenzoate) (**1b**) and its CD spectrum exhibited positive (237.4 nm, $\Delta\varepsilon$ +29.9) and negative (253.3 nm, $\Delta\varepsilon$ –20.0) Cotton effects, which were consistent with a negative chirality. Thus, the absolute configurations were determined as 3*R* and 5*R* (Fig. 3). The structure of **1** was shown to be (3*R*,5*R*)-3,5-dihydroxy-1-(3,4-dihydroxyphenyl)-7-(4-hydroxyphenyl)heptane. In the same way, the structure of **2** was elucidated as (3*R*,5*R*)-3,5-dihydroxy-1,7-bis(3,4-dihydroxyphenyl)heptane.

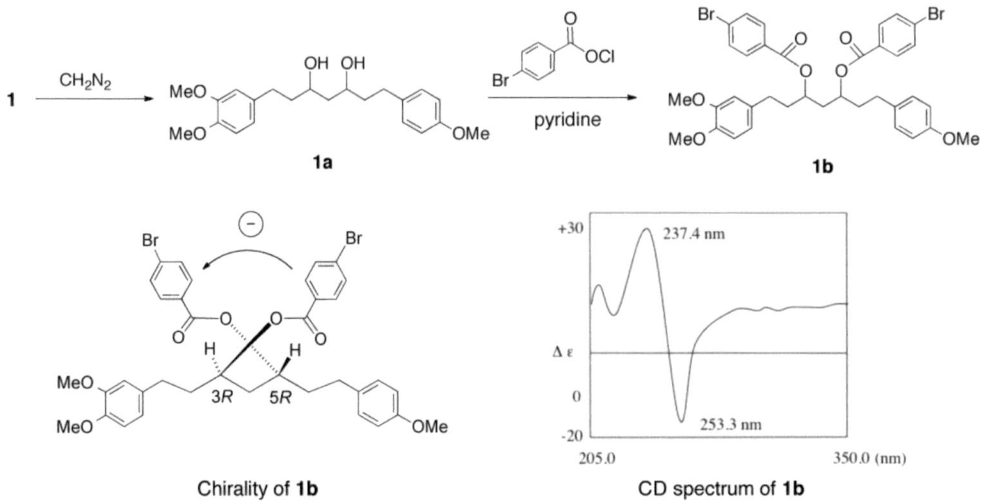

Figure 3. Determination of the absolute configurations at C-3 and C-5 of **1**

Compounds **3–9** are diarylheptanoid monoglucosides. Enzymatic hydrolysis of **3–9** with naringinase gave the diarylheptanoid derivatives and D-glucose. Identification of D-glucose, including its absolute configuration, was carried out by direct HPLC analysis of the hydrolysates. In the HMBC spectra, a long-range correlation was observed from each anomeric proton to the C-3 carbon in **3** and **5–9**, and to the C-5 carbon in **4**.

Diarylheptanoids are known to occur in only a limited number species of higher plants belonging to the families Zingiberaceae [7–10], Betulaceae [11], and Aceraceae [12]. This is the first isolation of diarylheptanoids from a plant of the family Taccaceae.

4. Ergostane glucosides

Compounds **10–21** are new ergostane glucosides (Fig. 4) [13–15]. Taccasterosides A–C (**10–12**) are novel bisdesmosideic oligoglucosides of (24*R*,25*S*)-3β-hydroxyergost-5-ene-26-oic acid (**10a**), whereas **13–20** are those of (24*S*,25*R*)-ergost-5-ene-3β,26-diol (**10b**). Compound **21** is an ergostane glucoside with the six-membered lactone on the side chain of the aglycone.

Taccasteroside A (**10**) was obtained as an amorphous solid. Acid hydrolysis of **10** with 1 M HCl in dixane/H_2O gave D-glucose and a C_{28}-sterol as the aglycone (**10a**). The structure of **10a**, except for the absolute configurations at C-24 and C-25, was identified as 3β-hydroxyergost-5-en-26-oic acid by analysis of its ^1H, ^{13}C, and 2D NMR spectra. In order to determine

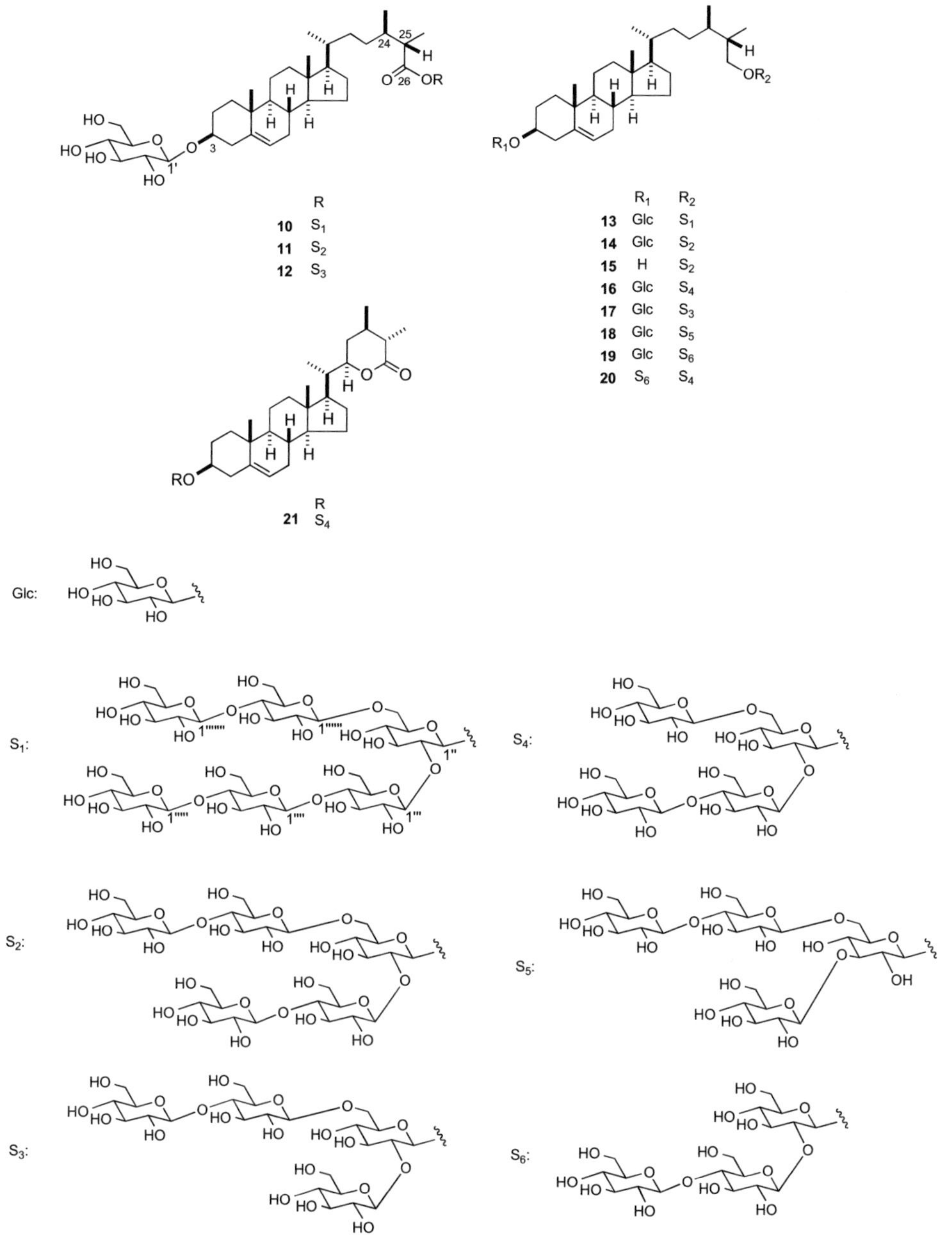

Figure 4. Structures of **10–21**

the absolute configuration at C-25, **10a** was reduced with $LiAlH_4$ to (24*R*,25*S*)-ergost-5-ene-3β,26-diol (**10b**). Then, **10b** was converted to the diastereomeric pairs of (*R*)-MTPA (**10a-R**) and (*S*)-MTPA (**10a-S**) esters with respect to the C-26 primary hydroxy group next to the C-25 chiral center and the differences in the ^{1}H NMR coupling patterns of the H_2-26 protons were inspected. The H_2-26 protons of **10a-R** were observed as a doublet-like signal at δ 4.20 (*J* = 6.3 Hz), whereas those of **10a-S** were observed as a doublet of doublets at δ 4.30 (*J* = 10.8, 6.6 Hz) and 4.09 (*J* = 10.8, 7.2 Hz). Application of these spectral data to the empirical rule reported by Yasuhara et al. [17] allowed us to confirm that the C-25 configuration was exclusively *S*. The configuration of C-24 position and other steroidal skeleton were established by the following chemical transformations. Compound **10b** was treated with *p*-toluenesulfonyl chloride to give the 26-*O*-tosylate of **10b** (**10b-T**), which was then reduced with $LiAlH_4$, affording (24*R*)-ergost-5-ene-3β-ol, that is, campesterol. The structure of **10a** was determined as (24*R*,25*S*)-3β-hydroxyergost-5-en-26-oic acid (Fig. 5).

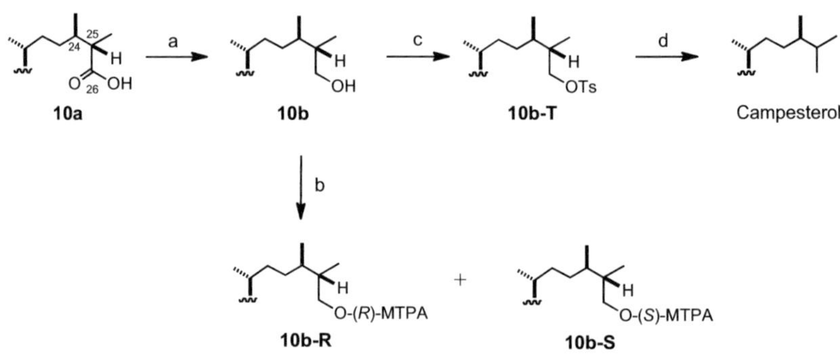

Reagents and conditions: a, $LiAlH_4$, THF, 0 °C, 5 h; b, (*R*)-MTPA or (*S*)-MTPA, EDC·HCl, 4-DMAP, CH_2Cl_2, r.t.,12 h; c, *p*-TsCl, pyridine, r.t., 6 h; d, $LiAlH_4$, THF, 0 °C, 5 h

Figure 5. Chemical transformations of **10a**

The severe overlap of the proton signals for the sugar moieties in **10** excluded the possibility of complete assignment in a straightforward way by conventional 2D NMR methods such as the ^1H-^1H COSY, 2D TOCSY, and HSQC spectroscopy. The exact structures of the sugar moieties and their linkage positions of the aglycone were resolved by detailed analysis of the 1D TOCSY and 2D NMR spectra. The ^1H NMR subspectra of individual monosaccharide units were obtained by using selective irradiation of easily identifiable anomeric proton signals, as well as irradiation of other nonoverlapping proton signals in a series of 1D TOCSY experiments [17–19]. Subsequent analysis of the ^1H-^1H COSY spectrum resulted in the sequential assignment of all the proton resonances due to the seven glucosyl units, including identification of their multiplet patterns and coupling constants. The HSQC and HSQC-TOCSY spectra correlated the proton resonances to those of the corresponding one-bond coupled carbons, leading to unambiguous assignments of the carbon shifts. The carbon chemical shifts thus assigned were compared with those of the reference methyl α-D- and β-D-glucosides [20], taking into account the known effects of *O*-glycosylation shifts. The comparison indicated that **10** contained three terminal β-D-glucopyranosyl moieties (Glc′, Glc′′′′, Glc′′′′′′′), three C-4 substituted β-D-glucopyranosyl moieties (Glc′′′, Glc′′′′, Gl*p*′′′′′′), and a C-2 and C-6 disubstituted β-D-glucopyranosyl moiety (Glc′′). The β-orientations of the anomeric centers of all the glucosyl moieties were supported by the relatively large *J* values of their anomeric protons (7.7–8.4 Hz).

http://dx.doi.org/10.5772/53668

In the HMBC spectrum, the anomeric proton of the terminal glucosyl unit (Glc′) at δ 5.07 exhibited a long-range correlation with C-3 of the aglycone at δ 78.2, indicating that one glucosyl unit was attached to the C-3 hydroxy group of the aglycone. Consequently, an oligoglucoside composed of six glucosyl units was presumed to be linkage with the C-26 carboxy group of the aglycone. Further HMBC correlations from H-1 of Glc″ at δ 6.30 to C-26 of the aglycone at δ 175.2, H-1 of Glc‴ at δ 5.20 to C-2 of Glc″ at δ 82.9, H-1 of Glc′′′′′′′ at δ 5.17 to C-4 of Glc′′′′′′ at δ 80.9, H-1 of Glc′′′′ at δ 5.16 to C-4 of Glc‴ at δ 81.5, H-1 of Glc′′′′′ at δ 5.13 to C-4 of Glc′′′′ at δ 80.9, and H-1 of Glc′′′′′′ at δ 4.93 to C-6 of Glc″ at δ 69.2 confirmed the hexaglucoside sequence as Glc-(1→4)-Glc-(1→4)-Glc-(1→2)-[Glc-(1→4)-Glc-(1→6)]-Glc, which was attached to C-26 of the aglycone (Fig. 6). Accordingly, the structure of **10** was elucidated as (24*R*,25*S*)-3β-[(β-D-glucopyranosyl)oxy]-ergost-5-en-26-oic acid *O*-β-D-glucopyranosyl-(1→4)-*O*-β-D-glucopyranosyl-(1→4)-*O*-β-D-glucopyranosyl-(1→2)-*O*-[*O*-β-D-glucopyranosyl-(1→4)-β-D-glucopyranosyl-(1→6)]-β-D-glucopyranosyl ester.

In the same way, the structures of **11–20** were elucidated as shown in Fig. 4.

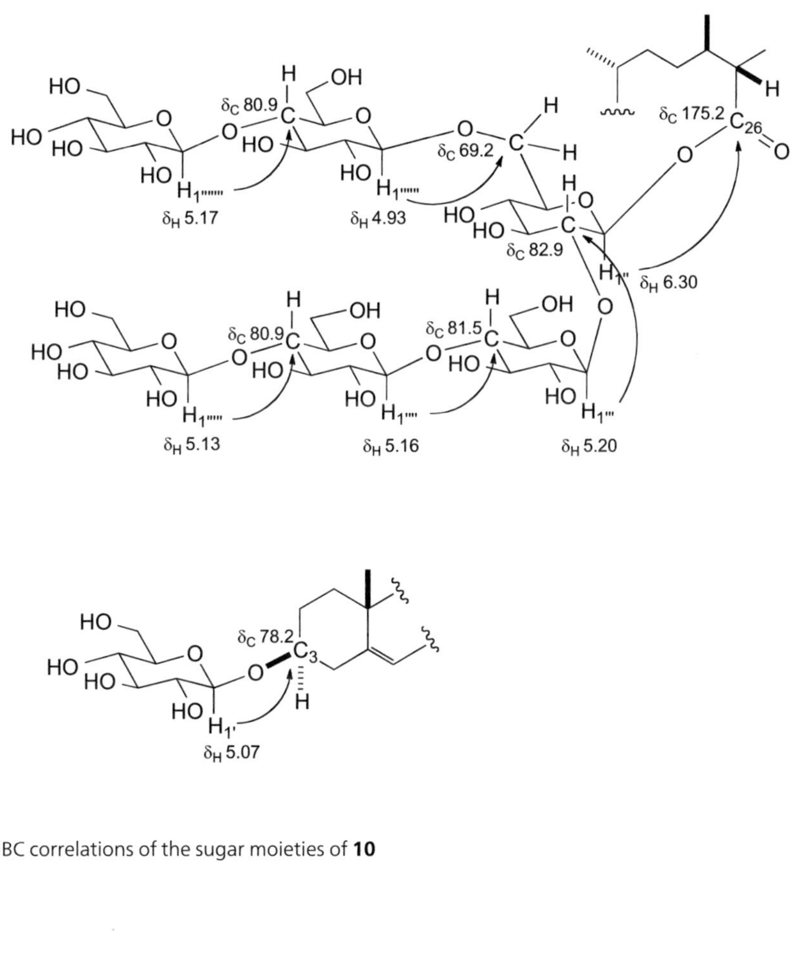

Figure 6. HMBC correlations of the sugar moieties of **10**

Phytosterols and their monoglucosides such as campesterol, stigmasterol, and β-sitosterol, and their 3-*O*-glucoside, widely occur in the plant kingdom. However, **10–20** are the first representatives of oligoglucosides of a phytosterol derivative to have sugar moieties with a total of four to seven glucose units. The bisdesmosidic nature of these structures, except for **15**, is also notable.

5. Withanolide glucosides

Compounds **22** and **23** are withanolide glucosides, named chantriolides A and B (Fig. 7) [21]. Chantriolides A and B were found to be minor components relative to the other secondary metabolites concomitantly isolated from *T. chantrieri*. However, it is notable that withanolides, which have been isolated almost exclusively from plants of the family Solanaceae previously [22, 23], have now been found in a species of the family Taccaceae in the study.

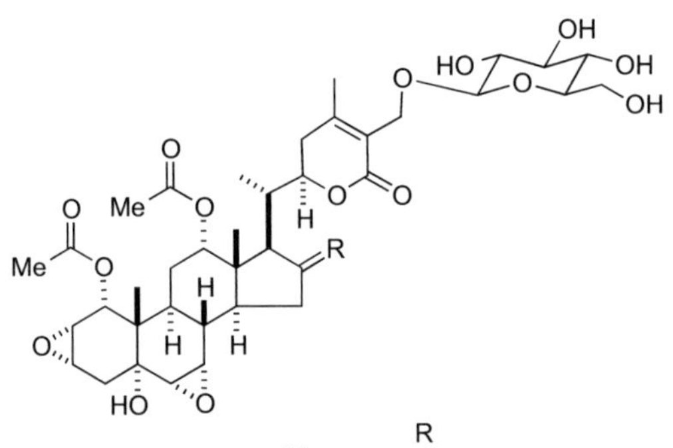

	R
22	=O
23	α-H, β-OH

Figure 7. Structures of **22** and **23**

6. Other glycosides

Spirostan glucosides (**24–28**), furostan glycosides (**29–32**), pseudofurostan glycosides (**33–37**), pregnane glycosides (**38–40**), and a phenolic glucoside (**41**) were also isolated from *T. chantrieri* rhizomes (Fig. 8) [15, 24–26].

The known naturally occurring 22,26-hydroxyfurostan glycosides exclusively exist in the form of glycoside, bearing a monosaccharide at C-26 [27]. The monosaccharide among the furostan glycosides reported thus far is limited to β-d-glucopyranose, except for one furostan glycoside from *Dracaena afromontana*, which has an α-l-rhamnopyranosyl group at C-26 [28]. Compound **31** is distinctive in carrying a diglucosyl group, *O*-glucosyl-(1→6)-glucosyl, in place of a monoglucosyl unit at C-26.

http://dx.doi.org/10.5772/53668

Compounds **33** is the corresponding $\Delta^{20(22)}$-furostan glycoside of **29**. This was confirmed by the fact that the peracetate (**33a**) of **33** agreed with the product (**29a**) obtained by treatment of **29** with Ac_2O in pyridine at 110 °C for 2.5 h, during which dehydration at C-20 and C-22, as well as the introduction of an acetyl group to all the hydroxy groups of the sugar moieties, occurred (Fig. 9).

The structure of **38**, including the absolute configuration at C-25, was found by the following chemical conversion. When the C-20 and C-22 bond of 33a was oxidatively cleaved by treating it with CrO_3 in AcOH at room temperature for 2 h, the resultant product was completely consistent with the peracetyl derivative of **38 (38a)** (Fig. 9).

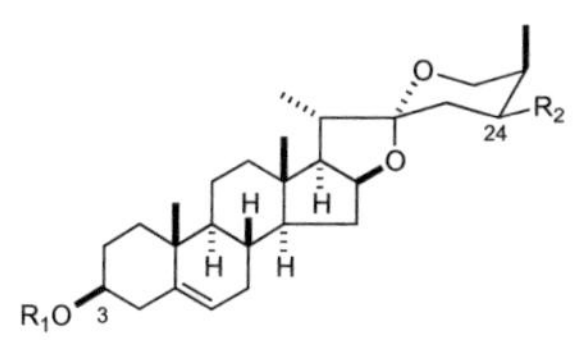

	R₁	R₂
24	S₁	H
25	S₁	OH
26	S₄	H
27	S₃	OH
28	S₃	H

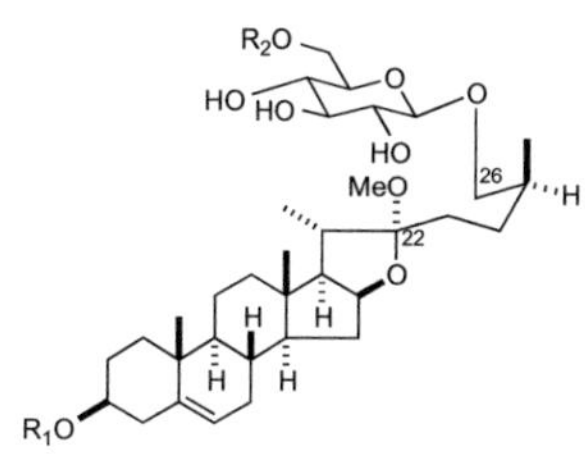

	R₁	R₂
29	S₁	H
30	S₂	H
31	S₁	Glc
32	S₃	H

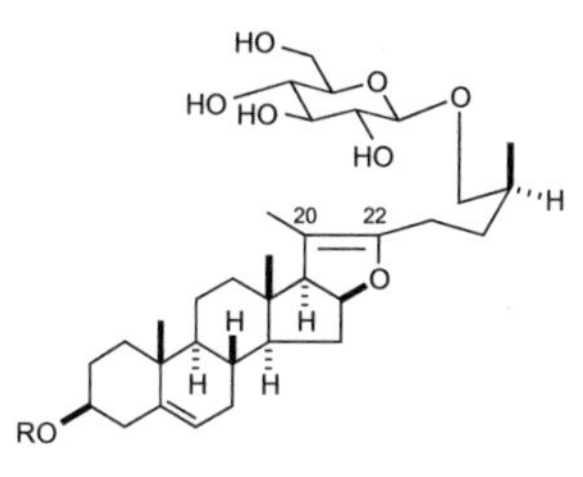

	R
33	S₁
34	S₂
35	S₃

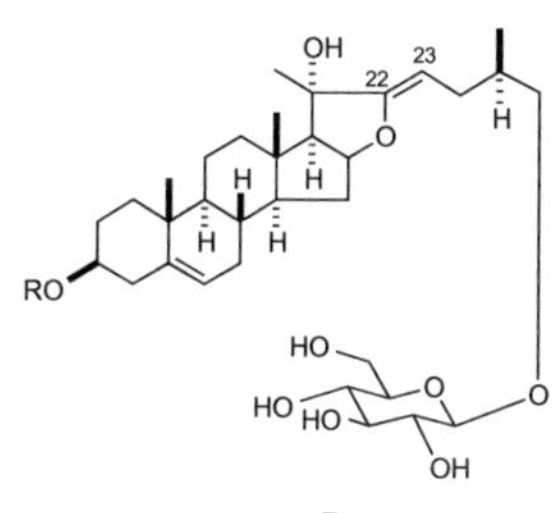

	R
36	S₁
37	S₃

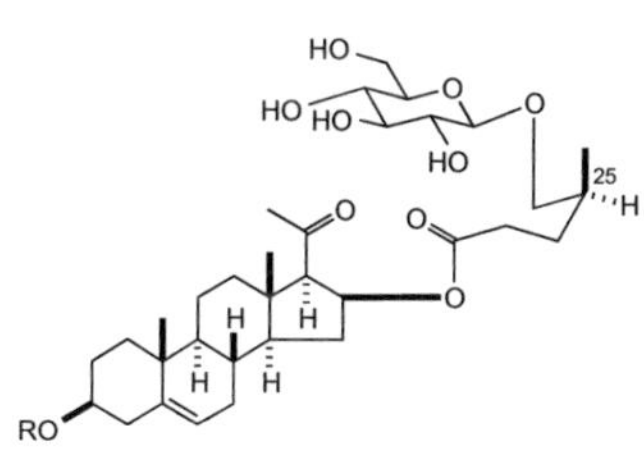

	R
38	S₁
39	S₃

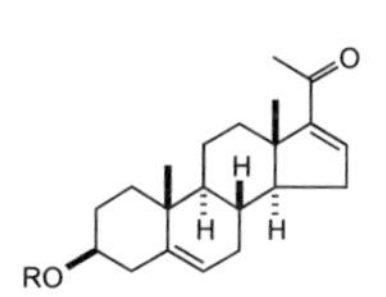

	R
40	S₁

Figure 8. Structures of **24–41**

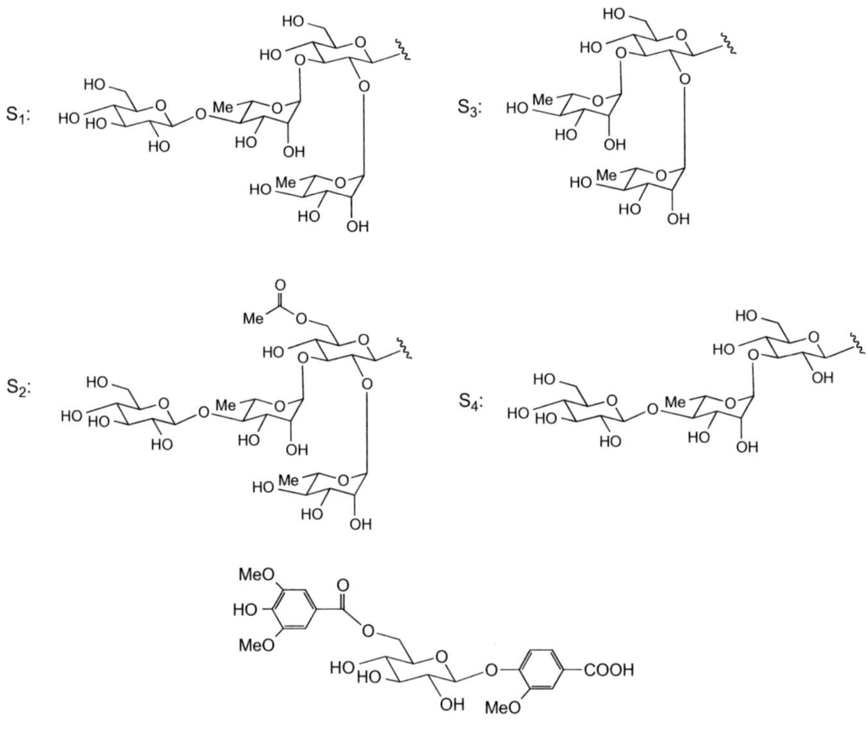

41

Figure 8. Continued.

A few compounds related to **38** and **39** have been isolated [29-31]; however, their C-25 configuration is not clearly presented in all the reports. In this investigation, we unequivocally determined the C-25 configuration of **38** to be *S* by a chemical correlation method. Compounds **38** and **39** could be defined as pregnane glycosides rather than furostan glycosides.

http://dx.doi.org/10.5772/53668

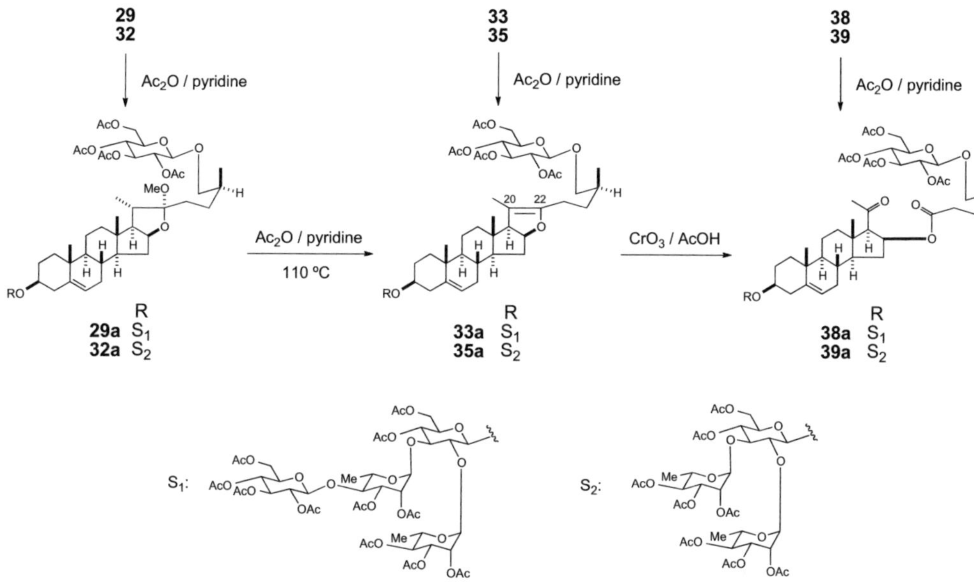

Figure 9. Chemical correlations of the furostan glycosides

7. Biological activity

7.1. Cytotoxic activity against HL-60 cells

The isolated compounds were evaluated for their cytotoxic activity against HL-60 human promyelocytic leukemia cells by a modified MTT assay method [32]. Diarylheptanoids (**1** and **2**), diarylheptanoid glucosides (**3**, **4**, **6**, and **7**), and spirostan glycosides (**24** and **28**) showed moderate cytotoxicity (IC_{50} 1.8–6.4 μg/mL) against HL-60 cells. Compounds **5**, **8–23**, **25–27**, and **29–41** did not show apparent cytotoxic activity against HL-60 cells at a sample concentration of 10 μg/mL.

7.2. Cytotoxic activity and structure–activity relationships of diarylheptanoids and diarylheptanoid glucosides against HL-60 cells, HSC-2 cells, and HGF

The diarylheptanoids and some derivatives, including **9b** prepared by treatment of **9** with CH_2N_2, were evaluated for their cytotoxic activities against HL-60 cells, HSC-2 human oral squamous carcinoma cells, and normal human gingival fibroblasts (HGF) (Table 1). The diarylheptanoids **1**, **2**, and **7a**, and the diarylheptanoid glucosides **3**, **4**, **6**, and **7**, each of which has three or four phenolic hydroxy groups, showed moderate cytotoxic activity against HL-60 cells with IC_{50} values ranging 1.8 to 6.4 μg/mL, while those possessing two phenolic hydroxy groups (**5**, **5a**, **8**, **8a**, **9**, and **9a**) did not exhibit apparent cytotoxic activity even at a sample concentration of 10 μg/mL. Notably, the diarylheptanoids whose phenolic hydroxy groups were all masked with methyl groups (**1a**, **2a**, and **9b**) were also cytotoxic. These observations suggest that the number of phenolic hydroxy groups contributes to the resultant cytotoxicity. Compounds **1a**, **2a**, and **9b** showed considerable cytotoxic activity against HSC-2 cells, whereas they had little effect on normal HGF.

compound	IC_{50} (μg/mL)		
	HL-60	HSC-2	HGF
1	2.1	54.0	162
1a	5.5	3.9	176
2	1.8	54.0	>250
2a	4.9	6.6	174
3	6.2	158	220
4	5.5	155	>250
5	>10	160	>250
5a	>10	–[b]	–[b]
6	3.0	92.0	189
7	4.5	209	>250
7a	4.1	–[b]	–[b]
8	>10	198	>250
8a	>10	–[b]	–[b]
9	>10	157	213
9a	>10	231	177
9b	6.4	23.0	173
etoposide	0.2	24.0	>200

[a]Key: HL-60 (human promyelocytic leukemia cells); HSC-2 (human oral squamous carcinoma cells); and HGF (normal human gingival fibroblasts). [b]not determined.

Table 1. Cytotoxic activities of compounds **1**-**9** and their derivates (**1a**, **4a**, **5a**, **7a**-**9a**, and **9b**), and etpside against HL-60 cells, HSC-2 cells, and HGF[a]

7.3. Cytotoxic activity and structure–activity relationships of steroidal glycosides against HL-60 cells

Spirostan glycosides (**24** and **28**) showed moderate cytotoxicity (IC_{50} 1.9 and 1.8 μg/mL) against HL-60 cells. Compounds **25** and **27**, the corresponding C-24 hydroxy derivatives of **24** and **28**, and **26**, the analogue of **24** without the terminal rhamnosyl group linked to C-2 of the inner glucosyl residue, did not show any cytotoxic activity at a sample concentration of 10 μg/mL. Furostan glycosides (**29–32**), pseudofurostan glycosides (**33–37**), and pregnane glycosides (**38–40**) also did not show cytotoxic activity. These data suggest that the structures of both the aglycone and sugar moieties contribute to the cytotoxicity.

http://dx.doi.org/10.5772/53668

7.4. Panel screening in the Japanese Foundation for Cancer Research 39 cell line assay

Diarylheptanoid **2** and spirostan glycosides **24**, which showed significant cytotoxic activity against HL-60 cells, were subjected to the Japanese Foundation for Cancer Research 39 cell line assay [33]. Subsequent evaluation of **2** and **24** showed that the mean concentration required for achieving GI_{50} levels against the panel of cells were 87 μM and 1.8 μM, respectively. Although **2** and **24** exhibited no significant differential cellar sensitivity, some cell lines such as colon cancer HCT-116 (GI_{50} 25 μM), ovarian cancer OVCAR-3 (GI_{50} 36 μM), OVCAR-4 (GI_{50} 39 μM), and stomach MKN-7 (GI_{50} 34 μM) were relatively sensitive to **2**.

8. Conclusion

Our systematic chemical investigations of *T. chantrieri* rhizomes revealed that this plant contains a variety of secondary metabolites, namely, diarylheptanoids, diarylheptanoid glucosides, steroidal glycosides with the aglycone structures of ergostane, withanolide, spirostan, furostan, pseudofurostan, and pregnane, as well as a phenolic glucoside. Some diarylheptanoids and steroidal glycosides showed cytotoxicity against human cancer cells. These compounds may be possible leads for new anticancer drugs.

On the other hand, a number of researchers have reported biological activities of diarylheptanoids and steroidal glycosides other than cytotoxicity. It has been reported that curcuminoids, well-known diarylheptanoid derivatives, showed antioxidant [34, 35], anti-inflammatory [35, 36], estrogenic [37, 38], and anticancer [39] effects. Steroidal glycosides have been shown to have antidiabetic [40, 41], antitumor [42], antitussive [43], antiherpes virus [44], and platelet aggregation inhibitory [45] activities. *T. chantrieri* rhizomes could be applied to treating a wide variety of ailments as an alternative herbal medicine.

Acknowledgements

We are grateful to Dr. Hiroshi Sakagami for evaluating the cytotoxic activities against HSC-2 cells and HGF.

Author details

Akihito Yokosuka and Yoshihiro Mimaki

Tokyo University of Pharmacy and Life Sciences, School of Pharmacy, Tokyo, Japan

References

[1] Tsukamoto Y. (ed.) The Grand Dictionary of Horticulture Vol. 1. Tokyo: Shogakukan; 1989; pp 148–149.

[2] Dictionary of Chinese Medicinal Materials Vol. 2. Shanghai: Shanghai Scientific and Technological Press; 1977; pp 1356–1357.

[3] Chen Z L, Wang B D, Chen M Q. Steroidal bitter principles from *Tacca plantaginea* structures of Taccalonolide A and B. Tetrahedron Letters 1987; 28: 1673–1676.

[4] Zhou J, Chen C, Liu R, Yang C. Studies on the chemical constituents of *Tacca chanteraeri* Andre. Zhiwu Xuebao 1983; 25: 568–573.

[5] Yokosuka A, Mimaki Y, Sakagami H, Sashida Y. New diarylheptanoids and diarylheptanoid glucosides from the rhizomes of *Tacca chantrieri* and their cytotoxic activity. Journal of Natural Products 2002; 65: 283–289.

[6] Harada N, Saito A, Ono H, Gawronski J, Gawronska K, Sugioka T, Uda H, Kuriki T. A CD method for determination of the absolute stereochemistry of acyclic glycols. 1. Application of the CD exciton chirality method to acyclic 1,3-dibenzoate systems. Journal of American Chemical Society 1991; 113: 3842–3850.

[7] Tezuka Y, Gewali M B, Ali M S, Banskota A H, Kadota S. Eleven novel diarylheptanoids and two unusual diarylheptanoid derivatives from the seeds of *Alpinia blepharocalyx*. Journal of Natural Products 2001; 64: 208–213.

[8] Ali M S, Tezuka Y, Awale S, Banskota A H, Kadota S. Six new diarylheptanoids from the seeds of *Alpinia blepharocalyx*. Journal of Natural Products 2001; 64: 289–293.

[9] Ali M S, Tezuka Y, Banskota A H, Kadota S. Blepharocalyxins C-E, three new dimeric diarylheptanoids, and related compounds from the seeds of *Alpinia blepharocalyx*. Journal of Natural Products 2001; 64: 491–496.

[10] tokawa H, Aiyama R, Ikuta A. A pungent diarylheptanoid from *Alpinia oxyphylla*. Phytochemistry 1981; 20: 769–771.

[11] Ohta S, Aoki T, Hirata T, Suga T. The structures of four diarylheptanoid glycosides from the female flowers of *Alnus serrulatoides*. Journal of the Chemical Society, Perkin Transactions 1 1984; 1635–1642.

[12] Nagai M, Kenmochi N, Fujita M, Furukawa N, Inoue T. Studies on the constituents of Aceraceae plants. VI.: Revised stereochemistry of (-)-Centrolobol, and new glycosides from *Acer nikoense*. Chemical and Pharmaceutical Bulletin 1986; 34: 1056–1060.

[13] Yokosuka A, Mimaki Y, Sashida Y. Taccasterosides A–C, novel C_{28}-sterol glucosides from the rhizomes of *Tacca chantrieri*. Chemical and Pharmaceutical Bulletin 2004; 52: 1396–1398.

[14] Yokosuka A, Mimaki Y, Sakuma C, Sashida Y. New glycosides of the campesterol derivative from the rhizomes of *Tacca chantrieri*. Steroids 2005; 70: 257–265.

[15] Yokosuka A, Mimaki Y. New glycosides from the rhizomes of *Tacca chantrieri*. Chemical and Pharmaceutical Bulletin 2007; 55: 273–279.

[16] Yasuhara F, Yamaguchi S, Kasai R, Tanaka O. Assignment of absolute configuration of 2-substituted-1-propanols by ^{1}H-NMR spectroscopy. Tetrahedron Letters 1986; 27: 4033–4039.

[17] Kuroda M, Mimaki Y, Ori K, Koshino H, Nukada T, Sakagami H, Sashida Y. Lucilianosides A and B, two novel tetranor-lanostane hexaglycosides from the bulbs of *Chionodoxa luciliae*. Tetrahedron 2002; 58: 6735–6740.

[18] Watanabe K, Mimaki Y, Sakuma C, Sashida Y. Eranthisaponins A and B, two new bisdesmosidic triterpene saponins from the tubers of *Eranthis cilicica*. Journal of Natural Products 2003; 66: 879–882.

[19] Mimaki Y, Harada H, Sakuma C, Haraguchi M, Yui S, Kudo T, Yamazaki M, Sashida Y. Contortisiliosides A–G: isolation of seven new triterpene bisdesmosides from *Enterolobium contortisiliquum* and their cytotoxic activity. Helvetica Chimica Acta 2004; 87: 851–865.

[20] Agrawel P K. NMR spectroscopy in the structural elucidation of oligosaccharides and glycosides. Phytochemistry 1992; 31: 3307–3330.

[21] Yokosuka A, Mimaki Y, Sashida Y. Chantriolides A and B, two new withanolide glucosides from the rhizomes of *Tacca chantrieri*. Journal of Natural Products 2003; 66: 876–878.

[22] Huang Y, Liu J K, Mühlbauer A, Henkel T, Huang Y, Liu J K, Mühlbauer A, Henkel T. Three novel Taccalonolides from the tropical plant *Tacca subflaellata*. Helvetica Chimica Acta 2002; 85: 2553–2558.

[23] Khan P M, Malik A, Ahmad S, Nawaz H R. Withanolides from *Ajuga parviflora*. Journal of Natural Products 1999; 62: 1290–1292.

[24] Yokosuka A, Mimaki Y, Sashida Y. Spirostanol saponins from the rhizomes of *Tacca chantrieri* and their cytotoxic activity. Phytochemistry 2002; 61: 73–78.

[25] Yokosuka A, Mimaki Y, Sashida Y. Two new steroidal glycosides from *Tacca chantrieri*. Natural Medicines 2002; 56: 208–211.

[26] Yokosuka A, Mimaki Y, Sashida Y. Steroidal and pregnane glycosides from the rhizomes of *Tacca chantrieri*. Journal of Natural Products 2002; 65: 1293–1298.

[27] Agrawel P K, Jain D C, Gupta R K, Thakur R S. Carbon-13 NMR spectroscopy of steroidal sapogenins and steroidal saponins. Phytochemistry 1985; 24: 2479–2496.

[28] Reddy K S, Shekhani M S, Berry D E, Lynn D G, Hecht S M. Afromontoside A new cytotoxic principle from *Dracaena afromontana*. Journal of the Chemical Society, Perkin Transactions 1 1984, 987-992.

[29] Dong M, Feng X Z, Wang B X, Wu L J, Ikejima T. Two novel furostanol saponins from the rhizomes of *Dioscorea panthaica*. Prain et Burkill and their cytotoxic activity. Tetrahedron 2001; 57: 501–506.

[30] Dong M, Feng X Z, Wu L J, Wang B X, Ikejima T. Two new steroidal saponins from the rhizomes of *Dioscorea panthaica* and their cytotoxic activity. Planta Medica 2001; 67: 853–857.

[31] Tran Q L, Tezuka Y, Banskota A H, Tran Q K, Saiki I, Kadota S. New spirostanol steroids and steroidal saponins from roots and rhizomes of *Dracaena angustifolia* and their antiproliferative activity. Journal of Natural Products 2001; 64: 1127-1132.

[32] Sargent J M, Taylor C G. Appraisal of the MTT assay as a rapid test of chemosensitivity in acute myeloid leukemia. British Journal of Cancer 1989; 60: 206-210.

[33] Yamori T, Matsunaga A, Sato S, Yamazaki K, Komi A, Ishizu K, Mita I, Edatsugi H, Matsuba Y, Takezawa K, Nakanishi O, Kohno H, Nakajima Y, Komatsu H, Andoh T, Tsuruo T. Potent antitumor activity of MS-247, a novel DNA minor groove binder, evaluated by an in vitro and in vivo human cancer cell line panel. Cancer Research 1999; 59: 4042-4049.

[34] Masuda T, Hidaka K, Shinohara A, Maekawa T, Takeda Y, Yamaguchi H. Chemical studies on antioxidant mechanism of curcuminoid: Analysis of Radical Reaction Products from Curcumin. Journal of Agricultural and Food Chemistry 1999; 47: 71-77.

[35] Motterlinia R, Forestia R, Bassia R, Greena C J. Curcumin, an antioxidant and anti-inflammatory agent, induces heme oxygenase-1 and protects endothelial cells against oxidative stress. Free Radical Biology and Medicine 2000; 28: 1303-1312.

[36] Chan M M Y, Huang H I, Fenton M R, Fong D. In vivo inhibition of nitric oxide synthase gene expression by curcumin, a cancer preventive natural product with anti-inflammatory properties. Biochemical Pharmacology 1988; 55: 1955–1962.

[37] Suksamrarn A, Ponglikitmongkol M, Wongkrajang K, Chindaduang A, Kittidanairak S, Jankam A, Yingyongnarongkul B, Kittipanumat N, Chokchaisiri R, Khetkam P, Piyachaturawat P. Diarylheptanoids, new phytoestrogens from the rhizomes of *Curcuma comosa*: Isolation, chemical modification and estrogenic activity evaluation. Bioorganic and Medicinal Chemistry 2008; 16: 6891-6902.

[38] Winuthayanon W, Piyachaturawat P, Suksamrarn A, Ponglikitmongkol M, Arao Y, Hewitt S C, Korach K S. Diarylheptanoid phytoestrogens isolated from the medicinal plant *Curcuma comosa*: Biologic actions in vitro and in vivo indicate estrogen receptor–dependent mechanisms. Environ Health Perspect 2009; 117: 1155–1161.

[39] Adamsa B K, Ferstlb E M, Davisb M C, Heroldb M, Kurtkayab S, Camalierc R F, Hollingsheadc M G, Kaurc G, Sausvillec E A, Ricklesd F R, Snyderb J P, Liottab D C, Shojia M. Synthesis and biological evaluation of novel curcumin analogs as anti-cancer and anti-angiogenesis agents. Bioorganic and Medicinal Chemistry 2004; 12, 3871–3883.

[40] Nakashima N, Kimura I, Kimura M, Matsuura H. Isolation of pseudoprototimosaponin AIII from rhizomes of *Anemarrhena asphodeloides* and its hypoglycemic activity in streptozotocin-induced diabetic mice. Journal of Natural Products 1993; 56: 345–350.

[41] Choi S B, Park S. A steroidal glycoside from *Polygonatum odoratum* (Mill.) Druce. improves insulin resistance but does not alter insulin secretion in 90% pancreatectomized rats. Bioscience, Biotechnology, and Biochemistry 2002; 66: 2036-2043.

[42] Wu R T, Chiang H C, Fu W C, Chien K Y, Chung Y M, Horng L Y. Formosanin-C, an immunomodulator with antitumor activity. International Journal of Immunopharmacology 1990; 12, 777–786.

[43] Miyata T. Antitussive action of Mai-Men-Dong-Tang: Suppression of ACE inhibitor- and tachykinin-inducing dry cough. Journal of Traditional Sino-Japanese medicine 1992; 13: 276-279.

[44] Ikeda T, Ando J, Miyazono A, Zhu X H, Tsumagari H, Nohara T, Yokomizo K, Uyeda M. Anti-herpes virus activity of Solanum steroidal glycosides. Biological and Pharmaceutical Bulletin 2000; 23, 363-364.

[45] Niwa A, Takeda O, Ishimaru M, Nakamoto Y, Yamasaki K, Kohda H, Nishio H, Segawa T, Fujimaru K, Kuramoto A. Screening test for platelet aggregation inhibitor in natural products. The active principle of Anemarrhenae Rhizoma. Yakugaku Zasshi 1988; 108: 555-561.

Chapter 5

Application of Saponin-Containing Plants in Foods and Cosmetics

Yukiyoshi Tamura, Masazumi Miyakoshi and
Masaji Yamamoto

Additional information is available at the end of the chapter

http://dx.doi.org/10.5772/53333

1. Introduction

Saponins are a class of natural products which are structurally constructed of aglycone (triterpene or steroid) and sugars (hexose and/or uronic acid). The name 'saponin' comes from soap as its containing plants agitated in water form soapy lather. Saponins are widely distributed in many plants and are relatively widespread in our foodstuffs and herbal preparations. Saponins traditionally used as a natural detergent. In addition to this physical property, plant-derived triterpenoid and steroidal saponins have historically received a number of industrial and commercial applications ranging from their use as sources of raw materials for the production of steroid hormones in the pharmaceutical industry, to their use as food additives and as ingredients in photographic emulsions, fire extinguishers and other industrial applications which take advantage of their generally non-ionic surfactant properties [1-3]. They also exhibit a variety of biological activities, and have been investigated toward the development of new natural medicines and prove the efficacy of traditional herbal medicines [4]. Other interesting biological applications for various specific saponins include their uses as anti-inflammatory [5], hypocholesterolemic [6] and immune-stimulating [7] whose properties are widely recognized and commercially utilized.

As to the application of saponins to foods and cosmetics, it is indispensable that sufficient amounts of plant resources are available, and that the content of saponins must be high. Furthermore, a plant must have a long history of human use as foodstuffs or ingredients of cosmetics, and their safety should be officially guaranteed.

The saponins of Quillaja bark and licorice root are widely utilized in the world. The *Quillaja saponaria* (Rosaceae) tree has remained of special interest, because of its bark containing 9-10

% saponins. A large amount of Quillaja saponin is utilized in photosensitized film as a surfactant. It is used also in beverages, food ingredients, shampoos, liquid detergents, toothpastes and extinguishers as an emulsifier and long-lasting foaming agent. Recently, the saponin mixture possesses the immunoadjuvant property and has pharmaceutical application as suspension stabilizer [8].

Nearly 50,000 tons of licorice roots (*Glycyrrhiza* spp., Leguminosae) are consumed on a year basis. Licorice extract and its major saponin, glycyrrhizin (yield: more than 2.5%), are used as a medicine and as a sweetener and flavor enhancer in foods and cigarettes [9].

It is known that the deterioration of cooked foods is caused mainly by yeast, and that many skin diseases are due to infection by dermatophytic fungi and yeasts. In an expansion of utilization of saponins in foods and cosmetics, we have examined antifungal and antiyeast saponins.

2. Screening of antiyeast saponins

Crude saponin fractions from several plants were subjected to an antiyeast screening test using *Candida albicans* and/or *Saccharomyces cerevisiae*. Preparation of saponin fraction for screening test was following methods. Each plant material was extracted with hot 50% of MeOH. A suspension of the MeOH-extract in H2O was chromatographed on a column of Diaion HP-20 eluting with 40%-, and MeOH. The MeOH eluate (crude saponin fraction) was subjected to the screening test.

Inhibitory activity against each yeast was determined using agar dilution method. The inhibitory activity of the samples was assessed as the minimum inhibitory concentration (MIC), the lowest concentration tested at which no growth was observed.

Table 1 shows the screening results of antiyeast activity tests of crude saponin mixtures from several plants. The saponin fraction from licorice root, quillaja bark, gypsophila root and soy bean seed showed no activity (MIC:>1000μg/ml) and that of hedera leaf, marronier seed, ginseng root, camellia seed, saponaria rhizome and tea seed showed a weak activity (MIC:500~1000μg/ml), wheras crude saponin fraction from pericarps of *Sapindus mukurossi* and the stems of Mohave yucca exhibited significant activity, the active principles of both these materials were further investigated in detail.

	C.a.	S.c.		C.u.	S.c.
Licorice root	>1000	>1000	Ginseng root	1000	1000
Quillaja bark	>1000	>1000	Camellia seed	1000	1000
Gypsophila root	>1000	>1000	Saponaria rhizome	NT	1000
Hedera leaf	1000	1000	Tea seed	500	500
Soy been seed	NT	>1000	Yucca stem	NT	250
Marronier seed	1000	1000	Sapindus pericarp	250	250

C.a: Candida albicans, S.c.: Saccharomyces cerevisiae, NT: not tested

Table 1. Antiyeast activities of crude saponin fractions (MIC μg/ml)

3. *Sapindus* pericarps

Addition of an antifungal and antiyeast ingredient to cosmetics is desirable for the protection of skin against, and prevention of, dandruff generation, dermatomycosis and cutaneous candidiasis.

Significant antiyeast activity was observed for the crude saponin fraction from the pericarps of *Sapindus mukurossi* (Sapindaceae), a tall tree that grows abundantly in China and Japan. Pericaps of this plant have been used as a natural detergent, and are utilized as foaming-stabilizing agents in chemical fire extinguishers in Japan. The pericarps have also been used as an antitussive, anti-inflammatory and anthelmintic agent as well as for treatment of dermatomycosis. In Japan, the pericarps is called "enmei-hi", which means "life prolonging pericarps", and in China, it has been called "wu-huan-zi", which means "non-illness fruit".

4. Antifungal and antiyeast oleanane-saponins of *Sapindus* pericarps

The percarps were extracted with hot 90% MeOH. A suspension of the MeOH-extract in H_2O was chromatographed on a column of highly porous polymer (Diaion H-20) eluting with H_2O and 50%- and 85%-MeOH, successively. 85%-MeOH eluate gave a saponin-mixture (mono- and bis-desmosides, SP-mix). Hederagenin (1) was obtained from SP-mix by usual acid hydrolysis. Saponins 2-7 were isolated from SP-mix, such as monodesmosides: saponin A (2), sapindoside B (3), saponin C (4), sapindoside A (5), mukurozi-saponin E1 (6) etc. and bisdesmosides: mukurozi-saponin Y1 (7) etc. [10]. The structures of these saponins are shown in Figure 1.

Antidermatophytic activities of these saponins are shown in Table 2. All the monodesmosides exhibited strong growth inhibition. It is noteworthy that activity of sapindoside A is almost as strong as that of griseofulvin, the well-known antidermatophytic antibiotic. Griseofulvin does not show inhibitory activity against a pathogenic yeast, *Candida albicans*, while these monodesmosides ehhibited significant inhibition. The bisdesmosides, mukurozi-saponin Y1 showed no activity.

It was found that while purified monodesmosides of pericarps are sparingly soluble in water, their solubility was greatly increased in the presence of bisdesmosides [10]. These phenomena are important for the biological activities of the pericarps.

5. Structure-antifungal activity relationship

Figure 1 showed antidermatophytic activity against *Tricophyton rubrum* was investigated for a variety of oleanane saponins. Saponins 8-10 were separated from roots of *Anemone rivularis* [11]. Saponins 11-13 were isolated from bupleurum roots [12], and saponins 14 and 15 were prepared from 11 and 12, respectively by the reference [13]. Saponin 16 was isolated from roots of *Kalopanax septemlobus* [14]. Saponin 17-20 were isolated from brans of *Chenopodium quinoa* [15, 16], and saponin 21 from rhizome of *Thladiantha hookeri* var. *pentadactyla* [17], derivative 1 (22) was prepared from 21, and derivative 2 (23) from 22 [16].

It was disclosed that for growth inhibition, the presence of free 28-COOH, 23-OH and 3-*O*-glycosyl groups is essential (Figure 2). A sugar moiety was prerequisite for the antifungal activity of oleanane saponin. All the bisdesmosides of hederagein, such as kalopanaxsaponin B (16), the 28-COOH of which is glycosylated, showed no activity. Mono- and bisdesmosides of oleanolic acid, such as saponin CP4 (8), which lack a 23-OH, also showed no growth inhibition. Saikosaponins, the active principles of *Bupleurum* radix, lack a 28-COOH, exhibiting no activity. Thalandioside H1 (21), a bisdesmoside which was isolated from *Thandiantha hookeri* var. *pentaphyla* in yield of 10% without any chromatography (Nie et al., 1989), showed no activity, while a monodesmoside of hederagein derived from this bisdesmoside, exhibited activity. Activity was also obserbed for hederagenin-3-*O*-α-L-arabinoside (24) which was prepared from 17 [18].

	Trichophyton mentagrophytes	***T. rubrum***	***Epidermophyton floccosum***	***Sabouraudites canis***	***Candida albicans***
SP-mix	25	25	25	12.5	50
2. saponin A	6.25	6.25	6.25	3.13	12.5
3. sapindoside B	6.25	6.25	3.13	3.13	12.5
4. saponin C	6.25	6.25	6.25	3.13	25
5. sapindoside A	3.13	1.56	3.13	1.56	12.5
6. mukurozi-saponin E1	6.25	6.25	6.25	3.13	12.5
7. Mukurozi-saponin Y1	>100	>100	>100	>100	>100
1. Hederagenin	>100	>100	>100	>100	>100
griseofulvin*	3.13	1.56	0.78	1.56	>100
* positive control					

Table 2. Antimicrobial activities of saponins and saponin mixture (**SP-mix**) against dermatophytes (**MIC**:μg/ml)

6. Antimicrobial activity of the saponin fraction of *Sapindus* pericarps

For commercial utilization as ingredient in cosmetics, the saponin fraction was prepared as follows. The methanolic extract was subjected to chromatography on Diaion HP-20. After removal of other water-soluble constituents by elution with water and then 50% of MeOH, the saponin fraction was obtained by elution with 80% MeOH.

The saponin fraction showed moderate antibacterial activity against Gram-positive bacteria, while no activity was obserbed against Gram-negative bacteria (Table 3).

A summarized in Table 4, the saponin fraction exhibited growth inhibition against food deteriorating yeasts, *Pichia nakazawae, Debaryomyces hansenii* and *Hansenula anomala*, as well as against *Malassezia furfur* which is associated with dandruff generation. The activity of saponin fraction against common fungi was not so strong, while it exhibited remarkable growth-inhibitory effects against the following dermatophytic fungi and pathogenic yeast, *Tricophyton rubrum, T. mentagrophytes, Sabouraudites canis,* and *Epidermophyton floccosum* (which are known as dermatophytic fungi) and against *Candida albicans,* a pathogenic yeast which causes cutaneous candidiasis.

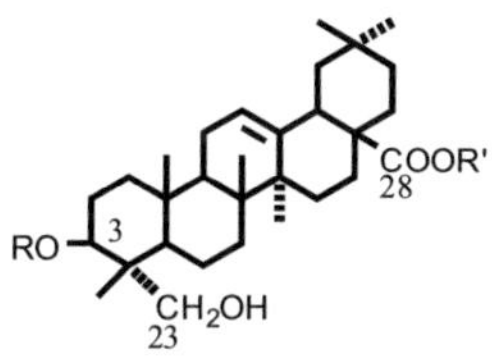

	R	R'
1. hederagenin	H	H
2. Saponin A	-Ara(p)-2-Rha-3-Ara(p)	H
3. Sapindoside B	-Ara(p)-2-Rha-3-Xyl	H
4. Saponin C	-Ara(p)-2-Rha-3-Ara(f)	H
5. Sapindoside A	-Ara(p)-2-Rha	H
6. Mukurozi-saponin E1	-Ara-(p)-2-Rha-3-Xyl-4-Ac	H
7. Mukurozi-saponin-Y1	-Ara(p)-2-Rha-3-Xyl	-Glc-2- Glc

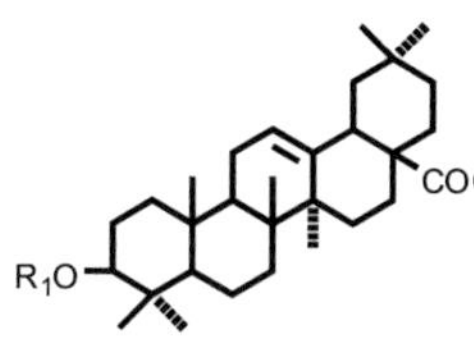

	R_1	R_2	MIC (μg/ml)
8. Saponin CP4	-Ara-Rha-Rib	H	>400
9. Huzhangoside A	-Xyl-Rha-Rib	H	>400
10. Huzhangoside B	-Ara-Rha-Rib	-(Glc)2-Rha	>400

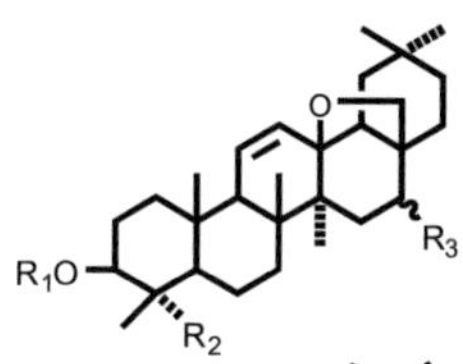

	R_1	R_2	R_3	MIC (μg/ml)
11. Saikosaponin a	-Fuc-Glc	CH_2OH	β-OH	>400
12. Saikosaponin b	-Fuc-Glc	CH_2OH	α-OH	>400
13. Saikosaponin c	-Glc-Rha \ Glc	Me	β-OH	>400

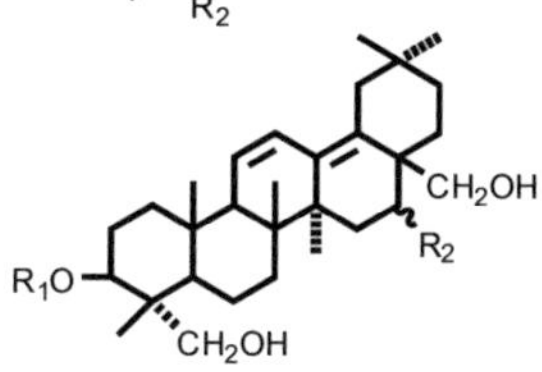

	R_1	R_2	MIC (μg/ml)
14. Saikosaponin b1	-Fuc-Glc	β-OH	>400
15. Saikosaponin b2	-Fuc-Glc	α-OH	>400

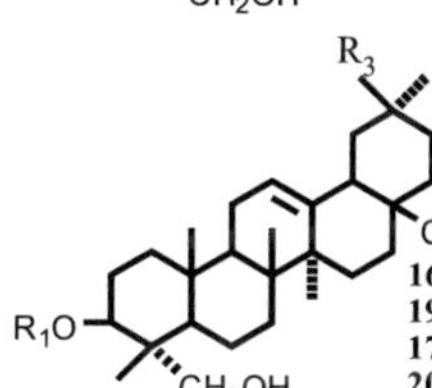

	R_1	R_2	R_3	MIC (μg/ml)
16. Kalopanax-saponin B	-Ara-Rha	$-(Glc)_2$-Rha	Me	>400
19. Quinoa-saponin 3	-Ara	-Glc	COOMe	>400
17. NH-saponin F	-Ara	-Glc	Me	>400
20. Quinoa-saponin 4	-Ara-Glc	-Glc	COOMe	>400
18. Quinoa-saponin 2	-Ara-Glc	-Glc	Me	>400

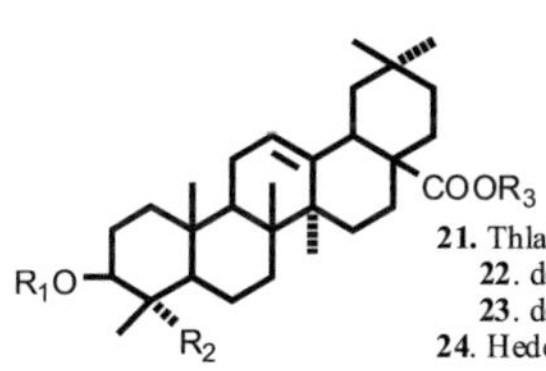

	R_1	R_2	R_3	MIC (μg/ml)
21. Thlandioside H1	-GlcA-Gal	CHO	-Xyl-Rha-(Xyl)2	>400
22. derivative 1	-GlcA-Gal	CH2OH	-Xyl-Rha-(Xyl)2	>400
23. derivative 2	-GlcA-Gal	CH2OH	H	>400
24. Hederagenin-3-Ara	-Ara(p)	CH_2OH	H	>400

Figure 1. Structure and antifungal activities of saponins on *Tricophyton rubrum*

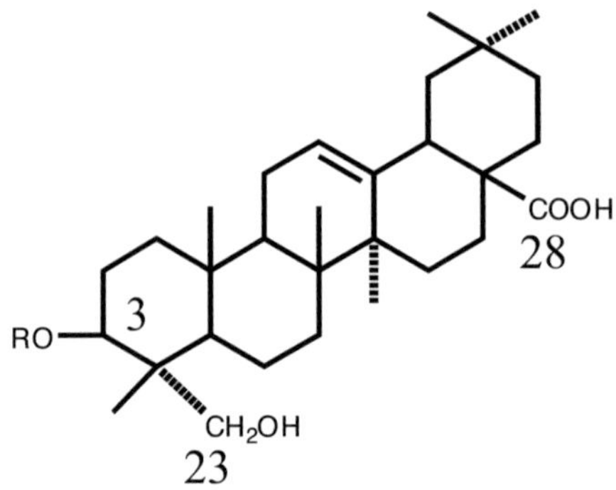

Figure 2. Structure-antimicrobial activity relationship of oleanane-type saponin analogues

Gram-positive, MIC:µg/ml		Gram-negative, MIC:µg/ml	
Staphylococcus			
aureus IID 671	400	*Escherichia coli* HUT 215	>400
epidermidis IID 866	400	*Pseudomonas aeruginosa* JCM 2776	>400
Streptococcus mutans IFO 13955	400	*Alcaligenes faecalis* IFO 13111	>400
Bacillus subtilis IFO 3007	400	*Proteus vulgaris* IFO 3851	>400

Table 3. Antibacterial activity of saponin mixture (SP-mix)

Yeast, MIC:µg/ml			
Saccharomyces cerevisiae IFO 0203	100	*Candida utilis* IFO 0396	100
Pichia nakazawae HUT 1688	50	*Hansenula anomala* HUT 7083	50
Malassezia furfur IFO 0656	200	*Debaryomyces hansenii* IFO 0018	>400
Fungi, MIC:µg/ml			
Aspergillus niger IFO 4343	>400	*Rhizopus nigricans* IFO 4731	>400
Mucor pusillus HUT 1185	100	*Penicillium citrinum* IFO 4631	>400

Table 4. Antiyeast and antifungal activity of saponin Mixture (**SP-mix**)

http://dx.doi.org/10.5772/53333

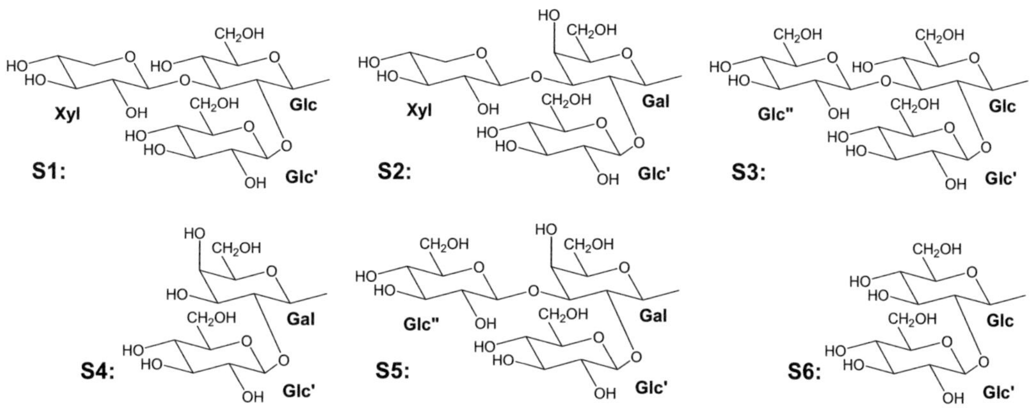

Figure 3. Saponins from Mohave yucca

7. *Sapindus* saponin fraction as an antidermatophytic ingredient in cosmetics

It is difficult to use *Sapindus* saponin fraction as a food ingredient without long-term toxicity test, because we have no history of this fraction or *Sapindus* extract as a foodstuff. Furthrmore, it tastes very bitter, changing the taste of foods. On the other hand, the extract has been used as a folk detergent,and is listed in the Japanese Cosmeic Ingredient Codex (JCIC), being authorized as an ingredient in cosmetics by the Ministry of Health and Welfare in Japan. We reconfirmed the safety of the saponin fraction by dermal toxicity tests. It did not show primary dermal irritant, sentitization, phototoxicity or photosensitization effects. The present study strongly suggests that the saponins of the pericarps as an ingredient in toiletries, are valuable not only as detergents, but also for the prevention of dermatomycosis, cutaneous candidiasis as well as for dandruff generation.

8. Mohave Yucca (Yucca schidigera)

Yucca species (Agavaceae), grows widely in North and Central America. Mohave yucca, *Y. schidigera*, has been used as a foodstuff and folk medicine by Native Americans as well as early California settlers to treat a variety of ailments including arthritis and inflammation [3], and is approved for use in food and beverages by the U.S. Food and Drug Administration (FDA) under Title 21 CFR 172.510, FEMA number 3121. Yucca products are currently used in a number of applications. Yucca powder and yucca extract are used as animal feed additives, as in reference [19]. Other applications include the use of the extract of this plant is now utilized as a long-lasting foaming agent in carbonated beverages, root beer, regular and low-alcohol beers, and in shampoos and foaming cosmetics. Recently, the potential of biological activities of saponins and phenolics from this plant was reviewed [20].

9. Antiyeast and antifungal spirostanoid saponins from Mohave yucca

The presence of steroidal saponins in this plant has been reported previously [21,22]. As to the saponin constituents of this plant, a monodesmoside named YS-1 is isolated and identified as in [23]. We have conducted the isolation and identification of individual saponins that had not been achieved prior to this study [24,25].

The EtOH extract of this plant was subjected to colomn chromatography on highly porous polymer, Diaion HP-20, which is styrene-divinylbenzene polymer. After successive elution with water and 60% and 80% MeOH, a saponin fraction which showed significant antiyeast activity against *Saccharomyces cerevisiae* was obtained by elution with 90% MeOH. This fraction was subjected to successive chromatography on silica gel and then octadesysilylated silica gel (ODS) and was finaly separated by HPLC on ODS to give fourteen yucca saponins 25-38.

Figure 3 shows the structure of all of these saponins and their sapogenins. The antiyeast activities of each saponin from *Y. schidigera* against six kinds of yeast, *Saccharomyces cerevisiae* (brewers yeast), *Candida albicans* (a pathogenic yeast) and *Hansenula anomala, Pichia nakazawae, Kloeckera apiculata* and *Debaryomyces hansenii* (food-deteriorating yeasts) were determined and are summarized in Table 5.

Those saponins having a branched-chain trisaccharide moiety without any oxygen functionalities at C-2 and –12 exhibited potent antiyeast activities, while saponins with 2β-hydroxyl (5,6,13, and 14) or 12-keto (4 and 12) groups showed very weak or no activity. A saponin (11) with a disaccharide moiety exhibited relatively low activities. The aglycons showed no antiyeast activity.

10. Antimicrobial activity of the saponin fraction

For the commercial utilization of Mohave yucca, the antimicrobial activity of the saponin fraction which was obtained by column chromatography of the extract on Diaion HP-20 (*vide supra*) was investigated. It showed no or only weak growth inhibition against both Gram-positive and Gram-negative bacteria (Table 6).

http://dx.doi.org/10.5772/53333

	S.c.[a]	C.a.[b]	H.a.[c]	P.a.[d]	K.a.[e]	D.h.[f]
25	3.13	6.25	3.13	3.13	12.5	6.25
26	12.5	12.5	3.13	3.13	>100	>100
27	12.5	12.5	6.25	3.13	>100	>100
28	>100	>100	>100	>100	>100	>100
29	100	100	>100	100	>100	>100
30	>100	>100	>100	>100	>100	>100
31	6.25	50	3.13	3.13	>100	6.25
32	25	>100	3.13	3.13	>100	50
33	6.25	>100	3.13	12.5	>100	6.25
34	12.5	25	3.13	6.25	50	6.25
35	12.5	12.5	6.25	3.13	>100	>100
36	100	>100	100	>100	>100	>100
37	100	>100	>100	>100	>100	100
38	>100	>100	>100	100	>100	>100

[a] *Saccharomyces cerevisiae*, [b] *Candid albicans*, [c] *Hansenula anomala*, [d] *Pichia nakazawae*, [e] *Kloeckera apiculata*, [f] *Debaryomyces hansenii*

Table 5. Antiyeast activity of *Yucca schidigera* saponins

Gram-positive bacteria, MIC (μg/ml)			
Staphylococcus		*Bacillus circulans* IFO 3329	>1,000
aureus IID 671	1,000	*Lactobacillus*	
aureus IFO 3060	1,000	*plantarum* IFO 3070	>1,000
epidermidis IID 866	>1,000	*rhamnosus* IFO 12521	>1,000
Bacillus		*Enterococcus faecalis* IFO 3971	>1,000
subtilis IFO 3007	1,000	*Streptococcus mutans* IFO 13955	>1,000
licheniformis IFO 12200	1,000		
Gram-negative bacteria, MIC (μg/ml)			
Escherichia coli HUT 215	>1,000	*Pseudomonas*	
Alcaligenes faecalis IFO 13111	1,000	*aeruginosa* JCM 2776	>1,000
Proteus vulgaris IFO 3851	1,000	*fluorescens* JCM 2779	>1,000
Klebsiella pneumoniae IFO14940	1,000		

Table 6. Antibacterial acrivity of yucca saponin fraction

Yeast, MIC (μg/ml)			
Saccharomyces		*Kloeckera apiculata* IFO 154	62.5
cerevisiae IMO 293	62.5	*Debaryomyces*	
cerevisiae HUT 2075	31.3	*hanenii* IFO 18	31.3
cerevisiae JCM 2223	62.5	*hanenii* IFO 27	62.5
Hansenulla sp.	31.3	*hanenii* IFO 47	31.3
anomala HUT 7083	31.3	*hanenii* IFO 7011	125
Cryptococcus sp.	31.3	*Zygosacharomyces*	
laurentii IFO 609	125	*rouxii* IFO 845	31.3
Pichia		*rouxii* IFO 1130	31.3
nalazawae HUT 1688	31.3	*Candida famata* IFO 664	31.3
carsonii IFO 946	31.3		
Fungi, MIC (μg/ml)			
Aspergillus		*Aspergillus*	
niger IFO 4343	>1,000	*awamoi* HUT 2014	>1,000
oryzae HUT 2065	>1,000	*awamoi* HUT 2015	>1,000
oryzae HUT 2175	125	*Mucor pusillus* HUT 1185	15.6
oryzae HUT 2188	>1,000	*Rhizopus*	
oryzae HUT 2192	>1,000	*formosaensis* IFO 4756	>1,000
sydowii HUT 4097	>1,000	*nigricans* IFO 4731	>1,000
		Penicillium expansum IFO 5453	>1,000
Dermatophytic yeast and fungi, MIC (μg/ml)			
Tricophyton		*Sabouraudites canis* IFO 7863	31.3
rubrum IFO 5807	15.6	*Epidermophyton floccosum* IFO 9045	31.3
mentagrophytes IFO 5809	31.3	*Candida albicans* TIMM 0134	62.5

* food deteriorating yeast ** film-forming yeast in soy sauce

Table 7. Antiyeast and antifungal acrivity of yucca saponin fraction

The antiyeast and antifungal activities are summarized in Table 7. The saponin fraction exhibited potent antiyeast activity. Infection of boiled rice such as "sushi" and "musubi" with *Hansenula anomala* and *Kloeckera apiculata* results in odor smelling like an organic solvent. Infection of cooked beans and processed fish meat with *Candida famata* and *Pichia carsonii* causes oders smelling like kerosene. *Pichia nakazawae, Debaryomyces hansenii* and *Zygosaccharomyces rouxii* are film-forming yeasts, damaging "soy sauce" and "miso", oriental fermented seasonings. The saponin fraction exhibited strong growth inhibition against these food-deteriorating yeasts.

The saponin fraction showed less activity against common fungi, while it significantly inhibited the growth of dermatophytic yeast and fungi.

Potassium sorbate has been utilized in foods as a preservative. Its antiyeast activity depends upon pH. Between pH 5.0 – 3.0, potassium sorbate completely inhibited the growth of yeast at the concentration of 0.05%, while at less acidic pH (near neutral), the activity decreased remarkably. In contrast to this, such pH dependence was not observed for the yucca saponin fraction. In the range of pH 6.3 – 3.0, it entirely inhibited the growth of yeasts at the concentration of 0.03%.

11. Effects of several culture conditions against antimicrobial activity of yucca extract

The inhibitory effects of yucca extract on the growth of the yeasts isolated from ume-zuke, a salted Japanese apricot fruit product were investigated with (2% or 5%) or without sodium chloride (Table 8). From the results of MICs of yucca extract without sodium chloride, the genera *Debaryomyces, Kloeckera, Pichia, Saccharomyces* and *Zygosaccharomyces* are sensitive to yucca extract, while the genera *Cryptococcus, Rhodotorula* and *Sporobolomyces* are tolerate to yucca extract. For the difference between these yeasts, latter yeast belong anamorphic basidiomycetous genera.

The inhibitory effect was enhanced and showed a broad antiyeast spectrum when yucca extract was used in combination with sodium chloride.

Table 9 shows the effects of several cultural conditions against antiyeast activity of yucca extract. The antiyeast activity of yucca extract was strengthened under the condition of chemical and physical conditions, low pH, alcohol, heating and high OP. While the high-polymer substances, such as polysaccharides and protein reduced antiyeast activity of yucca extract. It is interested that antiyeast activity of yucca extract was inhibited by free unsaturated fatty acids, palmitoleic acid, oleic acid and linoleic acid. On the other hand, saturated fatty acids, palmitic acid and stearic acid and oils composed of unsaturated fatty acids, olive oil, soybean oil and egg lecithin had no effect on the antiyeast activity of yucca extract.

Yeast	MIC (µg/ml) NaCl 0%	2%	5%	Yeast	MIC (µg/ml) NaCl 0%	2%	5%
Candida				***Pichia***			
C. albicans 221	1000	500	250	*P.anomala* 201	500	250	250
C. guilliermondii 212	>2000	1000	500	*P.anomala* 202	250	250	250
C. guilliermondii 213	>2000	2000	500	*P.anomala* 203	250	125	125
C. guilliermondii 222	1000	500	250	*P.anomala* 204	500	250	250
C. guilliermondii 224	1000	250	250	*P.anomala* 206	250	125	125
C. guilliermondii 227	>2000	>2000	2000	*P.anomala* 211	500	250	250
C. krusei 222	>2000	>2000	1000	*P.anomala* 216	500	250	125
C. lipolytica 223	62.5	62.5	62.5	*P.anomala* 219	500	250	250
C. parapsilosis 224	1000	500	500	*P.anomala* 223	500	250	250
C. tropicalis 225	>2000	>2000	1000	*P.anomala* 256	500	250	250
C. valida 226	1000	500	125	*P.anomala* 260	250	250	250
C. versatilis 228	500	250	250	*P.anomala* 261	500	250	250
C. zeylanoides 229	250	250	125	*P.anomala* 262	500	250	250
Cryptococcus				*P.anomala* 265	500	250	250
C. neoformans 231	>2000	>2000	1000	*P. farinosa* 207	250	250	125
Debaryomyces				***Rhodotorula***			
D.hansenii 201	1000	125	62.5	*R. rubra* 233	>2000	1000	500
D.hansenii 206	1000	1000	2000	***Saccharomyces***			
D.hansenii 214	1000	1000	1000	*S. cerevisiae* 203	500	250	62.5
D.hansenii 215	1000	1000	2000	*S. cerevisiae* 208	250	250	62.5
D.hansenii 220	2000	2000	>2000	*S. farmentati* 209	500	250	62.5
D.hansenii 225	1000	2000	2000	*S. fibullgera* 211	2000	1000	1000
D.hansenii 263	>2000	2000	1000	*S. servazzii* 210	2000	1000	1000
Geotrichum				***Shizosaccharomyces***			
G. candidum 218	500	125	NG	*S. pombe* 212	62.5	NG	NG
G. capitatum 219	2000	1000	NG	***Sporobolomyces***			
Hansenula				*S. albo-rubescens* 234	>2000	>2000	2000
H. saturnus 202	1000	500	250	***Torulaspora***			
Issatchenkia				*T. delbrieckii* 4188	500	125	62.5
I. orientalis 237	125	125	62.5	*T. delbrieckii* 4952	500	500	250

Yeast	MIC (μg/ml)			Yeast	MIC (μg/ml)		
	NaCl				NaCl		
	0%	2%	5%		0%	2%	5%
Kloeckera				***Zygosaccharomyces***			
K. apiculata 203	1000	1000	500	*Z. bailii* 213	2000	250	NG
K. apiculata 208	1000	500	500	*Z. rouxii* 214	500	250	250
K. apiculata 258	1000	1000	500	*Z. rouxii* 215	250	250	250
K. apiculata 266	>2000	>2000	2000	*Z. rouxii* 216	125	125	250
K. apiculata 4631	2000	1000	62.5				
K. apiculata 12219	2000	2000	500				
K. corticis 217	1000	1000	NG				
K. corticis 236	2000	250	NG				
K. corticis 12828	500	250	NG				
K. japonica 12220	500	500	250				

NG : No growth recognized without yucca extract

Table 8. Antiyeast activity of yucca extract against 64 yeasts isolated from foods and effect of NaCl on antiyeast activity of yucca saponin fraction

	low pH	heating	alcohol	polysaccharide	protein	lipid		high OP***
USFA*	TG**							
antiyeast activity	↑[a]	↑	↑	↓	↓	↓	→	↑

*unsatulated fatty acid, **triglycerides, ***osmotic pressure

a:↑strengthen, ↓reduce, →no change

Table 9. Effects of the cultural condition against antiyeast activity of yucca extract

12. Utilization of the yucca extract as an anti-food deteriorating agents

Yucca extract is non-toxic and non-mutagenic. It is recognized as safe for human food use by U.S.FDA (listed in 21 CFR 172.510). The extract is tasteless and odourless, exerting no influence on the taste of foods. It is readily soluble in water and stable on heating. Based on the present study, commercial application of the extract for extending the shelf life of cooked foods and fermented seasonings is now under development [26].

Figure 4 shows the application of yucca extract to sponge cake. Addition of 0.2% of yucca extract to sponge cake had effective on the growth of fungi and yeasts stored in room for one week.

The application of yucca extract to strawberry jam was showed in Figure 5. The jam mixed 0.02% and 0.04% of yucca extract and stored in room for one week shows no change, whereas control jam was contaminated by fungi.

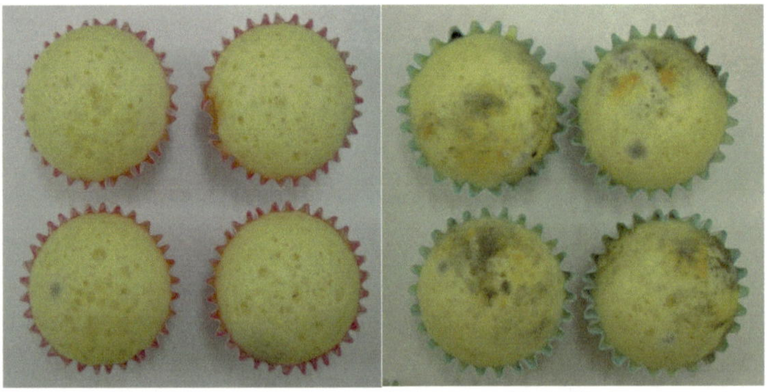

(Yucca (0.2%)) (Controll)

Figure 4. Application of yucca extract to sponge cake

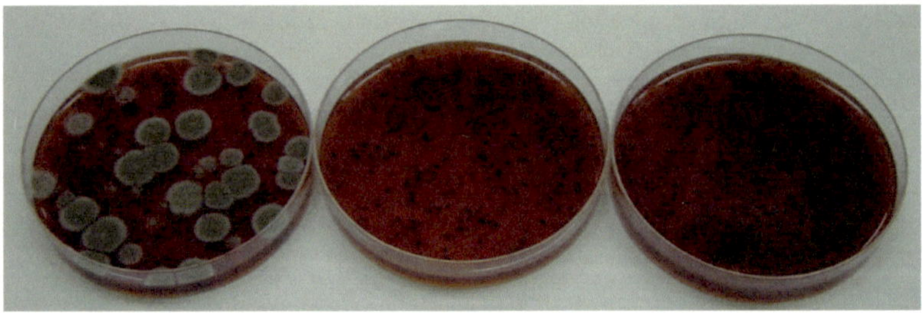

(Controll) (Yucca 0.02%) (Yucca 0.04%)

Figure 5. Application of yucca extract to strawberry jam

13. Conclusion

The microbial safety of foods and cosmetics continues to be a major concern to consumers, regulatory agencies and food industries throughout the world. Although synthetic antimicrobials are approved in many countries, the recent trend has been for use of natural preservatives, which necessitates the exploration of alternative sources of safe, effective and

http://dx.doi.org/10.5772/53333

acceptable natural preservatives. Many plant extracts possess antimicrobial activity against a range of bacteria, yeast and fungi, but the variations in quality and quantity of their bioactive constituents is major disadvantage to their industrial uses.

Based on the present study, mukurozi extract and yucca extract are considered to be effective for the preservation of foods and cosmetics. Both mukurozi and yucca plants have been consumed by humans for a long time. These plants also have wide application due to little pH or food component interaction.

Thus our works demonstrate that the saponin fraction from Sapindus pericarps and Mohave yucca stems can be recommended as alternative preservations for foods and cosmetics.

Author details

Yukiyoshi Tamura, Masazumi Miyakoshi and Masaji Yamamoto

Maruzen Pharmaceuticals Co. Ltd.,Hiroshima, Japan

References

[1] Leung AY, Encyclopedia of Common Natural Ingredients Used in Food, Drugs and Cosmetics, John Wiley and Sons, New York, 1980

[2] Hostettmann K, Marston, Saponins, Cambridge University Press, Cambridge, 1995

[3] Leung AY, Foster S. Encyclopedia of Common natural Ingredients Used in Food, Drugs and Cosmetics, 2nd ed., John Wiley and Sons, New York, 1996

[4] Waller GR, Yamasaki K. Proceedings of an American Chemical Society Symposium on Saponins: August 20-24, 1995, Chicago, Illinois

[5] Balandrin MF, Commercial Utilization of Plant-derived Saponins: An Overview of medicinal, Pharmaceutical and Industrial Applications, In: Waller GR and Yamasaki K. (eds) Saponins Used in Food and Agriculture: Plenum Press; 1996. p1-14

[6] Oakenfull D. Saponins in the treatment of hypercholesterolemia, In: Spiller GA (ed.) Handbook of Lipids in Human Nutrition. CRC Press; 1996. p107-112

[7] Klausner A. Adjuvants: a real shot in the arm for recombinant vaccines. Bio/Technology 1988; 6(7), 773-777

[8] Setten DC, Werken G. Molecular Structures of Saponins from *Quillaja saponaria* Molina. In: Waller GR and Yamasaki K. (eds) Saponins Used in traditional and Modern Medicine: Plenum Press; 1996. p185-193

[9] Hayashi H, Sudo H. Economic importance of licorice. Plant Biotechnology 2009; 26, 101-104

[10] Kimata H, Tanaka O. et al. Saponins of pericarps of *Sapindus mukurossi* Gaertn. and solubilization of monodesmosides by bisdesmosides. Chemical Pharmaceutical Bulletin 1983; 31(6), 1998-2005

[11] Mizutani K, Tanaka O. et al. Saponins from *Anemone rivularis*. Planta Medica 1984; 50(4), 327-331

[12] Ishii H, Yoshimura Y. et al. Isolation, characterization and nuclear magnetic response spectra of new saponins from the roots of *Bupleurum falcatum* L. Chemical Pharmaceutical Bulletin 1980; 28(8), 2367-2383

[13] Kimata H, Tanaka O. et al. Saponins of Juk-Siho and roots of *Bupleurum longeradiatum* Turcz. Chemical Pharmaceutical Bulletin 1982; 30(12), 4373-4377

[14] Shao CJ, Tanaka O. et al. Saponins from roots of *Kalopanax septemlobus* (Thunb.) Koidz., Ciqui: Structure of kalopanax-saponin C, D, E and F. Chemical Pharmaceutical Bulletin 1989; 37(2), 311-314

[15] Kizu H, Namba T. et al. Studies on Nepalese crude drugs. III. On the saponins of *Hedera nepalensis* K. Koch. Chemical Pharmaceutical Bulletin 1985; 33(8), 3324-3329

[16] Mizui F, Tanaka O. et al. Saponins from brans of quinoa, *Chenopodium quinoa* Willd. I. Chemical Pharmaceutical Bulletin 1988; 36(4), 1415-1418

[17] Nie R, Tanaka O. et al. A triterpenoid saponin from *Thladiantha hookeri* var. *pentadactyla*. Phytochemistry 1989; 28(6), 1711-1715

[18] Fujita M, Tanaka O. et al. The study on the constituents of *Clematis* and *Akebia* spp. II. On the saponins isolated from the stem of *Akebia quinata* Decne. (1). Yakugaku Zasshi 1974; 94(2), 194-198

[19] Cheeke PR, Biological Effects of Feed and Forage Saponins. In: Waller GR and Yamasaki K. (eds) Saponins Used in Food and Agriculture: Plenum Press; 1996. p377-385

[20] Cheeke PR, Oleszek W. Anti-inflammatory and anti-arthritis effects of Yucca schidigera: reviw. Journal of Inflammatory 2006;3:6.

[21] Wall ME, Eddy CR. Steroidal sapogenins, Journal of Biological Chemistry 1952; 198(2), 533-543

[22] Kaneda N, Staba JE. et al. Steroidal constituents of *Yucca schidigera* plants and tissue cultures. Phytochemistry 1987; 26(5), 1425-1429

[23] Kameoka H, Miyazawa M. 65th Spring National Meeting of the Chemical Society of Japan 1993; 28-31 March, Tokyo, Japan 1993

[24] Tanaka O, Tamura Y. et al. Application of saponins in foods and cosmetics: Saponins of Mohave yucca and *Sapindus mukurossi*. In: Waller GR and Yamasaki K. (eds) Saponins Used in Food and Agriculture: Plenum Press; 1996. p1-11

[25] Miyakoshi M, Yamasaki K. et al. Antiyeast steroidal saponins from *Yucca schidigera* (Mohawa Yucca), a new anti-food deteriorating agent. Journal of Natural Products 2000; 63(3), 332-338

[26] Otoguro C, Tamura Y. et al. Inhibitory effect of yucca extract on the growth of film-forming yeasts isolated from Ume-zuke, salted Japanese apricot fruit. Nihon Shokuhin Hozo Kagaku Kaishi. 1998; 24(1), 3-10

Section 3

Therapeutic Potential

Chapter 6

Energy Medicine

Christina L. Ross

Additional information is available at the end of the chapter

http://dx.doi.org/10.5772/52818

1. Introduction

Energy medicine (EM) is medicine based on physics instead of biochemistry. Energy medicine works with subtle forms of energy known as chi or prana that exist in and around the human body. EM treats with the understanding that all illness results from disturbances in this energy known as the human biofield. Physics does not override biochemistry, it drives it. Biology and chemistry behave according to the laws of physics. Physics is the study of energy. The human body is made of energy. It has structure (bones), plumbing (digestive tract), and electricity (nervous systems), all infused with energy. Energy is a property of all matter, therefore cells, molecules, and atoms are all made of energy. Science has begun to measure the subtle but important energy field around the human body and research is showing that when the natural flow of energy is obstructed, disordered, and depleted, the body becomes diseased [1]. Pharmaceuticals affect chemical signals in the body but EM affects electromagnetic signals in the body. EM heals using an integrated system that supervises the interaction of all the body's systems and is not only faster, but more efficient. A continuous, uninterrupted flow of energy through the biofield plays the main role in health and healing.

In 1989 the term *energy medicine* was coined by the International Society for the Study of Subtle Energy and Energy Medicine which studies the science of medical and therapeutic applications of subtle energies. Energy medicine came under government guidelines in 1992 when the National Institutes of Health (NIH) established the National Center for Complementary and Alternative Medicine [2]. According to the NIH, energy medicine is defined as a form of complementary and alternative medicine which has two distinct categories:

Veritable energy medicine, which uses mechanical vibration (sound) and electromagnetic radiation (light) in order to affect health and healing. Veritable EM involves the use of specific, measurable wavelengths and frequencies to treat patients. Many of the human body electrical systems and electromagnetic fields are well known, and veritable forms of EM are being used in well established models for patients in today's medicine. Examples of veritable forms of EM are the use of lasers and magnetic pulses which have been found to be therapeutic. Commonly used forms of veritable EM such as electrocardiogram (EKG), electroencephalogram (EEG), Computerized Tomography (CT or CAT) Scan, Magnetic Resonance Imaging (MRI) and ultrasound equipment are currently being used in traditional medical applications.

For many years it was thought that electromagnetic field (EMF) exposure would cause only harmful effects in the body, but it is now understood that the amount of energy (field strength or amplitude), and the frequency of the field is what determines whether it is harmful, therapeutic or benign [3]. In particular, ionizing radiation has been shown to cause harmful effects by breaking the electron bonds that hold molecules like DNA together[4, 5]. Ionizing radiation includes alternating current (AC) that is produced by power lines, electrical wiring, and electrical equipment. Some epidemiological studies have suggested there is an increased risk of cancer associated with magnetic field exposure near electrical power lines [3, 6, 7]. The energy in non-ionizing radiation, however, is not strong enough to break ion bonds in atoms and molecules [8, 9]. Depending on the frequency and amplitude, the beneficial effect of non-ionizing EMF has been reported to affect natural killer cells fighting cancer and viruses [10-16], traumatic brain injury, post-operative infections, as well as bacterial and viral related inflammatory responses that are major complications in today's medicine [17-19]. Extra low frequency electromagnetic field (ELF-EMF) in the 50 Hz range has been reported to prohibit bacterial growth and improve immune response against bacterial infection [20].

Veritable EM treatments also include pulsed electromagnetic field (PEMF) therapy. A Pulsed Electromagnetic Field device has been approved by the US Food and Drug Administration (FDA) for bone repair, although it remains widely unused due to physician misunderstanding and lack of knowledge concerning the treatment [21]. PEMF therapeutic devices can be applied in two different ways - either by capacitive or inductive coupling. In capacitive coupling there is no contact with the body, whereas direct coupling requires the placement of opposing electrodes in direct contact with the surface of the skin of the targeted tissue [22]. Inductive coupling does not require electrodes to be in direct contact with the skin because it produces a field (see Faraday's Law of Induction) that emanates in all directions. Research shows that therapeutic applications of PEMF at extra low frequency (ELF) levels (3-300 Hz) are beneficial to the immune system by suppressing inflammatory responses at the cell membrane level [23]. PEMF can pass through the skin and into the body's conductive tissue [24-26], resulting in reduced pain and the onset of edema shortly after trauma. Where edema is already present, treatment exhibits significant anti-inflammatory effects [27]. In a study of the effect of PEMF therapy on arthritis, three hours of exposure to a 50-Hz magnetic field revealed that experimentally-induced inflammation in rats was significantly inhibited as a result [28]. Strong beneficial effects have also occurred using 75 Hz frequency MF treatment in patients suffering from fractures of the ankle joints [29]. PEMF treatments also promote cell activation and endothelial cell proliferation through the cell membrane. ELF levels can increase the rate of formation of epithelial cells in partially healed wounds

http://dx.doi.org/10.5772/52818

[30] and also quicken the healing time of skin wounds [31]. Fields at 15 Hz were used to significantly accelerate wound healing in diabetic mice [32]. Skin wounds have electrical potentials that can be stimulated by ELF-EMF to aid in the healing process by dedifferentiating cells near the wound, thereby accelerating cell proliferation [23]. In a study examining the effects of whole body magnetic fields (50-165 Hz) on patients suffering from different forms of cancer, results showed the MF therapy had overall beneficial effects, particularly with respect to improved immune status and postoperative recovery [33]. Treatment consisted of 15 cycles, each 1-20 minutes in duration coupled with more traditional cancer therapies. PEMF has also been reported to reduce pain and inflammation after traumatic brain injury [34], decrease osteoarthritic inflammation [35], and reduce neuropathic pain [36], as well as control the growth of lymphocytes [37].

EMF treatments appear to improve certain psychological conditions as well. A study of twelve patients with posttraumatic stress disorder (PTSD) and major depression underwent PEMF treatment of either 1 Hz or 5 Hz as an adjunct to antidepressant medications. Seventy-five percent of the patients had a clinically significant antidepressant response after treatment, and 50 percent had sustained that response at 2-month follow-up as compared with controls. Comparable improvements were seen in anxiety, hostility, and insomnia [38]. Low-frequency PEMF therapy at 0.1 – 64 Hz has been shown to improve mobility function, pain, and fatigue in fibromyalgia patients [39] as well. It has been firmly established that tissues such as blood, muscle, ligaments, bone and cartilage respond to biophysical input, including electrical and electromagnetic fields. Research shows that certain field strengths and frequencies of PEMF appear to be disease-modifying [Table 1].

Condition	B or Freq *	Treatment Duration	Treatment Number	Key Finding
Alzheimer's [40]	5-8 Hz	30 min	2x	Significantly improves cognitive function
Arthritis [41]	50 Hz	60 min	3x	Reduction of pain and inflammation
Back Pain [42]	64 Hz	16 min	until pain stops	Statistically significant potential for reducing pain
Bacterial Infection [20]	50 Hz	4 – 6 h	1x	Increased immune response against bacteria
Cancer(breast, colon and prostate tumors) [43]	0.1 Hz to 114 kHz	4 months	2x/week	Tumor specific frequencies showed significant decrease in size
Carpal Tunnel Syndrome [44]	20 Hz	4 h	daily	Statistically significant short- and long- term pain reduction

Condition	B or Freq *	Treatment Duration	Treatment Number	Key Finding
Chronic Bronchitis [45]	30 mT	15- 20 min	15x	Proved effective in patients suffering from chronic bronchitis when coupled with standard drug therapies
Edema [27]	70 mT	15 - 30 min	6x	Significantly reduces acute edema
Fibromyalgia [39]	0.1-64 Hz	30 min	2x day/3 weeks	Improved function, pain, fatigue, and global status in FM patients
Gastroduodenitis [46]	100 Hz	6-10 min	8-10x	77 % of treatment patients experienced elimination of gastro-esophageal and duodenogastral refluxes compared to 29 % of controls
Mastitis [47, 48]	10-25 Hz	60 min	1x/2-3 mos	Significantly reduced post-op inflammation
Multiple Sclerosis [49]	1-25 Hz	2-24h/day	Up to 5 weeks	PEMF device significantly alleviated symptoms
Migraine Headache [50]	27.12 Hz	1 h/day	5days/wk/2 wks	Effective, short-term intervention for migraine, but not tension headaches
Nerve Regeneration [51]	2 Hz/0.3mT	1 h/day	10 days	Pre and post injury exposure suggests that PEMF influences regeneration indirectly
Neuritis [51]	10-100 Hz	6 min	10-12x	Produced beneficial effects in 93% of patients suffering from nerve problems
Oral Surgery [52]	5mT/30Hz	30 min	3-5 days prior to	Significantly reduce inflammation in clinical trials

http://dx.doi.org/10.5772/52818

Condition	B or Freq *	Treatment Duration	Treatment Number	Key Finding
Osteoarthritis [53]	25 G/5-24 Hz	25 G/5-24 Hz	18x	Rapid improvements of immuno-logical indices & alleviates symptoms
Pain and edema [54]	1mT or 5 mT	6 h/day	90 days	Significantly aids in clinical recovery
Post Traumatic Stress Disorder [38]	1Hz or 5Hz	40 sec or 8 sec/1 hr	20-30 days	Seventy-five percent of patients had a clinically significant antidepressant response
Rheumatoid Arthritis [55]	30 mT	30 min	15 – 20x	Reduces pain in chronic pain populations
Septic Shock [56]	50 Hz/2mT	6 h	1x	*E. coli* became more sensitive to antibiotics
Skin Ulcers [57]	75 Hz/2.7 mT	4 hr/day	for 3 months	Positive effects but only in small lesions
Tendonitis [58]	30 mT	60 min	10 – 20x	Significant beneficial effects
Whiplash [59]	64 Hz	8 min	4x	Considerable and statistically significant pain reduction
Wound Healing in diabetic mice [60]	15 Hz	8 h/day	24 days	Postoperative pain was significantly reduced for a decrease in the need for analgesic resolve

Table 1. Veritable EM therapies applied to various conditions. * B=magnetic field; G=Gauss; T=Tesla; Hz=Hertz; 1 mT=10 Gauss

How do veritable EMF therapies work?

The mechanism for action of EMF on cells and tissues is based on how cells can detect and generate electromagnetic fields in general. Biological systems such as cells communicate not only with each other but also interact with their environment [61, 62]. This is done through several mechanisms at many levels depending on the type of cell tissue and nature of the information being communicated. Most known mechanisms in the literature address cell-cell interaction as chemical or electrical signaling, but intercellular interaction can also be attributed to electromagnetic fields (EMFs) [63]. Burr *et al* published a report on stable voltage gradients in various biological systems back in 1935 [64]. Since then researchers have discovered that these stable gradients can be altered when the whole organism undergoes biological processes such as growth, localized injury and microbial invasion. Because EMFs radiate, they behave in a wave-like manner (Figure 1).

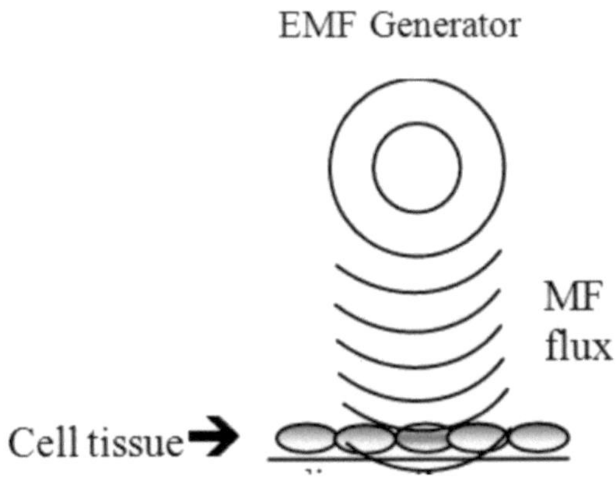

Figure 1.

The biological effects of low-frequency magnetic fields have been the subject of extensive studies since they can penetrate deep into tissues [65-72]. It has been shown that low-frequency EMF can act at the cellular level affecting various cell functions, including cell proliferation and differentiation [73-76], apoptosis [77-79], DNA synthesis [80, 81], RNA transcription [82], protein expression [83], protein phosphorylation [84], re-dox mediated rises in NFkB and cell damage [85, 86], microvesicle motility [87], ATP synthesis [88], hormone production [89], antioxidant enzyme activity [90], metabolic activity [91], and the inhibition of adherence [92]. It has been proposed that the initial interaction occurs outside the plasma membrane, but could also involve interactions with transmembrane proteins [93, 94]. For example, NIH3T3 cells exposed to a 50 Hz PEMF for over 2 h significantly increased the clustering of intermembrane proteins compared with controls [95]. Investigators concluded that the signal was likely being propagated and amplified through the intracellular signal transduction pathways [96]. An example of this is when the calcium stored in the intracellular compartment prompting mitochondria to produce free radicals (which increase DNA response) [97] can be controlled by PEMF[98], providing a first order effect in preventing the onset of inflammatory responses. The impact of EMF on calcium channel protein has been reported many times [99-102]. The genes that encode ion channels are important because they produce the gradients that determine downstream cell behavior. Future advances in this work will fully integrate bioelectric cascades. Increased understanding of how these mechanisms work will lead directly to devices that stimulate cell treatment directly to the damaged region producing the bioelectromagnetic changes needed to repair and regenerate tissues.

Effect of EMF on cytokine production

http://dx.doi.org/10.5772/52818

It is now well established that exogenous applied EMFs affect cell signaling and cytokine production. PEMF treatment appears to be disease-modifying in a model studying osteoarthritis [103]. Since transforming growth factor beta (TGF-β) is understood to upregulate gene expression for aggrecan (a cartilage-specific core protein), downregulate matrix metalloprotease and IL-1 activity, and upregulate inhibitors of matrix metalloprotease, the stimulation of TGF-β could be considered a mechanism by which PEMF favorably affects cartilage homeostasis.

Application of PEMF does not appear to alter the cell immunophenotype of fibroblast-like cell populations, but does appear to decrease the production of inflammatory cytokines IL-1β and TNF-α. PEMF also appears to increase anti-inflammatory cytokine IL-10 [104]. Both IL-1 and TNF-α concentration in the synovial fluid were significantly lowered while TGF-β was significantly higher compared with controls. Large bone formation was also observed one month after osteochondral graft implantation using PEMF treated grafts which favor early graft stabilation [105]. PEMF exposure at 75 Hz, 45 mT limited bone resorption in the subchondral bone while cytokine assessment in the synovial fluid indicated a more favorable articular environment for the graft.

EMF and Inflammation

EMF has many well documented physiological effects on cells and tissues including anti-inflammatory effects. MF therapies can provide noninvasive, safe and easy to apply methods to directly treat the source of pain, injury, inflammation and dysfunction [106]. Low-frequency EMF has a long term record of safety, backed by tissue culture, animal and clinical studies which have been conducted for over two decades [107]. Although the exact mechanism of anti-inflammatory effect is unclear, the cell membrane is most often considered the main target for EMF signals [106]. It has been reported that EMF affects membrane mediated signal transduction processes, especially the Ca^{2+} transport system [108]. Early events in signal transduction play a critical role in calcium influx in the lymphocyte. Because calcium is an important second messenger for a wide variety of important cellular processes such as RNA, DNA and protein synthesis; modulation of calcium signaling by electromagnetic fields has the potential to influence these cell functions [108]. Studies have demonstrated that EMF can stabilize the cell membrane by restoring membrane protein activity (Ca^{2+} -ATPase) and maintain intracellular Ca^{2+} levels [109, 110]. Biological systems in transition have been shown to be more sensitive to EMF exposure than in stationary systems. In one study immune compromised animals constituting systems in transition state were shown to be more sensitive to EMF exposure; whereas healthy animals, considered to be in relatively stable systems, exhibiting no sensitivity to the same field parameters [111]. Low-frequency, low-intensity EMF was reported to be beneficial in reducing inflammation without potential side effects indicating its value as a viable alternative for treating inflammatory responses. In living systems, from planarian flatworms to humans, mechanisms involved strongly suggest that therapeutic EMF applications stop inflammation first, then initiate healing [98].

2. Veritable EM Devices

PEMF Knee Device

The PEMF knee device is an FDA-approved device consisting of a cuff that surrounds the knee. It has a coil and heating pads that send magnetic pulses and heat through injured tissue. This device combines PEMF energy and thermal therapy to increase circulation, reduce swelling, relieve chronic pain and arthritis, as well as improve range of motion. It has been reported to benefit patients with osteoarthritis [112].

Transcutaneous Electrical Nerve Stimulation (TENS)

Transcutaneous electrical nerve stimulation (TENS) uses electric current to stimulate nerves to induce therapeutic treatment. These devices are usually connected to the skin using electrodes. A typical TENS device is able to modulate pulse width, frequency, and intensity of the electrical field it uses. TENS applied at frequencies above 50 Hz uses intensity below motor contraction (sensory intensity). TENS applied at frequencies below 10 Hz, use an intensity that produces motor contractions [113]. Studies show that TENS stimulates nerves in order to reduce both acute and chronic pain [114, 115].

PEMF Mats

PEMF mats produce a therapeutic pulsed electromagnetic field (PEMF) that surrounds the entire body. PEMF whole-body mats are promoted in many countries for a wide range of therapeutic applications. Randomized, sham-controlled, double-blind trials focusing on osteoarthritis of the knee (3 trials) or the cervical spine (1 trial), fibromyalgia (1 trial), pain perception (2 trials), skin ulcer healing (1 trial), multiple sclerosis-related fatigue (2 trials), or heart rate variability and well-being (1 trial) have been performed, with outcomes varying between improvement and ineffective [116]. PEMF mats are primarily advertised and distributed over the internet, and are often used without medical supervision. More research is needed to repeat outcomes. As of 2012 they have not been approved by the US Food and Drug Administration (FDA).

The second type of energy medicine is known as putative energy medicine.

Putative energy medicine is based on the idea that human beings are able to influence subtle forms of energy with their hands, intentions, or meditation. By focusing on these subtle energies, EM practitioners are able to feel vibrational frequencies with their hands and align the biofield through healing treatments [117]. Putative energy medicine is an all-inclusive term used for practices that include, but are not limited to Acupuncture, Alexander Technique, Bowen Technique, Chakra Balancing, Craniosacral Therapy, Eden Energy Medicine, Energy Psychology, Feldenkrais, Healing Touch (HT), Nambudripad's Allergy Elimination Techniques (NAET), Polarity Therapy (PT), Reiki, Rolfing, Therapeutic Touch (TT), Traditional Chinese Medicine (TCM), Trager Approach and yoga.

Putative EM is based on the understanding that a therapist instead of a device is able to facilitate healing by balancing disturbances in a patients' energy field. Practitioners are able to generate sub extremely low frequency (sub ELF) fields (0.3-30 Hz) from their hands through meditation and intention [118, 119]. This subtle energy entrains the biofield of the patient and initiates a healing effect. Instruction on body movement is also used to shift energy imbalances. Treatments are carried out in an integrative and holistic manner. The concept of holism in medicine dates back to 460 B.C. with Hippocrates, the father of medicine, positing the idea that every aspect of our body and mind are interrelated to every other aspect of our being [120]. Manipulation of the holistic field allows for healing throughout the entire being – body, mind and spirit.

How Putative EM Techniques work

The hands of EM practitioners produce coherent electromagnetic fields that affect the human biofield in many ways. A measuring device called the Superconducting Quantum Interference Device (SQUID) is a magnetometer used to detect very weak biomagnetic fields. SQUID has detected frequencies coming from the hands of practitioners in the sub extra low frequency electromagnetic field (sub ELF-EMF) range of 0.3 to 30 Hz [121]. The signal emitted by a practitioner is not steady or constant, but moves through the range of sub ELF-EMFs with an average range around 7 – 8 Hz. EM techniques are capable of producing healing results because they directly affect mechanical vibrations in the membrane and the cytoskeleton of human cells as well as the biofield in general. Many research studies have detected the frequency limit of cell oscillations to be only 30 Hz [122-126], which is the same frequency range coming from the hands of EM practitioners. This suggests a subtle resonance involved in the healing process. An interesting characteristic of energy emission from any living organism is that it stays somewhat organized in its fields. It has a tendency to remain stable and does not randomly dissipate [127]. Biofield vibrations are like tuning forks, acting as both transmitters and receivers of vibration coming from their environment. They resonate at specific harmonic pitches when we are healthy. When we are not healthy a non-coherent type noise vibrates from our cells and our biofield. Valerie Hunt, PhD, Professor Emeritus in the UCLA Department of Physiological Sciences has been conducting research in this field for over 40 years. She was the first to research the relationship between changes in bioenergy fields and human health. In mapping bioenergy fields, Hunt has found that each individual has a unique resting pattern she calls the *Signature Field*. "The Signature Field of a healthy human being is composed of balanced, coherent energy patterns running the full spectrum of frequencies (4 – 20 microns in wavelength [128]). This coherency shows up on a graph as smooth, gentle, shallow waves evenly distributed throughout the frequency spectrum". There are two types of patterns in the Signature Fields of people who have (or are soon going to develop) disease: deficiency patterns, and hyperactive patterns. They appear in graphs as thick, jagged waves concentrated in the high- or low-frequency bands (Figure 2).

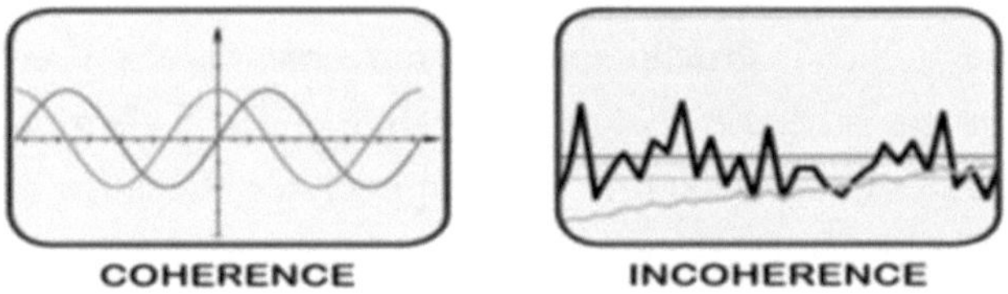

Figure 2.

Deficiency diseases like cancer and chronic fatigue syndrome have what Hunt calls "anti-coherent" patterns in the high frequency ranges, with almost no energy at all in the lower frequencies. Hyperactive conditions like colitis, hypertension, and skin problems show anti-coherent patterns in the low frequencies, with absent vibrations in the high frequencies [129]. The sub ELF-EMF frequency emitted from the hands of EM practitioners is capable of retraining the incoherent frequencies back to a healthy state. Gentle changes in body movement exhibited in EM therapies such as Alexander Technique, Feldenkrais and yoga retrain the cells and biofield back to a healthy vibrational state as well. The application of energy medicine, whether from a medical device or from the hands of a practitioner, is a viable alternative or complement to conventional medicine. Free flowing energy throughout the body eliminates physical health problems attributed to pain, disease and structural dysfunction [130]. EM significantly increases energy levels even if no specific problem exists [131]. It is used as both a preventative as well as a healing treatment.

Energy Medicine Therapies

More people are turning to energy medicine because of its holistic approach that includes not just the physiological, but mental, emotional and spiritual aspects of disease. Being diagnosed with a life threatening illness is very emotionally and psychologically disruptive; EM helps the patient find solace despite challenge. It also eases or counteracts the side effects of conventional therapies [131]. When it comes to selecting an EM therapy there are a variety of options. The following EM treatments are substantiated by peer reviewed published research:

Acupuncture uses meridians of Eastern medicine traditions which form a continuous, semi-conducting network. This Chinese medical procedure uses the stimulation of specific points on the body where the insertion of needles through the skin removes blockages in the flow of chi through the body's meridians to reinstate health. Acupuncture needles are metallic, solid, and hair-thin. Experienced differently, most people feel little or minimal pain while the needles are inserted. Some feel energized by treatment, others feel relaxed. Acupuncture has been shown to improve treatment related pain in cancer patients [132], pain management for women in labor [133], treatment of temporomandibular (TMJ) disorders [134], treat infertility, improve symptoms of menopause [135], improve insomnia [136], and improve chances of successful in vitro fertilization [137]. Relatively few complications have been reported from the use of acupuncture; however, acupuncture can cause potentially serious side effects if not delivered properly by a qualified practitioner. Make sure the practitioner is a certified Licensed Acupuncturist (L.Ac.).

Alexander Technique improves physical postural habits, particularly those that have become ingrained or are conditioned responses. The technique has been purported to improve athletic performance, self observation and impulse control, as well as relieve chronic stiffness, tension and stress. It changes movement habits in everyday activities, improving ease and freedom of movement, balance, support and coordination, teaching the use of appropriate amount of effort for a particular activity, increasing energy. It is not a series of treatments or exercises, but rather a reeducation of the mind and body. It can be applied to sitting, lying down, standing, walking, lifting, and other daily activities. Strong evidence exists for the effectiveness of Alexander Technique lessons for chronic back pain and moderate evidence in Parkinson's-associated disability [138].

Bowen is a gentle technique involving a series of moves held for several seconds and then released. The therapist gently pulls the skin on the back of the neck, knees, or affected body part away from the muscle or tendon beneath it and applies light pressure following a specific pattern. Bowen relieves both physical and psychosocial problems, including pain, sports injuries [139], shoulder problems [140], postpartum symptoms [141], fatigue, anger and depression [142].

Chakra balancing based on the seven energy centers along the center of the human body starting from the base of the spine to the top of the head. Chakras are responsible for keeping vital energy flowing through the biofield. They create openings for life energy to flow into and out of the aura. Their function is to vitalize the physical body and to bring about the development of our self-consciousness. They are associated with physical, mental and emotional interactions. An energy worker trained in chakra balancing will determine which chakras are functioning poorly and which chakras are over stressed in order to keep the body's energy balanced. When one or two chakras are performing at a reduced level, the remaining chakras have to work harder. Having a non-functioning or closed chakra can cause another chakra to blow, creating havoc in the biofield [143]. Blown chakras cause pain and initiate disease. Chakra balancing reprograms the chakra system to flow as nature intended.

Craniosacral therapy (CST) is a manipulation technique involving light touch to the cranium (skull) and sacrum (tailbone). It is based on the theory that the movement of bones within the skull and the lower back, as well as the rhythmic flow of cerebrospinal fluid (in and around the spinal cord), play a central role in the body's overall function. Obstruction of this flow of spinal fluid contributes to problems in the brain, spine and endocrine system. Research shows statistically significant improvements in the treatment of migraine headache using CST [144].

Eden Energy Medicine activates the body's natural healing ability by restoring weak or disturbed energy. Eden EM utilizes techniques from acupuncture, yoga, kinesiology, and qi gong. Energy is brought back into balance by tapping, massaging, pinching, twisting, or connecting specific energy points (acupoints) on the skin; by tracing or swirling the hand over the skin along specific energy pathways; through exercises or postures designed for specific energetic effects; by focused use of the mind to move specific energies; and/or by surrounding an area with healing energies. There is qualitative evidence that Eden EM relieves pain; stimulates immune function, relieves headaches, releases stress, improves memory, enhances digestion, relieve arthritis, neck, shoulder, and low back pain [145].

Energy Psychology (EP) addresses the relationship of energy systems to emotion, cognitive behavior and health [146]. Energy psychology uses imagery, narrative, and hyperarousal associated with traumatic memory or threatening situations to resolve traumatic memory [147]. When the brain reprocesses traumatic memory, the new association is retained by reducing it to hyperarousal. This leads to treatment outcomes that involve less time with fewer repetitions and higher impact. These techniques show less chance of retraumatization [147]. During EP treatments, mental/emotional/spiritual problems are healed through the biofield. The biofield is connected through the consciousness, thought processes and spirit, and includes the electrical activity of the nervous system, heart, meridians, biophotons (energy field particles), and chakras.

Feldenkrais Method uses gentle movement and directed attention to improve range of motion and enhance human functioning. Based on principles of physics, biomechanics and an empirical understanding of learning and human development, Feldenkrais exercises have been reported to be an effective way to improve balance and mobility, flexibility and coordination, helping to offset age-related declines in mobility and reduce the risk of falling among community-dwelling older adults [148].

Healing Touch (HT) is an energy medicine practice involving the relationship between the practitioner, the patient, intention, and the power of touch to facilitate healing. Like most EM treatments the patient is lying on a massage-type table, where the practitioner applies different forms of touch in order to assess the patient's biofield imbalances. HT is widely used to help ease pain, stress and anxiety [149]. Patients receiving music, imagery and touch therapy during angiograms or other cardiac procedures were 65 percent less likely to die in the following six months than patients who received no such intervention [150]. Other research shows that HT lowers blood pressure, heart and breathing rates, fatigue, mood disturbances, and pain in patients receiving chemotherapy [151]. HT is endorsed by the American Holistic Nurses' Association.

Nambudripad's Allergy Elimination Techniques (NAET®) is an EM treatment designed to alleviate allergies using a combination of energy balancing, testing and treatment procedures from acupuncture/acupressure, allopathy, chiropractic, nutritional, and kinesiological disciplines of medicine. Research suggests it is effective in treating allergies to milk, sugar, egg whites, pork meat and other foods causing eczema and dyspnea [152].

Polarity Therapy (PT) uses touch, verbal interaction, exercise, and nutrition [153] to balance and restore the natural flow of energy in the biofield. Blocked and stagnant energy is responsible for both emotional and physical pain as well as disease. Energy medicine treatments are patient-practitioner oriented, where both the giver and receiver of the energy treatment work in tandem to facilitate treatment. The practitioner grounds and centers his/her body, meaning all thoughts, emotions and physical sensations are neutralized

http://dx.doi.org/10.5772/52818

through intention. This mindset begins the healing process for both the practitioner and the client. PT balances the subtle energy of the biofield which can be detected and manipulated by movements of the practitioner's hands. The practitioner provides the resonating template for the patient's biofield to follow. Change occurs on a spiritual or unconscious level, and most people do not feel much other than becoming very relaxed. This mind-body state is optimal for healing and cell regeneration. After effects of the treatment last from hours to days with feelings of calm, focus, peace and serenity. PT bases its philosophy in the traditional system of Ayurvedic medicine, which defines patterns of health as energy moving through the Five Elements of Life – Ether, Air, Fire, Water and Earth. The practice of PT focuses on the balance of these elements as the foundation of good health. It integrates philosophies of Ayurvedic medicine, hermetic or ancient Egyptian medicine, Traditional Chinese Medicine (TCM), chakra balancing and the balance of yin and yang. PT understands that energy flows through the body along five pathways, enabled by positive and negative poles of the body. Five energy centers along the body represent the five elements of Ayurvedic tradition relating to different organs and functions in the body. Practitioners aim to correct disturbances and enable optimal physical, emotional as well as spiritual healing. Along with energy balancing sessions, cleansing diet and energy exercises are part of the therapy. PT has been shown to reduce cancer related fatigue [154], and improve the quality of life for caregivers of dementia and Alzheimer's patients [155] as well as improved stress reduction in burned out oncology professionals [131].

Reiki is an ancient Tibetan Buddhist practice in which practitioners serve as facilitators for life force energy (chi). Reiki is used to reduce stress, improve health and quality of life, and promote mental clarity. Practitioners use 12 – 15 specific hand positions each held for a few minutes on the patient's clothed body. Sessions last 30-90 minutes and the number of treatments may vary. Like other EM therapies, Reiki practitioners assert treatments can be effective over long distances. Formal scientific evidence has shown that Reiki can increase quality of life and reduce pain when used with standard medications [156]. Reiki has also been reported to relieve stress and improve psychological well being in patients with heart rate variability [157], and pain management issues [158].

Rolfing focuses on fascia tissue that connects all internal structures within the human frame. Connective tissue unites the structure of the body and divides it into individual functioning parts. Fascia is constantly changing and adapting in response to demands placed on the body. It reacts to trauma to a joint for instance by producing extra tissue to enhance stability and support; however, it can produce more than is necessary. In time, rather than stabilizing movement it can actually reduce mobility, leading to a changed posture and altered patterns of movement. After completing ten sessions a client can expect greater ease of movement and all over range of motion, along with better posture. Rolfing has been shown to significantly decrease pain and increase range of motion in adults who have cervical spine dysfunction [159].

Therapeutic Touch (TT) is similar to PT and HT, except practitioners usually do not actually touch the patient, but hold their hands 4-8 inches (10-18 cm) from the body in order to detect energy imbalances and correct them. TT has been shown to significantly reduce pain and increase the quality of life in fibromyalgia patients [160], significantly decrease pain and improve function in patients with osteoarthritis [161], produce significant reductions in behavioral symptoms of dementia [162], and chemical dependency in pregnant women who suffer from anxiety [163]. TT is mainly practiced by nurses.

Traditional Chinese Medicine (TCM) suggests that the basis for disease results from the disruption in the flow of subtle energy known as qi or chi. TCM works with imbalance in the forces of yin (feminine principle) and yang (masculine principle). Practices such as Chinese herbs, meditation, massage and acupuncture aid healing by restoring yin-yang and Qi to homeostasis. This same subtle energy is known as ki in the Japanese Kamp system.

Trager Approach is a combination of massage, meditation and movement education. The head, torso, arms and legs are manipulated with rhythmic pull and rotation techniques in order to release tension, increase mobility and clear the mind. Movement awareness is emphasized to promote relaxation and ease neuromuscular pain. The Trager Approach has been shown to reduce symptoms of chronic headache along with reduction of headache medication [164].

Yoga is an ancient Indian practice uniting the spirit, the body and mind accomplished through physical postures, controlled breathing exercises, and meditation, often accompanied by healthy lifestyle and search for higher consciousness. Yoga is not a religion but a philosophy and way of life. Hatha yoga is most commonly practiced in North America and Europe, using a sequence of postures or asanas held statically or moved through dynamically in sequence, using the breath and hand positions for balance. Ashtanga yoga builds strength, stamina and flexibility, more commonly known in the United States as power yoga. Bikram yoga is practiced in rooms heated to 100 °F (39 °C). Profuse sweating loosens muscles and tendons while promoting inner cleansing. This type of yoga should only be practiced after consulting with a physician. Research has shown the practice of yoga can reduce pain, and increase energy, flexibility, and function during physical activity, as well as relieve stress and anxiety in breast cancer survivors[165]. It has also been shown to reduce pain associated disability [166], reduce stress [167], and as a complementary therapy for major psychiatric disorders [168].

As with pharmaceuticals, the effectiveness of these treatments varies with each patient. It is important to speak with a practitioner before scheduling an appointment to discuss your needs and ask questions about what to expect during your visit. Most of these therapies are practiced with the patient fully clothed except for shoes, socks and jewelry. Although human biofields have as yet been proved measurable with conventional scientific equipment, medical journals have published articles suggesting the existence of such fields [169-171]. Please consult with a physician to determine any health issues (recent surgeries or trauma) which may not allow for physical manipulation. Many EM treatments are not recommended for people who have multi-personality disorder or schizophrenia as manipulation of the biofield can sometimes exacerbate delusion, hallucination and bring out multiple personalities at once.

http://dx.doi.org/10.5772/52818

In Summary

The growth and maintenance of correct vibrational patterning of tissues and organs is the hallmark of good health. Current biomedical interventions ultimately attempt to restore the body's optimal vibrational patterns. In order to accomplish this goal it is imperative to understand the key aspects of immune response with respect to cellular communication, as well as biochemical, bioelectrical, and bioelectromagnetic processes; and to develop technologies to facilitate the body's use of this information during the repair and regeneration process.

Author details

Christina L. Ross[1,2*]

Address all correspondence to: chrross@wakehealth.edu

1 Department of Energy Medicine, Akamai University, U. S. A.

2 Research Fellow, Wake Forest Institute for Regenerative Medicine, School of Medicine, Winston-Salem, U. S. A.

References

[1] Oschman, J. (2000). Energy Medicine: The Scientific Basis. Churchill Livingstone,. Edinburgh

[2] NCCAM,. (2010). http://nccam.nih.gov/health/whatiscam/.

[3] Administration, O., & S.a, H. (2012). Extremely Low Frequency (ELF) Radiation. http://www.osha.gov/SLTC/elfradiationretrieved February 15

[4] Buonanno, M., Toledo, S., & Azzam, E. (2011). Increased frequency of spontaneous neoplastic transformation in progeny of bystander cells from cultures exposed to densely ionizing radiation. PloS One. , 6(6), e21540.

[5] Mobbs, S., Muirhead, C., & Harrison, J. (2011). Risks from ionising radiation: an HPA viewpoint paper for Safegrounds. J Radiol Prot , 31(3), 289-307.

[6] Organization, W. H. (2012). Electromagnetic fields and public health. WHO fact sheet on electromagnetic hypersensitivity Retrieved February 15 http://www.who.int/mediacentre/factsheets/fs296/en/index.html

[7] Feychting, M., Ahlbom, A., & Kheifets, L. (2005). EMF and health. Annu Rev Public Health , 26, 165-89.

[8] Tenforde, T., & Kaune, W. (1987). Interaction of extremely low-frequency electric and magnetic fields with humans. Health Phys , 53, 585-606.

[9] Ng, K. H. (2003). Non-Ionizing Radiations- Sources, Biological Effects, Emissions and Exposures. Proceedings of the International Conference on Non-Ionizing Radiation at UNITEN ICNIR2003 Electromagnetic Fields and Our Health October 20- 22http://www.who.int/peh-emf/meetings/archive/en/keynote3ng.pdf

[10] Cadossi, R., Emilia, G., & Torelli, G. (1988a). Lymphocytes and pulsing magnetic field. *In A.A. Marino ed Modern Bioelectricity. Marcel Dekker, Inc: New York.*

[11] Cadossi, R., et al. (1988b). Effect of low-frequency low-energy pulsing electromagnetic fields on mice undergoing bone marrow transplantation. *Intl j of immunopath and pharm*, 1, 57-62.

[12] Cossarizza, A., et al. (1989). a Extremely low-frequency pulsed electromagnetic fields increase cell proliferation in lymphocytes from young and aged subjects. Biochem Biophys Res Commun , 160, 692-698.

[13] Cossarizza, A., et al. (1989b). Extremely low-frequency pulsed electromagnetic fields increase interleukin-2 (IL-2) utilization in IL-2 receptor expressionin mitogen-stimulated human lymphocytes from old subjects. *FEBS.*, 248(141-144).

[14] Cossarizza, A., et al. (1989c). DNA repair after irradiation in lymphocytes exposed to low-frequency pulsed eletromagnetic fields. *Radiat Res*, 118, 161-168.

[15] Mi, Y., Sun, C., Yao, C., Xiong, L., Wang, S., Luo, X., & Hu, L. (2007). Effect of steep pulsed electric fields on the immune response of tumor-bearing Wistar mice. *Sheng Wu Yi Xue Gong Cheng Xue Za Zhi*, 24(2), 253-256.

[16] Traitcheva, N., Angelova, P., Radeva, M., & Berg, H. (2003). ELF fields and photooxidation yielding lethal effects on cancer cells. *Bioelectromagnetics*, 148-150.

[17] Darouiche, R. (2001). Device-associated infections: a macroproblem that starts with microadherence. Clinical Infectious Disease , 33(9), 1567-1572.

[18] Harris, L., & Richards, R. (2006). Staphylococci and implant surfaces: A review. *Injury*, S3-S14.

[19] Saakatian-Elahi, M., Teyssou, R., & Vanhems, P. (2008). Staphylococcus aureus, the major pathogen in orthopaedic and cardiac surgical site infections. *Int J. Surg*, 6(3), 238-245.

[20] Akan, Z., Aksu, B., Tulunay, A., Bilsel, S., & Inhan-Garip, A. (2010). Extremely low-frequency electromagnetic fields affect the immune response of monocyte-derived macrophages to pathogens. *Bioelectromagnetics*, 603-612.

[21] Bassett, A., Carpenter, D., & Ayrapetyan, S. (1994). Therapeutic uses of electric and magnetic fields in orthopedics. *Biological Effects of Electric and Magnetic Fields: Beneficial and Harmful Effects,. II(San Diego: Academic Press):*, 13-48.

[22] Trock, D. (2000). Electromagnetic Fields and Magnets: Investigational Treatment for Musculoskeletal Disorders. Rheum Dis Clin North Am , 26(1), 51-62.

[23] O'Connor, M., Bentall, R., & Monahan, J. (1990). Emerging Electromagnetic Medicine conference proceedings. *Springer-Verlag, New York.*

[24] Stiller, M., et al. (1992). A portable pulsed electromagnetic field (PEMF) device to enhance healing of recalcitrant venous ulcers: a double-blind placebo-controlled clinical trial. Br J Dermatol , 27, 147-154.

[25] Hannan, C., et al. (1994). Chemotherapy of Human Carcinoma Xenografts during Pulsed Magnetic Field Exposure. *Anticancer Research,* 1521-1524.

[26] Traina, G., et al. (1998). Use of Electric and Magnetic Stimulation in Orthopaedics and Traumatology: Consensus Conference. *J Ortho Trauma,* 24(1), 1-31.

[27] Morris, C., & Skalak, T. (2007). Acute exposure to a moderate strength static magnetic field reduces edema formation in rats. Am J Physiol Heart Circ Physiol , 294, H50-H57.

[28] Mizushima, Y., Akaoka, I., & Nishida, Y. (1975). Effects of Magnetic Field on Inflammation. *Experientia,* 1141-1412.

[29] Gromak, G., & Lacis, G. (1987). Evaluations of the efficacy of using a constant magnetic field in treatments of patients with traumas. *Electromagnetic Therapies of Injuries and Diseases of the Support-Motor Apparatus., (International Collection of Papers, Riga, Latvia: Riga Medical Institute),* 88-95.

[30] Mertz, P., Davis, S., & Eaglestein, W. (1988). Pulsed electrical stimulation increases the rate of epithlialization in partial thickess wounds. Transactions of the 8th Annual Meeting ot the Bioelectrical Repair and Growth Society, (Washington, D.C) October , 9-12.

[31] Ottani, V., et al. (1988). Effects of pulsed extremely-low frequency magnetic fields on skin wounds in the rat. *Bioelectromagnetics,* 53-62.

[32] Callaghan, M., et al. (2007). Pulsed electromagnetic fields acclerate normal and diabetic wound healing by increasing endogenous FGF-2 release. *Plast Reconstr Surg,* 121(1), 130-141.

[33] Lubennikov, F., Lazarev, A., & Golubtsov, V. (1995). First Experience in Using a Whole-Body Magnetic Field Exposure in Treating Cancer Patients. *Vopr Onkol,* 41(2), 140-141.

[34] Rasouli, J., Lekhraj, R., White, N. M., Flamm, E. S., Pilla, AA, Strauch, B., & Casper, D. (2012). Attenuation of interleukin-1beta by pulsed electromagnetic fields after traumatic brain injury. Neurosci Lett , 519(1), 4-8.

[35] Fini, M., Torricelli, P., Giavaresi, G., Aldini, N. N., Cavani, F., Setti, S., Nicolini, A., Carpi, A., & Giardino, R. (2008). Effect of pulsed electromagnetic field stimulation on knee cartilage, subchondral and epyphiseal trabecular bone of aged Dunkin Hartley guinea pigs. Biomed Pharmacother , 62(10), 709-715.

[36] Weintraub, M., & Cole, S. P. (2004). Pulsed magnetic field therapy in refractory neuropathic pain secondary to peripheral neuropathy: electrodiagnostic parameters--pilot study. Neurorehabil Neural Repair , 18(1), 42-46.

[37] Jasti, A., Wetzel, B. J., Aviles, H., Vesper, D. N., Nindl, G., & Johnson, M. T. (2001). Effect of a wound healing electromagnetic field on inflammatory cytokine gene expression in rats. Biomed Sci Instrum , 37, 209-214.

[38] Rosenberg, P., et al. (2002). Repetitive Transcranial Magnetic Stimulation Treatment of Comorbid Posttraumatic Stress Disorder and Major Depression. *The Journal of Neuropsychiatry and Clinical Neurosciences*, 270-276.

[39] Sutbeyaz, S., et al. (2009). Low-frequency pulsed electromagnetic field therapy in fibromyalgia: a randomized, double-blind, sham-controlled clinical study. Clin J Pain , 25(8), 722-728.

[40] Arendash, G., Sanchez-Ramos, J., Mori, T., Mamcarz, M., Lin, X., Runfeldt, M., Wang, L., Zhang, G., Sava, V., Tan, J., & Cao, C. (2010). Electromagnetic field treatment protects against and reverses cognitive impairment in Alzheimer's disease mice. *J Alzheimers Dis*, 19, 191.

[41] Wagner, T., Rushmore, J., Eden, U., & Valero-Cabre, A. (2009). Biophysical foundations underlying TMS: setting the stage for an effective use of neurostimulation in the cognitive neurosciences. *Cortex*, 1025-1034.

[42] Lee, P., et al. (2006). Efficacy of pulsed electromagnetic therapy for chronic lower back pain: a randomized, double-blind, placebo-controlled study. J Int Med Res , 34(2), 160-167.

[43] Barbault, A., Costa, F., Bottger, B., Munden, R., Bomholt, F., Kuster, N., & Pasche, B. (2009). Amplitude-modulated electromagnetic fields for the treatment of cancer: discovery of tumor-specific frequencies and assessment of a novel therapeutic approach. J Exp Clin Cancer Res , 28(51-60)

[44] Weintraub, M., & Cole, S. (2008). A Randomized Controlled Trial of the Effects of a Combination of Static and Dynamic Fields on Carpal Tunnel Syndrome. Amer Acad Pain Med,. 9(5): , 493-504.

[45] Iurlov, V., Eksareva, T., & Dolodarenko, V. (1989). The Efficacy of the Use of Low-Frequency Electromagnetic Fields in Chronic Bronchitis. *Voen Med Zh*, 3, 35-36.

[46] Bukanovich, O., et al. (1996). Sinusoidally-modulated currents in the therapy of chronic gastroduodenitis in children. *Von Kurortol Fizioter Lech Fiz Kult*, 2, 22-26.

[47] Smith, A., Conneely, K., Kilaru, V., Mercer, K., Weiss, T., Bradley, B., Tang, Y., Gillespie, C., Cubells, J., & Ressler, K. (2011). Differential immune system DNA methylation and cytokine regulation in post-traumatic stress disorder. Am J Med Genet B Neuropsychiatr Genet , 156B(6), 700-708.

[48] Navaratil, L., Hlavaty, V., & Landsingerova, E. (1993). Possible Therapeutic Applications of Pulsed Magnetic Fields. *Cas Lek Cesk*, 132(9), 590-594.

[49] Lappin, M., et al. (2003). Effects of a pulsed electromagnetic therapy on multiple sclerosis fatigue and quality of life: a double-blind, placebo controlled trial. Altern Ther Health Med , 9(4), 38-48.

[50] Sherman, R., Acosta, N., & Robso, L. (1999). Treatment of migraine headaches with pulsing electromagnetic fields: A double blind, placebo controlled study. *Headache.*, 39(8), 567-575.

[51] Sisken, B. (1992). Nerve regeneration: implicaiton for clinincal application of electrical stimulation. Paper presented at the 1st World Congress for Electricity and Magnetism in Biology and Medicine, (Orlando, FL),June , 14-19.

[52] Hillier-Kolarov, V., & Pekaric-Nadj, N. (1992). PEMF Therapy as an Additional Therapy for Oral Diseases. *EuroBioelectromag Assoc, (1st Congress)*, 23-25.

[53] Hulme, J., et al. (2002). Electromagnetic Fields for the Treatment of Osteoarthritis. Cochrane Review, Cochrane Library, Oxford CD003523, 1

[54] Dallari, D. (2009). Effects of pulsed electromagnetic stimulation on patients undergoing hip revision prostheses: A randomized prospective double-blind study. *Bioelectromagnetics*, 423-430.

[55] Shupak, N. (2003). Therapeutic Uses of Pulsed Magnetic Field Exposure. Radio Science Bulletin (December): , 307, 9-32.

[56] Gaafar, E., et al. (2006). Stimulation and control of E. coli by using an extremely low-frequency magnetic field. *Romanian J. Biophys*, 16(4), 283-296.

[57] Jeran, M. (1987). PEMF Stimulation of Skin Ulcers of Venous Origina in Humans: Preliminary Report of a Double Blind Study. *Bioelectromagnetics*, 6(2), 181-188.

[58] Binder, A. (1984). Pulsed electromagnetic field therapy of persistent rotator cuff tendinitis. Lancet , 8379, 695-698.

[59] Thuilea, C., & Walzlb, M. (2002). Evaluation of electromagnetic fields in the treatment of pain in patients with lumbar radiculopathy or the whiplash syndrome. *NeuroRehabilitation*, 17(1), 63-67.

[60] Man, D. (1997). Effect of Permanent Magnetic Field on Postoperative Pain and Wound Healing in Plastic Surgery. *Second World Congress for Electricity and Magnetism in Biology and Medicine*.

[61] Levin, M. (2009). Bioelectric mechanisms in regeneration: unique aspects and furture perspectives. *Semin Cell Dev Biol*, 20(5), 543-556.

[62] Levin, M. (2012). Molecular bioelectricity in developmental biology: New tools and recent discoveries. *Bioessays*, 205-217.

[63] Cifra, M., Fields, J., & Farhadi, A. (2011). Electromagnetic cellular interactions. *Progress in Biophysics and Molecular Biology*, 223-246.

[64] Burr, H., & Northrop, F. (1935). The electrodynamic theory of life. *Quarterly Review of Biology*, 10(3), 322-333.

[65] Marino, A., & Becker, R. (1977). Biological effects of extremely low frequency electric and magnetic fields: a review. *Physiological Chemistry and Physics*, 131-147.

[66] Adey, W. (1980). Frequency and power windowing in tissue interaction with weak electromagnetic fields. *Proceedings of the IEEE*, 119-125.

[67] Robinson, K. (1985). The responses of cells to electrical fields: a review. *Journal of Cell Biology*, 101(6), 2023-2027.

[68] Frey, A. (1993). Electromagnetic field interactions with biological systems. FASB J , 7(2), 272.

[69] Hong, F. (1995). Magnetic field effects on biomolecules, cells and living organisms. Biosystems , 36(3), 187-229.

[70] Volpe, P. (2003). Interactions of zero-frequency and oscillating magnetic fields with biostructures and biosystems. Photochemical and Photobiological Sciences , 2(6), 637-648.

[71] Funk, R., & Monsees, T. (2006). Effects of electromagnetic fields on cells: physiological and therapeutical approaches and moleclular mechanisms of interaction. *Cell Tissues Organs*, 182(2), 59-78.

[72] Funk, R., Monsees, T., & Ozkucur, N. (2009). Electromagnetic effects: from cell biology to medicine. Progress in Histochemistry and Cytochemistry , 43(4), 177-264.

[73] Foletti, A., Lisi, A., Ledda, M., de Carlo, F., & Grimaldi, S. (2009). Cellular ELF signals as a possible to in informative medicine. Electromag Biol Med , 28(1), 71-79.

[74] Lisi, A., Foletti, A., Ledda, M., Rosola, E., Giuliani, L., D'Emilia, E., & Grimaldi, S. (2006). Extremely low frequency 7 Hz 100 uT electromagnetic radiation promotes differentiation in the human peithelial cell line HaCaT. *Electromag Biol Med*, 25(4), 269-280.

[75] Ventura, C., Maioli, M., Asara, Y., santoni, D., Mesirca, P., Remondini, D., & Bersani, F. (2005). Turning on stem cell cardiogenesis with extremely low frequency magnetic fields. FASB J , 19, 155-7.

[76] Ross, S. (2005). Combined DC and ELF magnetif fields can alter cell proliferation. *Bioelectromagnetics*, 11(1), 27-36.

[77] Tian, F., Nakahara, T., Yoshida, M., Honda, N., Hirose, H., & Miyakoshi, J. (2002). Exposure to power frequency magnetic fields suppresses X-ray induced apoptosis transiently in Ku80-deficient xrs5 cells. Biochem Biophys Res Commun , 292(2), 355-361.

[78] Tofani, S., Barone, D., Cintorino, M., De Santi, M., Ferrara, A., Orlassino, R., Ossola, P., Peroglio, F., Rolfo, K., & Ronchetto, F. (2001). Static and elf magnetic fields induce tumor inhibition and apoptosis. *Bioelectromagnetics*, 22(6), 419-428.

[79] Santini, M., Ferrante, A., Rainaldi, G., Indovina, P., & Indovina, P. (2005). Extremely low frequency (ELF) magnetic fields andapoptosis: a review. *Internat J Rad Biol*, 81(1), 1-11.

[80] Takahashi, K., Kaneki, I., Date, M., & Fukada, E. (1986). Effect of pulsing electromagnetic fields on DNA synthesis in mammalian cells in culture. Cellular and Molecular Life Sciences , 42(2), 185-186.

[81] Litovitz, T., Krause, D., Montrose, C., & Mullins, J. (1994). Temporally incoherent magnetic fields mitigate the response of biological systems to temporally cohreent magnetic fields. *bioelectromagnetics*, 15(5), 399-410.

[82] Goodman, R., Bassett, C., & Henderson, A. (1983). Pulsing electromagnetic fields induce cellular transcription. Science , 220(4603), 1283.

[83] Goodman, R., & Henderson, A. (1988). Exposure of salivary gland cells to low-frequency electromagnetic fields alters polypeptide synthesis. Proceed Nat Acad Sci USA , 85(11), 3928.

[84] Sun, W., Chiang, H., Fu, Y., Yu, Y., Xie, H., & Lu, D. (2001). Exposure to 50 Hz electromagnetic field induces the phosphorylation and activity of stress-activated protein kinase in cultures cells. Electromag Biol Med , 20(3), 415-423.

[85] Wolf, F., Torsello, A., Tedesco, B., Fasanella, S., Boninsegna, A., D'Ascenzo, M., Grassi, C., Azzena, G., & Cittadini, A. (2005). 50-Hz extremely low frequency electromagnetic fields enhance cell proliferation and DNA damage; possible involvement of redox mechanism. *Biochimica et Biophysica Acta (BBA) Molecular Cell Research*, 1743(1-2), 120-129.

[86] Regoli, F., Gorbi, S., Machella, N., Tedesco, S., Benedetti, M., Bocchetti, R., Notti, A., Gattorini, D., Piva, F., & Principato, G. (2005). Pro-oxidant effects of extremely low frequency electromagnetic fields in the land snail Helix aspersa. Free Radical biol and med , 39(12), 1620-1628.

[87] Golfert, F., Hofer, A., Thummler, M., Bauer, H., & Funk, R. (2001). Extremely low frequency electromagnetic fields and heat shock can increase microvesicle motility in astrocytes. *Bioelectromagnetics*, 71-78.

[88] Zrimec, A., Jerman, I., & Lahajnar, G. (2002). Alternating electric fields stimulate ATP synthesis in Escherichia coli. *Cell Mol Biol Letters*, 7(1), 172-175.

[89] Paksy, K., Thuroczy, G., Forgacs, Z., Lazar, P., & Gaati, I. (2000). Influence of sinusoidal 50-Hz magnetic field on cultured human ovarian granulosa cells. Electromag Biol Med , 19(1), 91-97.

[90] Kula, B., Sobczak, A., & Kuska, R. (2000). Effects of static and ELF magnetic fields on free-radical processes in rat liver and kidney. Electromag Biol Med , 19(1), 99-105.

[91] Milani, M., Ballerini, M., Ferraro, L., Zabeo, M., Barberis, M., Cannone, M., & Faleri, M. (2001). Magnetic field effects on human lumphocytes. *Electromag Biol Med,* 20(1), 81-106.

[92] Jandova, A., Hurych, J., Pokorny, J., Coeek, A., Trojan, S., Nedbalova, M., & Dohnalova, A. (2001). Effects of sinusoidal magnetic field on adherence inbition of leukocytes. *Electromag Biol Med,* 20(3), 397-413.

[93] Mc Leod, K., Rubin, C. T., & Donahue, H. J. (1995). Electromagnetic fields in bone repair and adaptation. Radio Sci , 30, 233-244.

[94] Otter, M., Mc Leod, K. J., & Rubin, C. T. (1998). Effects of electromagnetic fields in experimental fracture repair. Clin Orthop , 355, S90-104.

[95] Bersani, F., Marinelli, F., Ognibene, A., Matteucci, A., Cecchi, S., Santi, S., Squarzoni, S., & Maraldi, N. M. (1997). Intramembrane protein distribution in cell cultures is affected by 50 Hz pulsed magnetic fields. *Bioelectromagnetics,* 463-469.

[96] Gordon, G. (2007). Designed electromagnetic pulsed therapy: clinical applications. J Cell Physiol , 212(3), 579-582.

[97] Schild, L., Plumeyer, F., & Reiser, G. (2005). Ca(2+) rise within a narrow window of concentration prevents functional injury of mitochondria exposed to hypoxia/reoxygenation by increasing antioxidative defense. *FEBS J,* 272(22), 5844-5852.

[98] Ikehara, T., Yamaguchi, H., Hosokawa, K., Houchi, H., Park, K. H., Minakuchi, K., Kashimoto, H., Kitamura, M., Kinouchi, Y., Yoshizaki, K., & Miyamoto, H. (2005). Effects of a time-varying strong magnetic field on transient increase in Ca2+ release induced by cytosolic Ca2+ in cultured pheochromocytoma cells. Biochim Biophys Acta , 1724, 8-16.

[99] Lieb, R., Regelson, W., West, B., Jordan, R. L., & De Paola, D. P. (1980). Effect of pulsed high frequency electromagnetic radiation on embryonic mouse tissue palate in vitro. *J Dent Res,* 59(1649-1652).

[100] Mc Leod, B., Liboff, A. R., & Smith, S. D. (1992). Electromagnetic gating of ion channels. J Theor Biol , 158, 15-31.

[101] Baureus, Koch. C., Sommarin, M., Persson, B. R., Salford, L. G., & Eberhardt, J. L. (2003). Interaction between weak low frequency magnetic fields and cell membranes. *Bioelectromagnetics,* 395-402.

[102] Rosen, A. (2003). Mechanism of action of moderate intensity static magnetic fields on biological systems. Cell Biochem Biophys , 39, 163-173.

[103] Ciombor, D., Aaron, R. K., Wang, S., & Simon, B. (2003). Modification of osteoarthritis by pulsed electromagnetic field--a morphological study. Osteoarthritis Cartilage , 11(6), 455-462.

[104] Gómez-Ochoa, I., Gómez-Ochoa, P., Gómez-Casal, F., Cativiela, E., & Larrad-Mur, L. (2011). Pulsed electromagnetic fields decrease proinflammatory cytokine secretion (IL-1β and TNF-α) on human fibroblast-like cell culture. *Rheumatol Int,* 31(10), 1283-1289.

[105] Benazzo, F., Cadossi, M., Cavani, F., Fini, M., Giavaresi, G., Setti, S., Cadossi, R., & Giardino, R. (2008). Cartilage repair with osteochondral autografts in sheep: effect of biophysical stimulation with pulsed electromagnetic fields. J Orthop Res , 26(5), 631-642.

[106] Markov, M., & Colbert, A. P. (2001). Magnetic and electromagnetic field therapy. Journal of Back Musculoskeletal Rehab , 15, 17-29.

[107] Bassett, A. (1994). Biological effects of elctrical and magnetic fields. *Academic Press, Inc.,,. San Diego,* 13-48.

[108] Yost, M., & Liburdy, R. P. (1992). Time-varying and static magnetic fields act in combination to alter calcium signal transduction in the lymphocyte. *FEBS Letters,* 117-122.

[109] Selvam, R. K. G., Narayana, R., Raju, K., Gangadharan, A., Manohar, B., & Puvanakrishnan, R. (2007). Low frequency and low intensity pulsed electromagnetic field exerts its anti-inflammatory effect through restoration of plasma membrane calcium ATPase activity. *Life Sci,* 80, 2403-2410.

[110] Balcavage, W., Alvager, T., Swez, J., Goff, C. W., Fox, M. T., Abdullyava, S., & King, M. W. (1996). A mechanism of action of extremely low frequency electromagnetic fields on biological systems. Biochem Biophys Res Commun , 222, 374-378.

[111] Ubeda, A., Enrique, M. D., Pascual, M. A., & Parreno, A. (1997). Hematological changes in rats exposed to weak electromagnetic fields. *Life Sci,* 61, 1651-1656.

[112] Nelson, F., Zvirbulis, R., & Pilla, A. (2010). The use of a specific pulsed electromagnetic field (PEMF) in treating early knee osteoarthritis. *Trans 56th Annual Orthopaedic Research Society Meeting,. New Orleans, LA,* 1034.

[113] Robinson, A., & Snyder-Mackler, L. (2007). Clinical Electrophysiology: Electrotherapy and Electrophysiologic Testing (Third ed.). *Lippincott Williams & Wilkins.*

[114] Johnson, M., & Martinson, M. (2006). Efficacy of electrical nerve stimulation for chronic musculoskeletal pain: A meta-analysis of randomized controlled trials. *Pain,* 130(1), 157-165.

[115] Dubinsky, R., & Miyasaki, J. (2010). Assessment: efficacy of transcutaneous electric nerve stimulation in the treatment of pain in neurologic disorders (an evidence-based review): report of the Therapeutics and Technology Assessment Subcommittee of the American Academy of Neurology. *Neurology,* 74(2), 173-176.

[116] Hug, K., & Röösli, M. (2012). Therapeutic effects of whole-body devices applying pulsed electromagnetic fields (PEMF): A systematic literature review. *Bioelectromagnetics,* 95-105.

[117] Benor, D. (2002). Energy Medicine for the Internist. Medical Clinics of North America , 86(1), 105-125.

[118] Connor, M., Tau, G., & Schwartz, G. (2006). Oscillation of Amplitude as Measured by an Extra Low Frequency Magnetic Field Meter as a Physical Measure of Intentionality. *Toward a Science of Consciousness.*

[119] Connor, M., Flores, M., & Schwartz, G. (2004). The use of Triaxial ELF Magnetic Field Meter measurements as a predictor of capacity in Energy Medicine Practitioners in a research setting. World Qi Gong Congress,

[120] Hippocrates, (2012). The Hippocratic Oath. Translated by Michael North: National Library of Medicine, National Institutes of Health, retrieved(Hippocratic oath, nlm.nih.gov).

[121] Zimmerman, J. (1990). Laying on of hands healing and therapeutic touch: a testable theory. *J Bioelectromag Inst*, 2, 8-17.

[122] Korenstein, R., & Levin, A. (1990). Membrane fluctuations in erythrocytes are linked to mGATP-dependent dynamic assembly of the membrane skeleton. *Biophysical Journal*, 773-737.

[123] Tuvia, S., Almagor, A., Bitler, A., Levin, S., Korenstein, R., & Yedgar, S. (1997). Cell membrane fluctuation are regulated by medium macroviscosity: evidence for a metabolic driving force. Proceeding of National Academy of Science USA 94 , 5045-5049.

[124] Tuvia, S., Moses, A., Nathan, G., Levin, S., & Korenstein, R. (1999). adrenergic agonists regulate cell membrane fluctuations of human erythrocytes. *Journal of physiology*, 516(3), 781-792.

[125] Popescu, G., Badizadegan, K., Dasari, R., & Field, M. (2006). Coherence properties of red blood cell membrane motions. Journal of Biomedical Optics Letters. , 11(4), 040503.

[126] Popescu, G., Park-K, Y., Dasari, R., Badizadegan, K., & Feld, M. (2007). Coherence properties of red blood cell membrane motions. *Physical Review*, E 76, 031902.

[127] Dirac, P. (1930). The Principles of Quantum Mechanics. Clarendon Press, Oxford

[128] Rubik, B. (2002). The Biofield Hypothesis: its biophysical basis and role in medicine. J Altern Complem Medicine , 8(6), 703-713.

[129] Hunt, V. (2000). Infinite Mind: Science of the Human Vibrations of Consciousness. Malibu, CA: Malibu Publishing Co

[130] Hsieh, L., et al. (2006). Treatment of low back pain by acupressure and physical therapy: randomised controlled trial. BMJ , 25(332), 696-700.

[131] Pierce, B. (2007). The use of biofield therapies in cancer care. Clin J Oncol Nurs , 11(2), 253-258.

[132] Lin, J., & Chen, Y. The role of acupuncture in cancer supportive care. Am J Chin Med 40012. 2 , 219-229.

[133] Jones, L., Othman, M., Dowswell, T., Alfirevic, Z., Gates, S., Newburn, M., Jordan, S., Lavender, T., & Neilson, J. (2012). Pain management for women in labour: an overview of systematic reviews. Cochrane Database Syst Rev Mar 14;CD009234., 3

[134] Itoh, K., Asai, S., Ohyabu, H., Ima,i, K., & Kitakoji, H. (2012). Effects of trigger point acupuncture treatment on temporomandibular disorders: a preliminary randomized clinical trial. J Acupunct Meridian Stud , 5(2), 57-62.

[135] Baumelou, A., Liu, B., Wang, X., & Nie, G. (2011). Perspectives in clinical research of acupuncture on menopausal symptoms. Chin J Integr Med , 17(12), 893-897.

[136] Ganguly, G. (2011). Acupuncture may be helpful only for patients with comorbid insomnia secondary to chronic pain syndromes. J Clin Sleep Med , 7(4), 411.

[137] Huang, D., Huang, G., Lu, F., Stefan, D., Andreas, N., & Robert, G. (2011). Acupuncture for infertility: is it an effective therapy? *Chin J Integr Med,* 17(5), 386-395.

[138] Woodman, J., & Moore, N. (2012). Evidence for the effectiveness of Alexander Technique lessons in medical and health-related conditions: a systematic review. Int J Clin Pract , 66(1), 98-112.

[139] James, L. (2008). Bowen Technique for back pain and other conditions. *Positive Health.,* 143(38-39).

[140] Carter, B. (2001). A pilot study to evaluate the effectiveness of Bowen technique in the management of clients with frozen shoulder. Complement Ther Med , 9, 208-215.

[141] Stiles, K. (2003). Bowtech. *Massage Ther J,* 42, 94-104.

[142] Shapiro, G. (2004). The Bowen Technique for pain relief. *Positive Health Phys,* 48-51.

[143] Slater, V. (1995). Toward an understanding of energetic healing, Part 1: Energetic structures. J Holist Nurs , 13(3), 209-224.

[144] Curtis, P., Gaylord, S., Park, J., Faurot, K., Coble, R., Suchindran, C., Coeytaux, R., Wilkinson, L., & Mann, J. (2011). Credibility of low-strength static magnet therapy as an attention control intervention for a randomized controlled study of CranioSacral therapy for migraine headaches. J Altern Complement Med , 17(8), 711-721.

[145] Feinstein, D., & Eden, D. (2008). Six pillars of energy medicine: clinical strengths of a complementary paradigm. Altern Ther Health Med , 14(1), 44-54.

[146] Association, f.c.e.p. (2012). http://www.energypsych.orgRetrieved January 4,.

[147] Feinstein, D. (2008). a Energy psychology: a review of the preliminary evidence. Psychotherapy theory, research, practice, training , 45(2), 199-213.

[148] Ullmann, G., Williams, H., Hussey, J., Durstine, J., & Mc Clenaghan, B. (2010). Effects of Feldenkrais exercises on balance, mobility, balance confidence, and gait perform-

ance in community-dwelling adults age 65 and older. J Altern Complement Med , 16(1), 97-105.

[149] Wardell, D., & Weymouth, K. (2004). Review of studies of Healing Touch. *Journal of Nursing Scholarship Image*, 36(2), 147-154.

[150] Krucoff, M. (2005). Healing touch, music, relaxation a plus for heart surgery patients. *The Lancet*.

[151] Post-White, J., Kinney, M., Savik, K., Gau, J., Wilcox, C., & Lerner, I. (2003). Therapeutic massage and healing touch improve symptoms in cancer. Integr Cancer Ther , 2(4), 332-344.

[152] Terwee, C. (2008). Succesful treatment of food allergy with Nambudripad's Allergy Elimination Techniques (NAET) in a 3-year old: A case report. Cases J , 1(1), 166.

[153] Association, A.P.T., APTA. (2003). Standards for Practice. *Fourth Edition:*, 2.

[154] Mustian, K., Roscoe, J., Palesh, O., Sprod, L., Heckler, C., Peppone, L., Usuki, K., Ling, M., Brasacchio, R., & Morrow, G. (2011). Polarity Therapy for Cancer-Related Fatigue in Patients With Breast Cancer Receiving Radiation Therapy: A Randomized Controlled Pilot Study. Integr Cancer Ther , 10(1), 27-37.

[155] Korn, L., Logsdon, R., Polissar, N., Gomez-Beloz, A., waters, T., & Tyser, R. (2009). A Randomized Trial of a CAM Therapy for Stress Reduction in American Indian and Alaskan Native Family Caregivers. The Gerontologist , 32, 1-10.

[156] Olson, K., Hanson, J., & Michaud, M. (2003). A Phase II Trial of Reiki for the Management of Pain in Advanced Cancer Patients. *Journal of Pain and Symptom Management*.

[157] Baldwin, A., Wagers, C., & Schwartz, G. (2008). Reiki improves heart rate homeostasis in laboratory rats. J Altern Complement Med , 14(4), 417-422.

[158] Lucas, M., & Olson, K. (1997). Reiki To Manage Pain. *Cancer Prevention and Control*, 1, 108-113.

[159] James, H., Castaneda, L., Miller, M., & Findley, T. (2009). Rolfing structural integration treatment of cervical spine dysfunction. J Bodyw Mov Ther , 13(3), 229-238.

[160] Denison, B. (2004). Touch the pain away: new research on therapeutic touch and persons with fibromyalgia syndrome. Holist Nurs Pract , 18(3), 142-151.

[161] Gordon, A., Merenstein, J., Di Amico, F., & Hudgens, D. (1998). The effects of therapeutic touch on patients with osteoarthritis of the knee. Journal of Family Practice , 47, 271-277.

[162] Woodsa, D., Beckb, C., & Sinha, K. (2009). The Effect of Therapeutic Touch on Behavioral Symptoms and Cortisol in Persons with Dementia. 16(3), 181-189.

[163] Larden, C., Palmer, L., & Janssen, P. (2004). Therapeutic Touch Eases Anxiety for Pregnant, Chemically Dependent Women. *Journal of Holistic Nursing*, 22(4), 320-332.

[164] Foster, K., Liskin, J., Cen, S., Abbott, A., Armisen, V., Globe, D., Knox, L., Mitchell, M., Shtir, C., & Azen, S. (2004). The Trager approach in the treatment of chronic headache: a pilot study. *Altern Ther Health Med*, 10(5), 40-46.

[165] Galantino, M., Greene, L., Archetto, B., Baumgartner, M., Hassall, P., Murphy, J., Umstetter, J., & Desai, K. (2012). A qualitative exploration of the impact of yoga on breast cancer survivors with aromatase inhibitor-associated arthralgias. Explore , 8(1), 40-47.

[166] Büssing, A., Ostermann, T., Lüdtke, R., & Michalsen, A. (2012). Effects of yoga interventions on pain and pain-associated disability: a meta-analysis. J Pain , 13(1), 1-9.

[167] White, L. (2012). Reducing stress in school-age girls through mindful yoga. J Pediatr Health Care , 26(1), 45-56.

[168] Cabral, P., Meyer, H., & Ames, D. (2011). Effectiveness of yoga therapy as a complementary treatment for major psychiatric disorders: a meta-analysis. Prim Care Companion CNS Disord , 13(4), 8.

[169] Anderson, J., & Taylor, A. (2011). Effects of healing touch in clinical practice: a systematic review of randomized clinical trials. J Holist Nurs , 29(3), 221-228.

[170] Hart, L., Freel, M., Haylock, P., & Lutgendorf, S. (2011). The use of healing touch in integrative oncology. Clin J Oncol Nurs , 15(5), 519-525.

[171] Mills, P., & Jain, S. (2010). Biofield therapies and psychoneuroimmunology. *Brain Behav Immun*, 24(8), 1229-1230.

Chapter 7

Propolis: Alternative Medicine for the Treatment of Oral Microbial Diseases

Vagner Rodrigues Santos

Additional information is available at the end of the chapter

http://dx.doi.org/10.5772/54003

1. Introduction

Bees are arthropods of Hymenoptera order and are classified into two groups based on their type of life: solitary and social life. Propolis is produced by bees that live socially, from the harvesting of products derived from plants and used to seal and protect the hive against intruders and natural phenomena [1]. Propolis term derives from the Greek Pro, "opposite, the entry" and polis, "city or community" [2,3]. Propolis is a natural substance collected by *Apis mellifera* bees in several plant species. It has been used in folk medicine for centuries [2,4]. Characteristically, it is a lipophilic material, hard and brittle when cold, but soft, flexible and very sticky when warm. Hence the name "beeswax" [5]. It has characteristic odor and shows adhesive properties of oils and interact strongly with skin proteins [6]. The composition of propolis is complex [7,8]. Some factors, such as the botanical origin of propolis and its time of collection can influence the chemical composition of this resinous material [9]. The color of propolis varies from yellowish green to dark brown, depending on location - savannah, tropical forests, desert, coastal and mountainous regions - where it is produced. [10,11,12]. Propolis is used by bees to protect against the entry of microorganisms, fungi and bacteria in the hive, and as a sealing material for preventing the entry of light and moisture inside. It is also used to line the comb, to allow the deposition of eggs by the queen, and to embalm small dead animals (beetles and insects) that usually bees could not take into the hive, preventing its putrefaction.3,5,7].

Interest in the pharmacological action of natural products has grown and found significant popular acceptance. Among these products, propolis has been highlighted due to its applicability in the food industry and cosmetics, to be used as the active ingredient in several products, among which include toothpastes and skin lotions [13]. Also available in the form of a capsule (pure or combined), extract (hydroalcoholic or glycolic acid), mouthwash (combined with melissa, sage, mallow and / or rosemary), lozenges, creams and powders (for use in or gargling internal use, once dissolved in water) [2].

Regarding the ethnobotanical aspect, propolis is one of the few "natural remedies" that continue to be used for a long period by different civilizations [14]. Propolis is widely used in popular medicine, especially in communities with inadequate public health conditions[15]. It was noticed that it can be more effective and less toxic than certain compounds. Significant decrease in H_2O_2-induced DNA damage in cultures treated with propolis demonstrated antioxidant activity of phenolic components found in propolis may contribute to reduce the DNA damage induced by H_2O_2 [16].

2. History

Propolis is a natural remedy that has been used extensively since antiquity. The Egyptians, who knew very well the anti-putrefactive properties of propolis, used it for embalming [17]. It was recognized for its medicinal properties by Greek and Roman physicians, such as Aristotle, Dioscorides, Pliny and Galen. The drug was used as an antiseptic and healing in the treatment of wounds and as a mouthwash, and its use in the Middle Ages perpetuated among Arab doctors [2]. Also, it was widely used in the form of ointment and cream in the treatment of wounds in battle field, because of their healing effect. This healing propolis property known as "Balm of Gilead," is also mentioned in the Holy Bible [18]. From the pharmacological point of view, propolis has been used as solid; in an ointment based on vaseline, lanolin, olive oil or butter, and in the form of alcoholic extract and hydroalcoholic solution. The proportion propolis/carrier may vary, in order to obtain bacteriostatic or bactericidal results [19]. In the 1980s and 1990s, a great number of publications occurred worldwide, highlighting Japan in number of published papers followed by Brazil and Bulgaria [6]. In Dentistry, there are studies investigating the pharmacological activity of propolissome situations, such as gingivitis, periodontitis, oral ulcers, pulp mummification in dogs' teeth and dental plaque and caries in rats [19]. Also, it has been used in dressings of pre and post-surgical treatment, oral candididosis, oral herpes virouses and oral hygiene. There was also the investigation of antiseptic and healing properties of propolis in subjects admitted to various hospitals and the results were extremely positive [20]. Thus, this natural product revealed great interest for the treatment of oral diseases [21]. Internationally, the first licensed commercial product containing propolis was registered in Romania in 1965. Worldwide, in the same period analyzed, it was found a total of 239 commercial licenses. In the 1980s, commercial licenses were predominant in the former USSR and satellite countries. Currently, 43% of commercial licenses are Japanese origin and 6.2% of them are products for dental treatment. In Japan, the scientific productivity reported for propolis increased 660% between the 1980 and 1990 [22]. The global interest in propolis research increased considerably in relation to its various biological properties [23-27]. Another incentive for conducting research on propolis is a high value on the international market, mainly in Japan, where a bottle of ethanol extract is sold at prices ten times higher than that prevailing in Brazil. Brazil is considered the third largest producer of propolis in the world, behind Russia and China only. Japan's interest for the Brazilian propolis is due to its therapeutic and organoleptic properties, and also the presence of minor amounts of heavy metals and other environmental pollutants [28,29]. In the last thirty years, various studies and scientific research were performed to clarify the medicinal properties attributed to propolis [30,31].

3. Classification / rating

There was an attempt to classify the Brazilian propolis into twelve types according to physical-chemical properties and geographical reports. However, to date, only three types of propolis had their botanical origin identified. The main types of botanical origin are South (three), Northeast (six) and Southeast (twelve), and they were reported as resins from *Populus sp.*, *Hyptis divaricata* and *Baccharis dracunculifolia* (Figure 5), respectively. An attempt to classify propolis produced in Brazil according to botanical origin and chemical composition [32] has recognized 12 different types. It was suggested that *Hyptis divaricata* is the resin source of northeastern propolis, *Baccharis dracunculifolia* of southeastern propolis and poplar (*Populus nigra*) of southern propolis. This study by Park et al. [32] is indicative that just stating that a certain sample corresponds to 'Brazilian propolis' hardly means anything indicative of physical, chemical and biological characteristics, because a wide diversity of propolis types exist in a country as large as Brazil, housing a wide plant diversity and a complex honeybee genetic variation [3]. The different compounds present in Brazilian propolis were identified and quantified using high performance liquid chromatography (HPLC) technique. Established the process of separation by liquid chromatography, capable of identifying the major components of propolis samples (primary marker). Through the technique of HPLC and quantification of compounds identified by it, it was established a classification for Brazilian propolis based on the presence of markers (Table 1 and Table 2). The main feature of this classification relates to the speed in which this product bee can reach the market, from the field to the pharmaceutical and cosmetic industries, encouraging the use of these typing for the manufacture of their medicines and cosmetics, with established quality control, since all of these markers were separated in a concentration range types. That is, the classification is quantitative. Another important factor is that the classification will be possible to manufacture pharmaceuticals, cosmetics and oral hygiene products knowing the propolis type used and the quantities of bioactive components, features never reported before in publications and patents on propolis [33]. The Brazilian Cerrado is one of the richest areas in *Baccharis* sp. These plants are a group of woody perennial shrubs, which are dioecious with male and female inflorescences appearing on separate plants. Of the 30 different species of *Baccharis*, *Baccharis dracunculifolia* is the dominant source of propolis in southeastern Brazil (Sao Paulo State and Minas Gerais State), where most of propolis based products sold are produced [34]. Recently, it was founded a red type of propolis in hives located in mangrove areas in the Northeast. It was observed that bees collect exudate from the surface of red *Dalbergia ecastophyllum* (Linnaeus, Taubert) (Figure 6). Analysis and comparision of plant exudates and propolis samples demonstrate that the chromatographic profiles are exactly the same as the one found for *D. ecastophyllum* [35]. The best way to find the plant origin of propolis would be by comparing the chemical composition of propolis with the alleged plant origin [36]. World Propolis constituents of are shown in Table 3.

4. Chemical composition

Table 1 and Table 2 show the chemical markers constituents of green and red Brazilian propolis, respectively, while Table 3 shows the chemical composition of various types of world propolis. The highest concentration of phenolic compounds was obtained using solvents with lower concentrations of ethanol and higher concentrations of crude propolis, but the highest concentration of flavonoids in the extract was obtained with higher concentrations of ethanol in the solvent [11]. Over 300 chemical compounds are described in various propolis origins [22]. Among the chemicals constituents, we can include waxes, resins, balsams, oils and ether, pollen and organic material. The proportion of these substances varies and depends on the place and period of collection [5,37]. The collected propolis in a bee hive, also known as crude propolis, in its basic composition, contains about 50% of plant resins, 30% of beeswax, 10% essential oils, 5% pollen, 5% debris of wood and earth [7,14,6]. Propolis also contains various organic acids, considerable amount of minerals (including, manganese, zinc, calcium, phosphorus, copper), vitamins B1, B2, B6, C and E, acids (nicotinic acid and pantothenic acid) and aminoacids [5,7,11,38]. These constitutive features may vary by region and period of the year [39, 40].

Nº	Compounds	mg/g
1	Coumaric acid	3.56
2	Cinnamic acid	1.66
3	Quercetin	1.38
4	Kaempferol	1.77
5	Isorhamnetin	0,91
6	Sakuranetin	5.57
7	Pinobanskin-3-acetate	13.92
8	Chrysin	3.51
9	Galangin	9.75
10	Kaempferide	11.60
11	Artepillin C (3,5-diprenyl-4-hydroxycinnamic acid)	82.96

BGP from *Baccharis dracunculifoila* (SBN97). HPLC test (Park et al.) [32].

Table 1. Chemical constituents markers of Brazilian green propolis sample

http://dx.doi.org/10.5772/54003

Number	Compounds	Contents (mg/g)
01	Rutin	0.7
02	Liquiritigenin	1.8
03	Daidzein	0.3
04	Pinobanksin	1.7
05	Quercetin	0.5
06	Luteolin	1.2
07	Dalbergin	0.4
08	Isoliquiritigenin	4.8
09	Formononetin	10.2
10	Pinocembrin	3.3
11	Pinobanksin-3-acetate	1.7
12	Biochanin A	0.5

from *Dalbergia ecastophyllum* (Alencar et al.) [41]

Table 2. Flavonoids and other chemical constituents of Brazilian red propolis

Compounds (percentage of content)			Authors
Fatty and aliphatic acids (24–26%)	Flavonoids (18–20%)	Microelements (0.5–2.0%)	
Butanedioic acid (Succinic acid)	Astaxanthin	Aluminum (Al)	
Propanoic acid (Propionic acid)	Apigenin	Copper (Cu)	Burdok et al. [7]
Decanoic acid (Capric acid)	Chrysin	Magnesium (Mg)	Maciejewicz et al [43]
Undecanoic acid	Tectochrysin	Zinc (Zn)	Park et al. [32]
Malic acid	Pinobanksin	Silicon (Si)	Kumazawa et al.[44]
D-Arabinoic acid	Squalene	Iron (Fe)	Salatino et al. [3]
Tartaric acid	Pinostrobin chalcone	Manganese (Mn)	Ozkul et al.[45]
Gluconic acid	Pinocembrin	Tin (Sn)	Eremia et al.[46]
α-D-Glucopyranuronic	acid Genkwanin	Nickel (Ni)	Machado et al.[47]
Octadecanoic acid (Stearic acid)	Galangin	Chrome (Cr)	Vandor-Unlu et al.[48] Wang et al.[49]
β-D-Glucopyranuronic acid	Acacetin		
9,12-Octadecadienoic acid	Kaemferide		
Tetradecanoic acid	Rhamnocitrin		
Pentanedioic acid	7,4'-dimethoxyflavone		
Glutamic acid	5-hydroxy-4'7-dimethoxyflavone		

Compounds (percentage of content)			**Authors**
2,3,4-trihydroxy butyric acid	5,7-dihydroxy-3,4'dihydroxyflavone		
Phosphoric acid	3,5-dihydroxy-7,4'-dimethoxyflavone		
Isoferulic acid			
	Sugars (15–18%)	Others (21–27%)	
	Sorbopyranose	Cyclohexanone	
	D-Erythrotetrofuranose	3-methyl,antitricyclo undec-3-en 10-one	
	D-Altrose	Cyclohexane	
	D-Glucose	Cyclopentene	
	Arabinopyranose	5-n-propyl-1,3 dihydroxybenzene	
	d-Arabinose	Butane	
	α-D-Galactopyranose	2(3H)-Furanone	
	Maltose	L-Proline	
	α-D-Glucopyranoside	2-Furanacetaldehyde	
	D-Fructose	2,5-is-3-phenyl-7-pyrazolopyrimidine	
Aromatic acids (5–10%)	Esters (2–6%)	Cliogoinol methyl derivative	
Benzoic acid	Caffeic acid phenethyl ester	Fluphenazine	
Caffeic acid	4,3-Acetyloxycaffeate	4,8-Propanoborepinoxadiborole	
Ferulic acid,	Cinnamic acid	1,3,8-Trihydroxy-6-methylanthraquinone	
Cinnamic acid	3,4 dimethoxy-trimethylsilyl ester	1-5-oxo-4,4-diphenyl-2-imidazolin-2-yl guanidine	
	3-Methoxy-4-cinnamate	3,1,2-Azaazoniaboratine/ Piperonal	
	Cinnamic acid	4 methoxy 3 TMS ester 3-Cyclohexene	
	2-propenoic acid methyl ester	1H-Indole	
Alcohol and terpens (2–3.3%) 1H-	Vitamins (2–4%)	Indole-3-one	
Glycerol	A, B1, B2, E, C, PP	2-Furanacetaldehyde	
Erythritol		Guanidine	
α-Cedrol		2(3H)Furanone	
Xylitol		1,3,8-trihydroxy-6-meyhylanthraquinone	
Germanicol			
Stigmast-22-en-3-ol			
Pentitol			

Compounds (percentage of content)	Authors
Ribitol	
Vanilethanediol	
Bicyclohept-3-en-2-ol	
Farneso	

Table 3. Propolis constituents according to Shawicka et al.[42].

However, the plant determines the chemical composition of propolis [4,39,40]. Today there are various substances known in propolis with distinct chemical structures from following classes: alcohols, aldehydes, aliphatic acids, aliphatic esters, amino acids, aromatic acids, aromatic esters, flavonoids, hydrocarbohydrates esters, ethers, fatty acids, ketones, terpenoids, steroids and sugars [21].The first studies to identify the active elements of propolis were performed in 1911 by researchers in Germany [50]: vanillin, cinnamic acid and alcohol. In the 1970s, [51] succeeded in isolating and identifying eleven elements, especially the most important type flavonoids, mainly flavones, flavonols and flavonones, terpenes, alpha-aceto butilenol and isovanillin. At the same time, [52] it was identified the unsaturated aromatic acids such as caffeic and ferulic acids. In the same decade, Kadakov et al.[53] reported the presence of thirteen amino acids in samples of propolis. The therapeutic effects are attributed to various phenolic compounds whichmake up the green propolis, which are widely distributed in plant kingdom. These flavonoids can be considered the main compounds [7,8], and also some phenolic acids and their esters, phenolic aldehydes, alcohols and ketones [54]. Flavonoids and caffeic acid phenethyl ester (CAPE) are phenolic compounds which have the ability to inhibit the growth and cell division and to increase membrane permeability interfering with microbial cell motility [13]. Despite being the most studied components of propolis, flavonoids are not solely responsible for the pharmacological properties. Several other components have been related to the medicinal properties of propolis [55]. Propolis from Europe and China contains many flavonoids and phenolic acids esters. Flavonoids are present only in small quantities in Brazilian propolis. The major components of propolis of Brazilian origin are terpenoids and ñ-coumarin prenylated acid derivatives [39]. In Southeastern Brazil there is plenty of the botanical species for production of green resin, which is the *Baccharis dracunculifolia,* also called "Rosemary's field", or "broom", which is a plant species typical of the Americas, due to the necessity of acid soil to grow. Rosemary easily develops in Brazil, both in planted areas and in abandoned spaces [34, 3,56]. The biodiversity needs to be investigated as a source of new bioactive substances, such as cinnamic acid derivatives, especially artepilin C, flavonoids and other pharmacological or functional properties [36].The renewed interest on the composition of Brazilian propolis is due to the fact that Brazil has a very diverse flora, tropical climate and Africanized *Apis mellifera* bees species that produce propolis during the period from April to September [5,32]. The typical constituents of Brazilian green propolis from *Baccharis dracunculifolia* are derived prenylated cafeochemic acid and cinnamic acid derivatives, such as artepilin C and baccharin. Brazilian green propolis is chemically different because it contains not only prenylateds of cinnamic acid, but also triterpenoid [57]. In dealing with the chemical composition and biological activity of green propolis, one can not point to a component of a particular substance or class of substances that could be responsible for their distinct pharmacological activities. Isoliquiritigenin, liquiritigenin and naringenin, isoflavones, isoflavans and pterocarpans were detected in Cuban Red Propolis, Brazilian Red Propolis (BRP) and *Dalbergia ecastophylum* extract (DEE), whereas polyisoprenylated benzophenones guttiferone E/xanthochymol and oblongifolin A were detected only in BRP. Pigments responsible for the red color of DEE and red propolis were also identified as two C30 isoflavans, the new retusapurpurin A and retusapurpurin B [10]. Obviously, different samples at different combinations of substances are essential for the biological activity of propolis [58,14]. It is important to note that all investigations on the antibacterial activity of specific substances isolated from propolis showed that a single component does not have an activity greater than the total extract [59]. The chemical properties of propolis are of great relevance considering its pharmacological value as a natural mixture and as a powerful source of new antimicrobial agents, antifungal, antiviral and individual compounds [58, 60].

5. Therapeutic properties of propolis

Currently, it is known that Brazilian propolis shows several biological activities, such as antimicrobial, antiinflammatory, immunomodulatory, among others [12]. The composition of propolis is very complex. We can observe the following: antibacterial activity, conferred by the presence of flavonoids, aromatic acids and esters in its composition; bactericidal action resulting from the presence of cinnamic acid and coumarin; *in vitro* antiviral activity (herpes simplex, influenza), due to the action of flavonoids and aromatic acids derivatives, antiulcer (assistance in healing), immunostimulating, hypotensive and cytostatic actions [21]. The methods of extraction of propolis may influence its activity, from different solvents at different soluble extract components [6,61]. The composition of propolis can vary according to the geographic locations from where the bees obtained the ingredients. Two main immunopotent chemicals have been identified as caffeic acid phenethyl ester (CAPE) and artepillin C. CAPE and artepillin C have been shown to exert immunosuppressive function on T lymphocyte subsets but paradoxically they activation macrophage function. On the other hand, they also have potential antitumor properties by different postulated mechanisms such as suppressing cancer cells proliferation via its anti-inflammatory effects; decreasing the cancer stem cell populations; blocking specific oncogene signaling pathways; exerting antiangiogenic effects; and modulating the tumor microenvironment[62]. The good bioavailability by the oral route and good historical safety profile makes propolis an ideal adjuvant agent for future immunomodulatory or anticancer regimens. However, standardized quality controls and good design clinical trials are essential before either propolis or its active ingredients can be adopted routinely in our future therapeutic armamentarium [62].

5.1. Anti-inflammatory activity

As an anti-inflammatory agent, green propolis is known to inhibit the prostaglandin synthesis, activate the thymus gland, help the immune system by promoting the phagocytic activity, stimulating cellular immunity, and increasing healing effects on epithelial tissue. Additionally, the propolis contains elements such as iron and zinc, which are important for the synthesis of collagen [63,35]. Recently it was reported that Artepillin C has an inhibitory effect on nitric oxide and prostaglandin E2 by modulating NF-êâ using the macrophage cell line RAW 264.7 [64]. The anti-inflammatory activity observed in green propolis seems to be due to the presence of prenylated flavonoids and cinnamic acid. These compounds have inhibitory activity against cyclooxygenase (COX) and lipooxygenase. It also appears that the caffeic acid phenethyl ester (CAPE) has anti-inflammatory activity by inhibiting the release of arachidonic acid from cellular membrane, removing the activities of COX-1 and COX-2 [65, 66]. Propolis also exhibits anti-inflammatory effects against models of acute and chronic inflammation (formaldehyde and adjuvant-induced arthritis, carrageenin and PGE 2, induced paw edema and granuloma pellete cotton). The exact mechanism of anti-inflammatory action of propolis is still unclear [2]. Treatment with 50 μM CAPE significantly reduced the levels of leptin ($p<0.05$), resistin ($p<0.05$) and tumor necrosis factor (TNF)-alpha ($p<0.05$) which are known to aid adipocytokines production in adipocytes. CAPE has inhibitory effects on 3T3-L1 mouse fibroblast differentiation to adipocytes. In 3T3-L1 cells, treatment of CAPE decreased the triglyceride deposition similar to resveratrol, which is known to have an inhibitory effect on 3T3-L1 differentiation to adipocytes. In conclusion, we found that CAPE suppresses the production and secretion of adipocytokines from mature adipocytes in 3T3-L1 cells [67]. The crude hexane and dichloromethane extracts of propolis displayed antiproliferative/cytotoxic activities with IC50 values against the five cancer cell lines ranging from 41.3 to 52.4 μg/ml and from 43.8 to 53.5 μg/ml, respectively. Two main bioactive components were isolated, one cardanol and one cardol, with broadly similar in vitro antiproliferation/cytotoxicity IC(50) values against the five cancer cell lines and the control Hs27 cell line, ranging from 10.8 to 29.3 μg/ml for the cardanol and < 3.13 to 5.97 μg/ml (6.82 - 13.0 μM) for the cardol. Moreover, both compounds induced cytotoxicity and cell death without DNA fragmentation in the cancer cells, but only an antiproliferation response in the the non-transformed human foreskin fibroblast cell line

(Hs27, ATCC No. CRL 1634) used as a comparative control.However, these compounds did not account for the net antiproliferation/cytotoxic activity of the crude extracts suggesting the existence of other potent compounds or synergistic interactions in the propolis extracts. This is the first report that *A. mellifera* propolis contains at least two potentially new compounds (a cardanol and a cardol) with potential anti-cancer bioactivity. Both could be alternative antiproliferative agents for future development as anti-cancer drugs [68].

5.2. Antimicrobial activity

5.2.1. Antibacterial and antifungal activity

Previous studies have shown that green propolis extracts inhibit the *in vitro* growth of *Streptococcus mutans* [5,69,8,59]. This microorganism is etiologically related to the formation of dental caries in humans and animals. Propolis showed efficient antimicrobial activity against *Pseudomonas* sp and *Staphylococcus aureus* [70]. Propolis antimicrobial effect is directly proportional to its concentration [54]. Propolis ethanolic extracts exhibited significant antimicrobial activity against many pathogens from the oral cavity, including *Porphyromonas gingivalis*,

Prevotella intermedia, Tannerella forsythia, Fusobacterium nucleatum [(69,24,71], which is the main microbiota involved in periodontal disease related to plaque. Gram-positive bacteria are more sensitive than Gram-negative bacteria to propolis extracts [72]. So far, no data is available to answer this observation. Gram-negative bacteria have a cell wall chemically more complex and a higher fat content, which may explain the higher resistance [73,74]. Antibacterial activity of green propolis derives mainly of flavonoids, aromatic acids, esters present in resins, galangin, pinostrobin, and pinocembrin which have been known as the more effective agents against bacteria. Ferulic acid and caffeic acid also contribute to the bactericidal action of propolis [5]. A simple analogy can not be made to the mode of action of classic antibiotics. There are no reports considering the resistance to bacterial constituents of propolis, and these properties may influence the success of antibiotic therapy in the oral cavity [63]. The solvent used for propolis extraction (ethanol, chloroform, methanol, propylene glycol, for example) can influence its antimicrobial activity. In fact, oily preparations have high antimicrobial activity, while solutions of glycerin showed little inhibition of Gram-positive and ethanolic solutions and propylene glycol showed good activity against yeasts [74]. Several studies have reported synergistic activity of propolis associated with various antibiotics, including activity against strains resistant to benzylpenicillin, tetracycline and erythromycin. These studies concluded that propolis has significant synergistic action, which may constitute an alternative therapy for microbial resistance, but dependent on its composition [75,9,76]. Propolis has also shown fungistatic and fungicidal activity *in vitro* against yeasts identified as cause of onychomycosis [35]. Although propolis is not widely used in conventional health care, is recommended for use as home remedies in the treatment of oral candidosis, denture stomatitis and skin lesions by numerous books and articles in the popular press [77,78]. Although some studies have focused on showing the antifungal activity of propolis extract, few have shown their effects on morphology and structure of *Candida albicans* [79,80]. Combinations of some drugs, antimycotic with propolis (10%) increase their activity against the yeast *Candida albicans*. The greatest synergistic effect against various strains were obtained when propolis is combined with other antifungal agents [5]. Siqueira et al.[81] demonstrated the antifungal activity of aqueous and alcoholic extracts of the green propolis and the alcoholic extract of red propolis was observed against *Trichophyton rubrum, Trichophyton tonsurans* and *Trichophyton mentagrohytes* samples, using as controls itraconazole and terbinafine. The data obtained showed that the green propolis alcoholic extract's antifungal activity was from 64 to 1024 μg/mL. The antifungal activity of red propolis alcoholic extract was more efficient than the green propolis alcoholic extract for all three species studied. The antifungal potential of the alcoholic extracts of green and red propolis demonstrated suggest an applicable potential as an alternative treatment for dermatophytosis caused by these species [82, 81]. On the other hand the diterpenes: 14,15-dinor-13-oxo-8(17)-labden-19-oic acid and a mixture of labda-8(17),13E-dien-19-carboxy-15-yl oleate and palmitate as well as the triterpenes, 3,4-seco-cycloart-12-hydroxy-4(28),24-dien-3-oic acid and cycloart-3,7-dihydroxy-24-en-28-oic acid were isolated from Cretan propolis. All isolated compounds were tested for antimicrobial activity against some Gram-positive and Gram-negative bacteria as well as against some human pathogenic fungi showing a broad spectrum of antimicrobial activity [83]. Concerning the antimicrobial activity of propolis phenols, *Candida albicans* was the most resistant and *Staphylococcus aureus* the most sensitive from Portugal, Braganca and Beja`s propolis. The reference microorganisms were more sensitive than the ones isolated from biological fluids [84]. Tables 4, 5, 6, and 7 show results from *in vitro* antimicrobial activity of ethanolic extract and gel containing Brazilian green propolis. Imaging studies with electron microscopy suggest the rupture of the cell wall of *Candida albicans* as one of the mechanisms of action of Brazilian green propolis (Figure 1) [78].

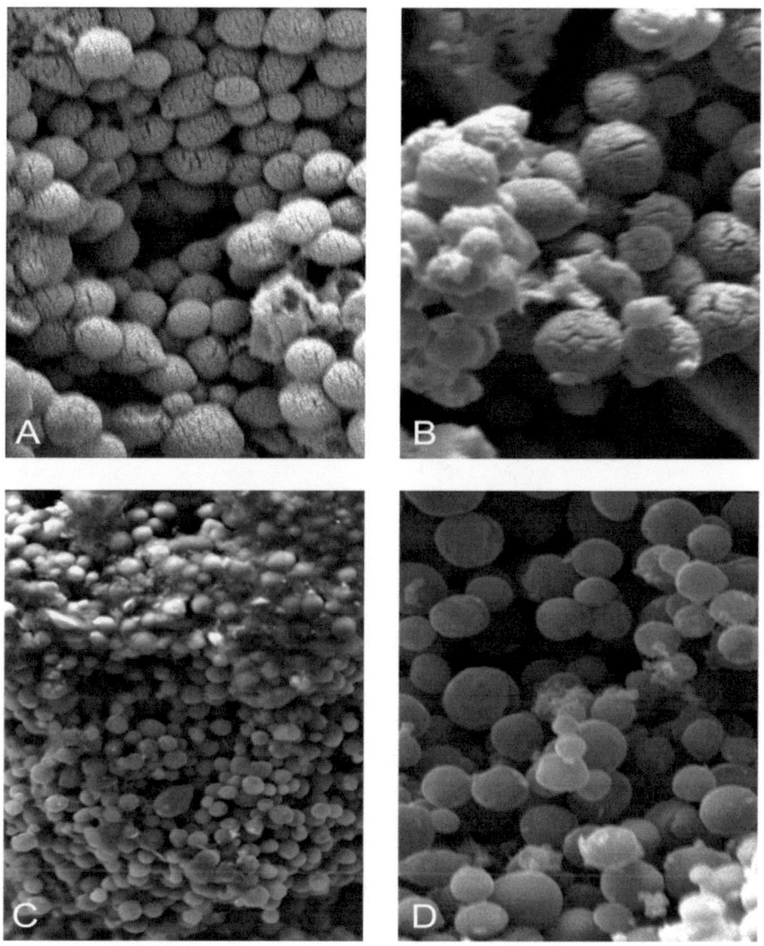

Figure 1. Micrographs showing *C. albicans* treated for 24h with subinhibitory concentrations of Brazilian Green Propolis extract (BGP). Scanning electron micrographs: Treated (panels A, B, and C) and untreated (panel D). A and B: cell wall detachment. C: cell agglomeration. Mello et al. [78].

Microorganisms	MIC (ìg/mL)	MBC (ìg/mL)	Inhibition zones (M±SD =mm)
C. albicans	20-50	100-300	16.3±0.52
C. tropicalis	20-50	100-300	12.3±0.08
C. glabrata	20-50	100-300	15.6±0.50
C. krusei	20-50	100-400	28.3±0.15
C. parapsilosis	20-50	100-400	18.6±0.08
C. guilliermondii	20-50	100-400	12.6±0.57
S. mutans	25-50	200-400	18.3±1.15
S. sobrinus	25-50	200-400	28.6±0.57
P. intermedia	20-50	200-400	17.5±2.50
T. forsythensis	30-60	300- 500	14.0±0.00
B. fragilis	25-50	300-500	15.3±1.15
S. aureus	25-50	200-400	16.3±2.08
P. gingivalis	30-50	200-400	14.0±0.00
F. nucleatum	30-60	200-400	15.2±0.26
F. necrophorum	30-60	200-400	17.3±0.57
A. actinomycetemcomitans	30-60	200-400	14.6±0.57

Table 4. Minimum Inhibitory Concentration (MIC); Minimum Bactericidal Concentration (MBC), Means and Standard Deviation (M±SD) of diameter inhibition zones obtained in agar diffusion test using Brazilian Green Propolis Extract (BGP) against *Candida* spp., Gram positive and Gram negative oral pathogenic bacteria. (Tests in triplicate).Paula et al. [59]

Microorganisms	Propolis MIC (ìg/ml)	Nystatin MIC (ìg/ml)	Chlorexidine MIC (ìg/ml)	Tetracycline MIC (ìg/ml)
C. albicans	14.00	16.00	_	_
C. tropicalis	14.00	16.00	_	_
S. mutans	28.00	_	8.00	1.00
S. aureus	14.00	_	32.00	4.00
A. israelii	1.75	_	32.00	4.00
E. faecalis	7.00	_	- 16.00	2.00
A. actnomycetemcomitans	3.50	_	8.00	1.00

Table 5. Minimum Inhibitory Concentration (MIC) of propolis ethanolic extract and control obtained for each strain tested. Tests in quadruplicates. (Paula et al.) [59].

	Propolis ointment %	Tetracycline 1%								
Bacteria	**48 hs activity**	**7 days activity**	**48h**	**7days**						
	5%	10%	15%	20%	5%	10%	15%	20%		
S. mutans	13.33±3.09	19.00±2.00	19.66±2.08	23.33±1.52	9.66±1.52	15.66±2.58	14.33±2.08	18.33±1.52	14.33±0.57	9.33±1.52
S. aureus	13.00±1.00	17.66±2.08	18.66±2.08	21.66±0.57	9.66±0.57	12.33±1.15	14.00±1.00	15.00±2.00	18.33±2.51	11.00±1.53
A. israelii	12.00±1.00	14.66±2.08	15.00±2.08	21.66±2.51	7.33±1.15	9.66±2.08	11.66±2.08	13.66±1.52	14.00±1.73	10.00±1.00
E. faecalis	14.66±1.15	18.33±0.57	21.00±1.00	24.00±1.00	9.66±0.57	11.00±1.00	12.66±0.57	15.00±1.00	9.66±2.08	7.66±1.15
A.a.	14.33±1.52	18.00±2.00	21.66±2.08	25.33±2.08	8.66±2.51	11.00±2.00	14.33±1.52	13.66±1.52	18.00±2.00	12.00±1.00

Table 6. Susceptibility of oral bacteria to Brazilian propolis adhesive formulation. Inhibition zones values in mm (M ±SD; n=3). Negative control was inactive..A.a. = *A. actinomycetemcomitans* (Santos et al.) [71]

Fungi	**Propolis ointment %**	**Nystatin 5%**								
	48 h activity	**7 day activity**	***48 h***	***7day***						
	5%	10%	15%	20%	5%	10%	15%	20%		
C. albicans	16.33±1.52	21.66±1.57	23.00±1.00	26.00±1.00	12.33±1.52	17.00±1.00	16.66±1.52	20.66±0.57	12.00±2.00	8.66±1.52
C. tropicalis	16.66±2.51	24.33±2.03	23.00±2.00	26.00±2.00	13.33±2.08	19.33±0.57	17.66±0.57	19.00±1.00	14.66±1.52	10.66±1.52

Table 7. Susceptibility of *Candida* species to Brazilian propolis adhesive formulation. Inhibition zones values in mm (M ±SD; n=3). Negative control was inactive. (Santos et al.) [71]

5.2.2. Antiviral activity

There are many reports on the antiviral activity of propolis. In a study performed in Ukraine compared the efficacy of ointment with propolis Canadian ointments acyclovir and placebo (vehicle) in treating subjects with type 2 Herpes applicant. The preparation of propolis containing flavonoids found to be more effective than the other two in wound healing and reduction of local symptoms [98]. The cytotoxic and antiherpetic effect of propolis extracts against HSV-2 was analysed in cell culture, and revealed a moderate cytotoxicity on RC-37 cells. However both propolis extracts exhibited high anti-herpetic activity when viruses were pretreated with these drugs prior to infection. Selectivity indices were determined at 80 and 42.5μg/mL for the aqueous and ethanolic extract, respectively, thus propolis extracts might be suitable for topical therapy in recurrent herpetic infection [99]. Huleihel & Isanu [100] reported potent antiviral activity of propolis against Herpes simplex-1 infection *in vitro* and *in vivo*. They suggested that the propolis can prevent absorption of the virus within the host cells and interfere with viral replication cycle. *In vitro* studies suggest that the green propolis has potent antiviral activity against variants X4 and R5 HIV-1. Similar activity was observed with CD4 + lymphocytes in operation, at least in part, as an inhibitor of viral entry [101,35]. Also, the antiviral activity of components of propolis, such as esters of cinnamic acids replacements was studied in vitro [5, 9, 102]. The antiviral effect of propolis extracts and selected constituents, e.g. caffeic acid, *p*-coumaric acid, benzoic acid, galangin, pinocembrin and chrysin against herpes simplex virus type 1 (HSV-1) was analysed in cell culture by Schnitzler et al.[103]. The 50% inhibitory concentration IC50 of hydro ethanolic propolis extracts for HSV-1 plaque formation was determined at 0.0004% and 0.000035%, respectively. Both propolis extracts exhibited high levels of antiviral activity against HSV-1 in viral suspension tests, plaque formation was significantly reduced by >98%. Both propolis extracts exhibited high anti-HSV-1 activity when the viruses were pretreated with these drugs prior to infection. Among the analysed compounds, only galangin and chrysin displayed some antiviral activity. However, the extracts containing many different components exhibited significantly higher antiherpetic effects as well as higher selectivity indices than single isolated constituents. Propolis extracts might be suitable for topical application against herpes infection [104]

5.3. Antioxidative activity

The antioxidative activity deserves special interest because propolis could be topically applied successfully to prevent and treat skin damaged [85, 86, 87]. Phenolic compounds found in high concentrations in Brazilian green propolis, including Artepillin C, have a wide range of biological properties including the ability to act as an anti-oxidizing free radicals and nitric oxide radicals and also the ability to interfere with the inflammatory response through inhibition of iNOS and COX-2 activities [88]. Although studies of propolis ethanol extracts are very common, it is reported that the aqueous extract has good antioxidant activity, associated with high content of phenolic compounds [89,90,91, 92]. Some studies have indicated propolis inhibiting superoxide anion formation, which is produced during autoxidation of â-mercaptoethanol [93,2]. The antioxidative activity of propolis and its main phenolic compounds, caffeic acid, p-coumaric acid, ferulic acid, and caffeic acid phenethyl ester, were investigated in yeast *Saccharomyces cerevisiae*. Yeast cells showed decreased intracellular oxidation, with no significant differences seen for the individual phenolic compounds. Ethanol Extract Propolis (EEP) antioxidative activity was also investigated at the mitochondrial proteome level and changes in the levels of antioxidative proteins and proteins involved in ATP synthesis were seen [94]. Brazilian green propolis is derived of *B. dracunculifolia* and protective effects of *B. dracunculifolia* glycolic extract against oxidative stress in isolated rat liver mitochondria (RLM) were investigated by Guimaraes et al.[95]. So, *B. dracunculifolia* exhibit potent antioxidant activity protecting liver mitochondria against oxidative damage and such action probably contribute to the antioxidant and hepatoprotective effects of green propolis [95]-. CAPE are involved with the renal damage protection induced by Cd (II) owing to its antioxidant capacity and anti-inflammatory effect [96]. Preadministration of Brazilian Propolis Ethanol Extract (50 or 100 mg/kg) to the stressed rats protected against the hepatic damage and attenuated the increased hepatic lipid peroxide and NO(x) contents and myeloperoxidase activity and the decreased hepatic non-protein SH and ascorbic acid contents and superoxide dismutase activity, possibly through its antioxidant and antiinflammatory properties [97].

5.4. Antitumoral activity

Several researchers reported the antitumoral property of propolis *in vitro* and *in vivo* [105,106, 30, 68]. Propolis isolated components showed antiproliferative activity in tumor cells [6]. Artepilin C, the major component of Brazilian green propolis, has antiangiogenic activity. Propolis may suppress tumor growth *in vivo*, but these mechanism effects is not completely understood [107, 39, 60]. Propolis shows antitumor properties, and its anticarcinogenic and antimutagenic potential is promising, but the mechanisms involved in chemoprevention are still unclear [108]. On other hand, CAPE and chrysin may be useful as potential chemotherapeutic or chemopreventive anticancer drugs [42]. However, the human aldo-keto reductase (AKR) 1C3, also known as type-5 17â-hydroxysteroid dehydrogenase and prostaglandin F synthase, has been suggested as a therapeutic target in the treatment of prostate and breast cancers was inhibited by Brazilian propolis-derived cinnamic acid derivatives that show potential antitumor activity, and it was found that baccharin a potent competitive inhibitor (K(i) 56 nM) with high selectivity [109]. There are currently several authors studied the antitumor activity of propolis, especially its components. Some initial studies are, however, some authors already have in-depth evaluation of about the propolis activity onto various animal or human types of tumor cell lines [110-115].

5.5. Immunomodulatory activity

The immunomodulatory activity of propolis is one of the most studied areas in conjunction with its anti-inflammatory property [116-120]. The immunomodulatory action of propolis seems to be limited to macrophages, with no influence on the proliferation of lymphocytes [121]. The inhibitory effect of green propolis (5-100μg/mL) on splenocyte proliferation was observed *in vitro* [122], and previous studies demonstrated that flavonoids have an immunosuppressive effect in lymphoproliferative response [123-125]. Since, propolis contains flavonoids, that may explain the reported effect [6,10]. Another explanation for the inhibitory effect on lymphocyte proliferation from the observation that both CAPE has inhibitory effects on transcription of nuclear factor-êB (NF-êB) (p65) and nuclear factor of activated T-cells (NFAT). Consequently, CAPE inhibited IL-2 gene transcription, IL-2R (CD25) expression and proliferation of human T cells, providing new insights into the molecular mechanisms involved in inflammatory and immunomodulatory activities of this natural component [6]. Green propolis exhibited immuno-stimulatory and immunomodulatory effects on CD4/CD8T cells and on macrophages *in vitro* and *in vivo* mice [126]. Propolis administration to melanoma-bearing mice submitted to stress stimulated IL-2 expression, as well as Th1 cytokine (IL-2 and IFN-ã) production, indicating the activation of antitumor cell-mediated immunity. Also, propolis stimulated IL-10 expression and production, which may be related to immunoregulatory effects indicating its antitumor action *in vivo* [127]. On other hand, Orsatti and Sforcin [128] demonstrated the propolis immunomodulatory action in chronically stressed mice, upregulating TLR-2 and TLR-4 mRNA expression, contributing to the recognition of microorganisms and favoring the initial steps of the immune response during stress. A new line of research involving propolis is the possible application as a vaccination adjuvant, although most commercial vaccines use aluminum salts to this end. A sample of green Brazilian propolis was tested, together with other adjuvant compounds, to immunize mice against inactivated swine herpes virus (SuHV-1). When administered together with aluminum hydroxide, the propolis extract increased both cellular and humoral responses [103].

6. Toxicity

It must be emphasized that propolis has the advantage of being a natural product, with a higher molecular diversity. It has many therapeutic substances compatible with the metabolism of mammals in general, which reduces the possibility of causing adverse reactions to oral tissue as compared to industrial products tested [13]. The aqueous and alcoholic extracts of propolis do not cause irritation to the tissues [17] and are considered relatively toxic [7]. Experimental mouthwash solutions containing propolis showed no significant inhibitory activity of microorganisms as effective as chlorhexidine, but found lower cytotoxicity on human gingival fibroblasts; propolis is relatively non-toxic and studies have exhibited a no-effect level in a mice study of 1400 mg/kg weight/day leading the authors to propose that a safe dose in humans would be 1.4 mg/kg weight/day, or approximately 70 mg/day [63]. On other hand, Pereira et al. [29] demonstrated high effectiveness of mouthwash containing propolis in control of dental plaque and gingivitis in humans and not observed no toxic or side effects in the administration of the rinse during 90 days. Propolis is considered safe in small doses. Therefore, adverse effects are common at doses above 15g/day. The most commonly experienced adverse effects are allergic reactions, as well as irritation of the skin or mucous membranes [129]. Caution should be used in the treatment of individuals with asthma and eczema and nettle rash [2].

7. Standardization

A universal chemical standardization of propolis would be impossible. Therefore, a detailed investigation of its composition, botanical origin and biological properties is significant [6]. It was postulated that different propolis may have different chemical and pharmaceutical properties. In this sense, standardization of propolis is required. Most studies on the chemistry of propolis include those directed to the European propolis composed of *Populus* sp. These studies have been conducted by paired with Gas Chromatography Mass Spectrometry (GC-MS). Therefore, due to the lower reproducibility of these methods, the use of High- Performance Liquid Chromatography (HPLC) is currently recommended [22,130,131]. An alternative method, using electro-spray, was recently tested to determine the patterns and content of polyphenolic components of propolis [132]. Nuclear magnetic resonance is one of the best detection methods because it recognizes components sensitive or insensitive to Ultraviolet Light (UL) [133,134]. Standardization can prevent product adulteration. Therefore, the methods used to extract components of propolis require adequate standardization [22, 87,135].

8. Oral clinical studies

Several clinical studies have demonstrated propolis efficacy in clinical trials, but the majority of studies involve topical application [20, 136-138]. The great diversity and the complexicity of chemical components makes difficult to standardize and to research the mechanisms of action. It is known the propolis anti-inflammatory, anti-microbial, analgesic, antioxidant, and antitumorproperties. Recently, some authors have demonstrated the properties of some components, however, one can not consider when using propolis but as a whole. The antimicrobial activity, for example, may be effective when considering the synergism between the components. Moreover, there was always the concern of several authors to develop oral mouthwashes- based propolis to control oral microbiota [138-140]. Koo et al.[141] demonstrated the effect of a mouthrinse containing selected propolis on 3-day dental plaque accumulation and polysaccharide formation and observed the Dental Plaque Index(PI) for the experimental group was 0.78 (0.17), significantly less than for the placebo group, 1.41 (0.14). On other hand, the experimental mouthrinse reduced the PI concentration in dental plaque by 61.7% compared to placebo ($p < 0.05$). The clinical efficacy of an alcohol-free mouthwash containing 5.0% (W/V) Brazilian green propolis (MGP 5%) for the control of plaque and gingivitis were demonstrated by Pereira et al.[29] (Tables 8, 9, 10, and 11). Twenty five subjects, men and women aging between 18 and 60 years old (35 ± 9), were included in a clinical trial`s phase II study of the patients who had a minimum of 20 sound natural teeth, a mean plaque index of at least 1.5 (PI), and a mean gingival index (GI) of at least 1.0. They were instructed to rinse with 10mL of mouthwash test for 1 minute, immediately after brushing in the morning and at night. After 45 and 90 days using mouthwash, the results showed a significant reduction in plaque and in gingival index when compared to samples obtained in baseline. These reductions were at 24% and 40%, respectively ($P < 0.5$). There were no important side effects in soft and hard tissues of the mouth.

	Baseline	45 days	90 days	Reduction %		
MGP5%	N=22 1.17 (0.20)	N=22 0.64 (0.24)	N=21 0.70 (0.18)	Baseline- 45 days 45*	Baseline- 90 days 40*	45 days – 90 days

Table 8. Mean scores of Gingival Index (DP) and percent reduction between periods (Pereira et al., 2011) [29].∗ Friedman test (ANOVA) $P < .05$.

	Baseline	45 days	90 days	Reduction-%		
MGP5%	*n* = 22 0.30 (0.17)	*n* = 22 0.08 (0.06)	*n* = 21 0.07 (0.03)	Baseline–45 days 73*	Baseline–90 days 77*	45 days–90 days 13 (ns)**

Table 9. Mean scores of Severity Gengival Index (DP) and percent reduction between periods (Pereira et al., 2011) [29]. *Friedman test (ANOVA) $P < .05$. ∗∗Not significant.

	Baseline	45 days	90 days	Reduction-%		
				Baseline–45 days	Baseline–90 days	45 days–90 days∗
MGP5%	n = 22 2.39 (0.69)	n = 22 1.77 (0.61)	n = 21 1.82 (0.62)	26*	24*	———

Table 10. Mean scores of Plaque Index (DP) and percent reduction between periods (Pereira et al., 2011) [29].∗Friedman test (ANOVA) $P < .05$.

	Baseline	45 days	90 days	Reduction-%		
MGP5%	n = 22	n = 22	n = 21	Baseline–45 days	Baseline–90 days	45 days–90 days
	0.44 (0.19)	0.26 (0.14)	0.26 (0.15)	41*	41*	———

Table 11. Mean scores of Severity Plaque Index (DP) and percent between periods (Pereira et al., 2011) [29].∗ Friedman test (ANOVA) $P < .05$.

In this study, the MGP 5% showed evidence of its efficacy in reducing PI and GI. However, it is necessary to perform a clinical trial, double-blind, randomized to validate such effectiveness [29]. Regression of 95% gingivitis and suppuration in all the teeth irrigated with Brazilian Green Propolis gel (BGPg), as well as a pocket depths and all treated patients with the BGPg showed periodontitis/gingivitis regression. This result suggest that 10% BGPG used could be used as an adjuvant therapeutic method assigned for the treatment of periodontal disease (Figure 2) [142]. Ethanol Propolis Extract (EPE) inhibited all the *Candida albicans* strains collected from HIV-seropositive and HIV-seronegative Brazilian patients with oral candidiasis. No significant difference was observed between Nystatin and EPE. But significant differences were observed between EPE and other antifungals. *C. albicans* showed resistance to antifungal agents. This fact suggests commercial EPE could be an alternative medicine for candidosis treatment from HIV-positive patients (Figure 3) [143]. Brazilian commercial ethanol propolis extract, also formulated to ensure physical and chemical stability, was found to inhibit oral candidiasis in 12 denture-bearing patients with prosthesis stomatitis candidiasis association is show in Table 12 and Figure 4 [144]. Also, denture stomatitis presents as a chronic disease in denture-bearing patients, especially under maxillary prosthesis. Despite the existence of a great number of antifungal agents, treatment failure is observed frequently. So, the clinical efficacy of a Brazilian propolis gel formulation in patients diagnosed with denture stomatitis was evaluated. Thirty complete-denture wearers with denture stomatitis were enrolled in this pilot study. At baseline, clinical evaluation was performed by a single clinician and instructions for denture hygiene provided. Fifteen patients received Daktarin® (Miconazole gel) and 15 received Brazilian propolis gel. All patients were recommended to apply the product four times a day during one week. Clinical evaluation was repeated by the same clinician after treatment. All patients treated with Brazilian propolis gel and Daktarin® had complete clinical remission of palatal candidiasis edema and erythema. [77]. Noronha [31] found the efficacy of a Brazilian green propolis mucoadhesive gel (BPGg) in preventing and treating the oral mucositis and candidiasis in patients harboring malignant tumors and receiving radiotherapy. All patients who used the gel applied 24 hours before the first radiotherapy session, three times a day, during the whole period(six weeks) of radiotherapy, did not develop mucositis and candidosis over the entire period of radiotherapy.

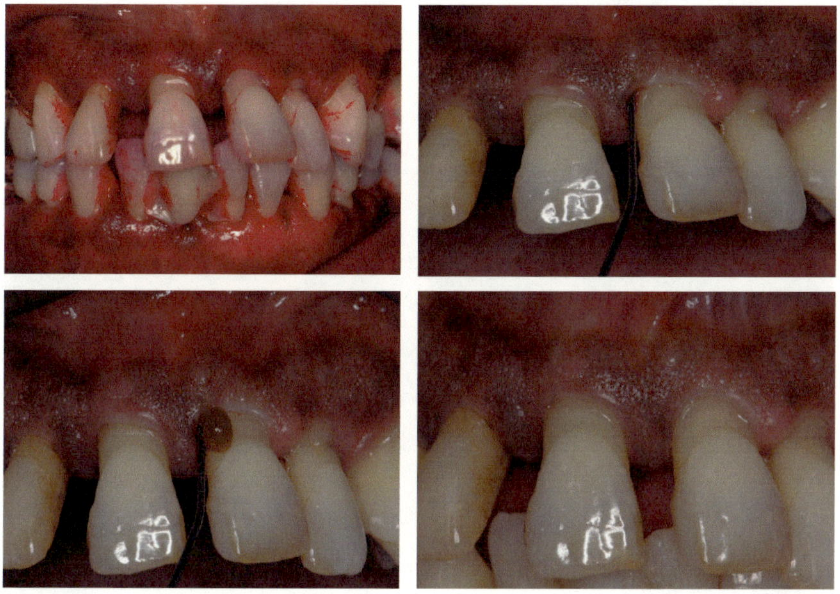

Figure 2. Periodontitis treatment with mucoadhesive green propolis gel. **A**) Evidencing of dental plaque with basic fuchsin. **B**) Confirmation of insertion loss and presence of periodontal pockets with periodontal probe. **C**) Applying mucoadhesive green propolis gel intra-periodontal pocket. **D**) Clinical aspect of the periodontium after treatment with gel containing propolis (Cairo do Amaral et al. [142].

The prevalence of candidosis in denture wearers is as well established as its treatment with antifungal agents (AAs). However, little research has been done regarding the effects of AAs on denture base surfaces. Then, da Silva et al.[150] evaluate the effects of fluconazole (FLU), nystatin (NYS) and propolis orabase gel (PRO) on poly (methyl-methacrylate) (PMMA) surfaces. So, PRO was able to induce changes in PMMA surface properties, such as roughness, which could be related to microbial adhesion [146]. Recurrent aphthous stomatitis (RAS) is a common, painful, and ulcerative disorder of the oral cavity of unknown etiology. No cure exists and medications aim to reduce pain associated with ulcers through topical applications or reduce outbreak frequency with systemic medications, many having serious side effects. Propolis is a bee product used in some cultures as treatment for mouth ulcers. A randomized, double-blind, placebo-controlled study, patients were assigned to take 500 mg of propolis or a placebo capsule daily. Subjects reported a baseline ulcer frequency and were contacted biweekly to record recurrences. Data were analyzed to determine if subjects had a decrease of 50% in outbreak frequency. The data indicated a statistically significant reduction of outbreaks in the propolis group (Fisher's exact test, one sided, $p = 0.04$). Patients in the propolis group also self-reported a significant improvement in their quality of life ($p = 0.03$). This study has shown propolis to be effective in decreasing the number of recurrences and improve the quality of life in patients who suffer from RAS [145].

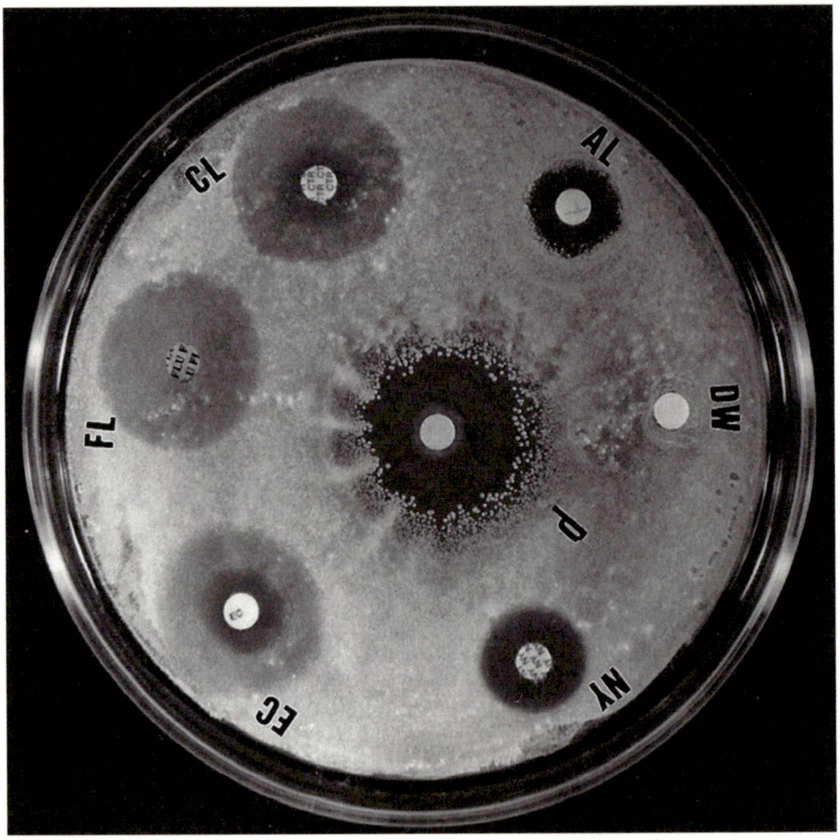

Figure 3. Inhibition zones of in vitro culture of *Candida albicans* collected from HIV-positive patients exposed to Ethanol Propolis Extract (EPE= P), and antifungal agents: CL= clotrimazole; FL= fluconazole; EC= Econazole; NY =Nystatin; AL= Alcohol; DW= Destiled water. (Martins et al., 2002) [143].

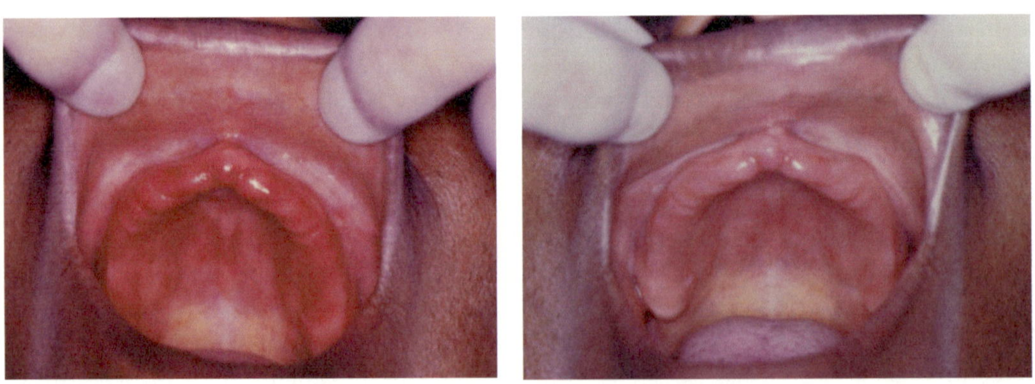

Figure 4. Clinical aspects of oral candidosis in patients with Total Removable Dental Prothesis (TRDP). **A**) Before propolis use. **B**) After propolis use. Source: Prof. Vagner Santos archives (2005) [146].

Patient	Age (years)	Race	Gender	Prosthesis	Local lesions	Antifungal agent	Result
ISS Hard	29	B	F	TRDP	palate/soft palate	Nys	+
SVCL	34	W	F	TRDP	Hard palate	Nys	+
AFF	36	W	M	TRDP	Hard palate	Nys	+
GMR	37	W	M	TRDP	Hard / soft palate	Nys	++
MIC	39	B	F	TRDP	Hard palate	NYS	+
AFS	71	B	F	TRDP	Hard palate	Nys	++
EGSM	29	W	F	TRDP	Hard /soft palate	EPE	+
TMS	31	B	F	TRDP	Hard palate	EPE	++
LMC	33	W	M	TRDP	Hard palate	EPE	+
HL	38	W	M	TRDP/PRDP	Hard palate/ alveolar mucosa	EPE	+
SFS	39	W	F	TRDP	Hard /soft palate	EPE	++
MCTS	43	W	M	TRDP/PRDP	Hard palate/ alveolar mucosa	EPE	+
MJNM	46	W	F	TRDP	Hard palate	EPE	++
	46	B	F	TRDP	Hard palate	EPE	+
HBS	48	B	M	TRDP	Hard palate	EPE	+
JJAF	50	W	F	TRDP	Hard palate	EPE	+
GRA	56	W	F	TRDP	Hard palate	EPE	++
NMBA	63	W	F	TRDP	Hard palate	EPE	++

Table 12. Clinical aspects of patients with oral candidiasis from Clinic of Semiology and Pathology of Dentistry School UFMG participating in this study and Results of *in vivo* patients treatment of oral candidiasis with 20% Brazilian green ethanol propolis extract (EPE) and Nystatin (Nys). Use posology: 4 time/day for 7 days, topic application in local lesion and prosthesis surface F, female; M, male; TRDP, total removable dental prosthesis; PRDP, partial removable dental prosthesis; B, black; W, white. (Santos et al., 2005) [146]

9. Future perspectives

The potential pharmacological activity investigation of natural products, especially antimicrobial activity, has attracted the attention of several researchers. Increase of bacterial resistance to traditional antimicrobial agents and side effects are often seen [147, 28]. Many mouthwashes with alcohol are used as adjuvants in the control of dental plaque and gingivitis, but undesirable side effects are observed, despite its efficacy. This stimulates the research of alternative products, such as the use of toothpastes and mouthwashes based on natural products, because there is the need for prevention and treatment options that are safe, effective and economical. Mouthwash based on herbal extracts and propolis are for sale in the Brazilian and world market, without, however, have undergone clinical studies proving their effectiveness and documenting possible undesirable side effects. Previous studies have demonstrated the efficacy of propolis extracts as an antimicrobial agent useful for dental caries and periodontal pathogens microorganisms in *in vitro* studies [24,78,59,148,149]. Propolis standardization is necessary and several authors from different countries are involved in the study of pharmacological activity and mechanism of action of various types of propolis. The separation of organic compounds and their mechanism of action on cells may lead to new products that can be important in controlling tumor growth, and infection control. However one should not forget that the effect of synergism observed in raw propolis is responsible for its excellent antimicrobial activity making it a unique product against bacterial and fungal resistance. Moreover, pre-clinical and clinical phase I, II, III studies are necesssary in order to better determine the effect on patients and safety. Several components of propolis have shown efficacy in the growth inhibition of *in vitro* tumor cells and *in vivo* tumors. This may be the way to the discovery of drugs against cancer, however, the clinical confirmations should be prioritized. The diversity of pharmacological properties of propolis may also be extended to studies against autoimmune diseases in order to ameliorate the clinical evolution. Also, studies against systemic diseases that affect largely population world as is the case of diabetes and hypertension. But for that attention should turn to as separation of compounds that can be a great gain for treatment of these diseases.

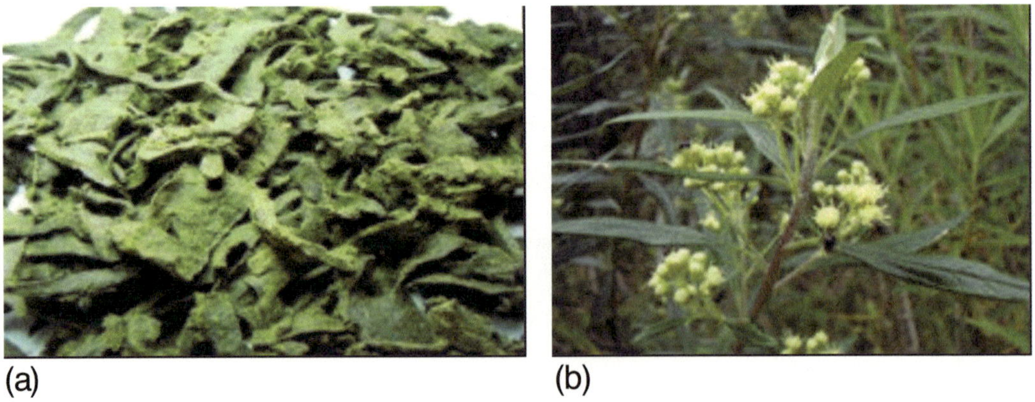

Figure 5. (a) Physical aspect of Brazilian green crude propolis. (b) Plant caracteristic of *Baccharis dracunculifolia*. (Prof. Vagner Santos archives, 2012).

Propolis component	Pharmacological properties	Author/year
Green Propolis extract	Apoptosis and cell propliferation	Giertsen et al, 2011 [153]
Moronic acid	Epstein-Barr virus suppresion	Chang et al., 2010 [154]
Polyphenols	Neurological diseases	Farooqui and Farooqui, 2012 [15]
Red propolis extract	Adipocyte differentiation	Iio et al., 2010 [155]
Caffeic acid phenethyl ester Cardanol, cardol	Antitumoral / anticancer, citotoxicity	Chuu et al., 2012 [156] Sawaya et al., 2011 [39] Chan et al., 2012 [152] Watanabe et al., 2011 [159] Teerasripreecha et al, 2012 [68]
epicatechin, *p*-coumaric acid, morin, 3,4-dimethoxycinnamic acid, naringenin, ferulic acid, cinnamic acid, pinocembrin, and chrysin , 3-prenyl-4-hydroxycinnamic acid	Antioxidant	Guimaraes et al., 2012 [95] Guo et al., 2011 [87] Sawaya et al, 2011 [39]
3-prenyl-4-hydroxycunnamic acid, 2,2-dimethyl-6-carboxyethenyl,2H-1-benzopyran; 3,5-diprenyl-4-hydroxycinnamic acid derivative 4 (DHCA4) 2,2-dimethyl-6-carboxyethenyl-2H-1-benzopyran (DCBEN	Antiparasitic *Trypanosoma cruzi; Leishmania amazonensis*	Sawaya et al., 2011 [39] Salomao et al., 2008 [160] Salaomao et al., 2011 [161]
Green, red and brown propolis extracts; Artepillin C; Crysin	Anti-inflamatory	Marcucci et al., 2000 [11] Ha et al., 2010 [158] Sawaya et al., 2011 [39] Moura et al., 2011 [57] Orsatti et al., 2012 [128]
Green, Red, Brown propolis extract; p-coumaric acid (PCUM), 3-(4-hydroxy-3-(oxo-butenyl)-phenylacrylic acid (DHCA1); Caffeic acid, caffeoylquinic acid, diterpenic acids, flavonoids	antimicrobial	Martins et al., 2002 [143] Paula et al., 2006 [59]; Santos et al., 2007 [71] Dias et al., 2012 [162]; Mattigatti et al., 2012 [163] Sawaya et al., 2011 [39] Choudhari et al., 2012 [157]

Table 13. Recent advances in propolis components studies.

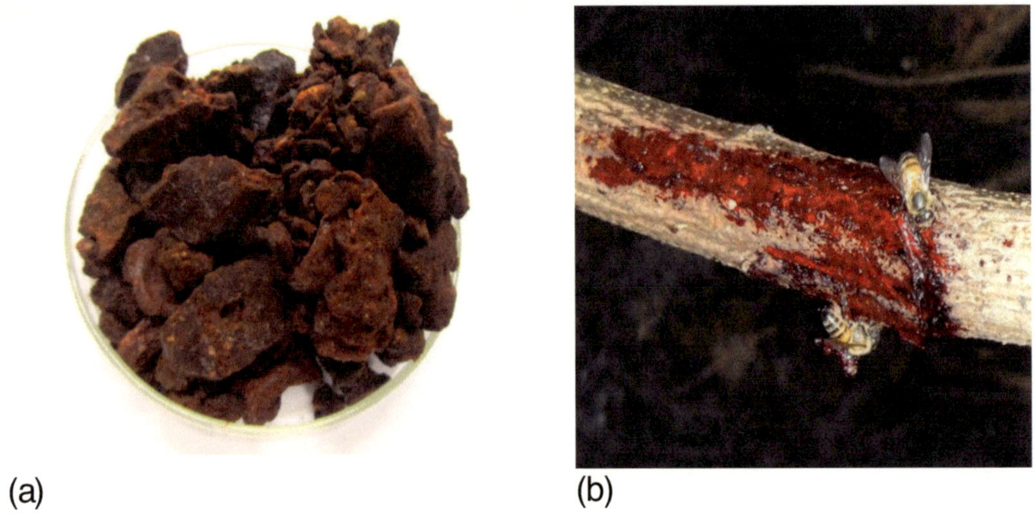

Figure 6. (a) Physical aspect of Brazilian red propolis. (Prof. Vagner Santos archives, 2012) (b) Dalbergia ecastophylum plant aspect. http://www.google.com.br/imgres?q=Dalbergia+ecastophyllum&num=10&hl=pt BR&biw=1280&bih=673&tbm= isch&tbnid=WIUAFEd2jCOSxM:&imgrefurl=http://meliponariojandaira.blogspot.com/2011/02/abelhas-indigenas-sem-ferrao.

Acknowledgements

Research Foundation of Minas Gerais State (FAPEMIG), National Council of Scientific and Tecnologic Development (CNPq) for financial support in all of our research group and also for supporting the publication of this chapter. Special thanks to Gustavo Araujo and Rafael Tomaz.

Author details

Vagner Rodrigues Santos

Address all correspondence to: vegneer2003@yahoo.com.br

Universidade Federal de Minas Gerais, Faculty of Dentistry, Department of Clinical, Pathology and Surgery, Laboratory of Microbiology and Biomaterials, Brazil

References

[1] Souza BM, Palma MS. Peptides from Hymenoptera venoms. In: Lima M.H. (ed). Animal Toxins: State of Art - Perspectives in Health and Biotechnology. EditoraUFMG. 2009.p 345-367.

[2] Castaldo S, Capasso F. Propolis, an old remedy used in modern medicine. Fitoterapia. 2002; 73(Suppl 1) S1- S6.

[3] Salatino, A; Teixeira, E.W.; Negri, G.; Message, D. Origin and Chemical Variation of Brazilian Própolis. Evidence-Based Complementary and Alternative Medicine 2005; 2(1) 33–38.

[4] Bankova V. Recent trends and important developments in propolis research. Evidence-Based Complementary Alternative Medicine 2005; 2(1) 29-32.(a)

[5] Marcucci MC. Propolis: chemical composition, biological properties and therapeutic activity. Apidologie 1995; 26(2) 83–99, 1995.

[6] Sforcin JM. Propolis and the immune system: a review. Journal Ethnopharmacology 2007; 113(1) 1-14.

[7] Burdock GA. Review of the biological properties and toxicity of bee propolis (propolis). Food and Chemical Toxicology 1998; 36(4) 347–363.

[8] Boyanova L, Kolarov R, Gergova G, Mitov I. In vitro activity of Bulgarian propolis against 94 clinical isolates of anaerobic bacteria. Anaerobe 2006; 12(4) 173-77.

[9] Fernandes FF, Dias ALT, Ramos CL, Ikegak M, Siqueira AM, Franco MC The "in vitro" antifungal activity evaluation of propolis G12 ethanol extract on *Cryptococcus neoformans*. Revista do Instituto de Medicina Tropical de Sao. Paulo 2007; 49(2) 93-95.

[10] Piccinelli AL, Lotti C, Campone L, Cuesta-Rubio O, Campo Fernandez M, Rastrelli L Cuban and Brazilian red propolis: botanical origin and comparative analysis by high-performance liquid chromatography-photodiode array detection/electrospray ionization tandem mass spectrometry. Journal of Agricultural Food and Chemistry. 2011; 59 (12) 6484-91.

[11] Marcucci, M.C.; Ferreres, F.; Custódio, A. Evaluation of phenolic compounds in Brazilian própolis from different geographic regions. Z. Naturforsch. 2000; 55 (1) 76-86.

[12] Bankova, V. Chemical diversity of propolis and the problem of standardization. Journal of Ethnopharmacology 2005; 100 (1) 114-117. (b)

[13] Simões CC, Araújo DB, Araújo RPC. Estudo in vitro e ex vivo da ação de diferentes concentrações de extratos de própolis frente aos microrganismos presentes na saliva de humanos. Brazilian Journal of Pharmacognosy 2008; 18(1) 84-89.

[14] Menezes H. Própolis: uma revisão dos recentes estudos de suas propriedades farmacológicas. Arquivos do Instituto de Biologia 2005; 72(3) 405-411.

[15] Farooqui T, Farooqui AA. Beneficial effects of propolis on human health and neurological diseases. Frontiers in Bioscience (Elite Ed) 2012; 4(1) 779-793.

[16] Aliyazicioglu Y, Demir S, Turan I, Cakiroglu TN, Akalin I, Deger O, Bedir A. Preventive and protective effects of Turkish propolis on H_2O_2-induced DNA damage in foreskin fibroblast cell lines. Acta Biological Hungarica. 2011; 62(4) 388-396.

[17] Ghisalberti EL. Propolis: a review. Bee World 1979; 60: 59–84.

[18] Park YK, Alencar SM, Moura FF, Ikegaki FFM. Atividade biológica da própolis. Revista OESP – Alimentação 1999; 27:46-53.

[19] Geraldini, C.A.C.; Salgado, E.G.C.; Rode, S.M. Ação de diferentes soluções de própolis na superfície dentinária - avaliação ultra-estrutural. Faculdade de Odontologia Sao Jose dos Campos 2000; 3(2) 28-32 .

[20] Grégio AMT, Lima AAS, Ribas MO, Barbosa APM, Pereira ACP, Koike F, Repeke CEP. Efeito da Propolis *Appis mellifera* sobre o processo de reparo de lesões ulceradas na mucosa bucal de ratos. Estudos em Biologia 2005; 27: 58.

[21] Manara LRB, Anconi SI, Gromatzky A, Conde MC, Bretz WA. Utilização da própolis em Odontologia. Revista da Faculdade de Odontologia de Bauru 1999; 7(3-4) 15-20.

[22] Peña RC. Propolis standardization: a chemical and biological review. Ciencias de Investigacao Agraria 2008; 35: 11-20.

[23] Pereira AS, Seixas FRM, Aquino-Neto FR. Própolis: 100 anos de pesquisa e suas perspectivas futuras. Quimica Nova 2002; 25(1) 321-326.

[24] Santos FA, Bastos EMA, Rodrigues PH, Uzeda M, Carvalho MAR, Farias LM, Moreira ESA. Susceptibility of *Prevotella intermédia/ Prevotella nigrescens* and *Porphyromonas gingivalis* to propolis (bee glue) and other antimicrobial agents. Anaerobe 2002; 8(1) 9-15.

[25] Boyanova L, Gergova G, Nikolov R, Derejian S, Lazarova E, Latsarov N, Mitov I, Krastev Z. Activity of Bulgarian própolis against 94 *Helicobacter pylori* strains in vitro by agar-well diffusion, agar dilution and disc diffusion methods. Journal Medical Microbiology 2005; 54(pt5) 481-483.

[26] Auricchio MT, Bugno A, Almodóvar AAB, Pereira TC. Avaliação da atividade antimicrobiana de preparações de própolis comercializadas na cidade de São Paulo. Revista do Instituto Adolfo Lutz 2007; 65(2) 209-212.

[27] Parker JF; Luz MMS. Método para avaliação e pesquisa da atividade antimicrobiana de produtos de origem natural. Revista Brasileira de Farmacognosia 2007; 17(1) 102-107.

[28] Libério SA, Pereira AL, Araújo MJ, Dutra RP, Nascimento FR, Monteiro-Neto V, Ribeiro MN, Gonçalves AG, Guerra RN. The potential use of propolis as a cariostatic agent and its actions on mutans group streptococci. Journal of Ethnopharmacology 2009; 125(1): 1-9.

[29] Pereira EM, da Silva JL, Silva FF, De Luca MP, Ferreira EF, Lorentz TC, Santos VR. Clinical Evidence of the Efficacy of a Mouthwash Containing Propolis for the Control of Plaque and Gingivitis: A Phase II Study. Evidence- Based Complementary and Alternative Medicine 2011; 2011:750249. Epub 2011 Mar 31. PMID: 21584253 [PubMed]

[30] Banskota AH, Tezuka YY, Kadota S. Recent progress in pharmacological research of propolis. Phytoterapy Research 2001; 15(7) 561-571.

[31] Noronha VRAS. Evidencias preliminares da eficácia de gel contendo propolis na prevenção e tratamento de mucosite e candidose bucais em pacientes submetidos a radioterapia em região de cabeça e pescoço. Thesis. Minas Gerais Federal University, 2011.

[32] Park YK, Alencar SM, Aguiar CL. Botanical origin and chemical composition of Brazilian propolis. Journal of Agricultural and Food Chemistry 2002; 50 (9) 2502-2506.

[33] Miguel MG, Antunes MD. Is propolis safe as an alternative medicine? Journal of Pharmacy and Bioallied Sciences 2011; 3(4) 479-495.

[34] Park YK, Paredes-Guzman JF, Aguiar CL, Alencar SM, Fujiwara FY. Chemical constituents in Baccharis dracunculifolia as the main botanical origin of southeastern Brazilian propolis. Journal Agricultural Food Chemistry 2004; 52 (1) 100-1103.

[35] Lustosa SR, Galindo AB, Nunes LCC, Randau KP, Rolim Neto PJ. Própolis: atualizações sobre a química e a farmacologia. Brazilian Journal of Pharmacognosy 2008; 18: 447-454.

[36] Silva BB, Rosalen PL, Cury JA, Ikegaki M, Souza VC, Esteves A, Alencar SM. Chemical composition and botanical origin of red própolis, a new type of Brazilian propolis. Evidence-Based Complementary and Alternative Medicine 2008; 5(3) 313-316.

[37] Park YK, Ikegaki M, Alencar SM, Moura FF. Evaluation of Brazilian propolis by both physicochemical methods and biological activity. Honey Bee Science 2000; 21(2): 85-90.

[38] Ahn MR, Kunimasa K, Ohta T, Kumazawa S, Kamihira M, Kaji K, Uto Y, Hori H, Nagasawa H, Nakayama T. Suppression of tumor-induced angiogenesis by brazilian propolis: major component artepilin C inhibits in vitro tube formation and endothelial cell proliferation. Cancer Letters 2007; 252(2) 235-243.

[39] Sawaya AC, Barbosa da Silva Cunha I, Marcucci MC Analytical methods applied to diverse types of Brazilian propolis. Chemistry Central Journal 2011, 5(1) 27.

[40] Fischer G, Cleff MB, Dummer LA, Paulino N, Paulino AS, Vilela CO, Campos FS, Storch T, Vargas GD, Hübner SO, Vidor T. Adjuvant effect of green propolis on humoral immune response of bovines immunized with bovine herpesvirus type 5. Veterinary Immunology and Immunopathology 2007; 116(1) 79–84.

[41] Alencar SM, Oldoni TL, Castro ML, Cabral IS, Costa-Neto CM, Cury JA, Rosalen PL, Ikegaki M. Chemical composition and biological activity of a new type of Brazilian propolis: red propolis. Journal of Ethnopharmacology 2007; 113(2) 278-83.

[42] Sawicka D, Car H, Borawska MH, Nikliński. The anticancer activity of propolis. Folia Histochemica Cytobiologica 2012; 50(1) 25-37.

[43] Maciejewicz W. Isolation of flavonoid aglycones from propolis by a column chromatography method and their identification by GC-MS and TLC methods. Journal of Liquid Chromatography and Related Technolology 2001; 24 (1) 1171-1179.

[44] Kumazawa S, Goto H, Hamasaka T, Fukumoto S, Fujimoto T, Nakayama T. A new prenylated flavonoid from propolis collected in Okinawa, Japan. Biosciences Biotechnology and Biochemistry 2004; 68(1) 260-262.

[45] Ozkul Y, Silici S, Eroğlu E. The anticarcinogenic effect of propolis in human lymphocytes culture. Phytomedicine. 2005; 12(10) 742-747.

[46] Eremia N, Dabija T. The content micro- and macroelements in propolis. Bulletin USAMV-CN 2007; 63–64.

[47] Machado GM, Leon LL, De Castro SL. Activity of Brazilian and Bulgarian propolis against different species of Leishmania. Memorial do Instituto Oswaldo Cruz 2007; 102(1) 74–77.

[48] Vandar-Unlu G, Silici S, Unlu M. Composition and *in vitro* antimicrobial activity of Populus buds and poplar-type propolis. World Journal of Microbiology and Biotechnology 2008; 24 (1) 1011–1017.

[49] Wang HQ, Sun XB, Xu YX, Zhao H, Zhu QY, Zhu CQ. Astaxanthin upregulates heme oxygenase-1 expression through ERK 1/2 pathway and its protective effect against beta-amyloid-induced cytotoxicity in SH-SY5Y cells. Brain Research 2010; 1360(1) 159–167.

[50] Veronese R. Própolis na clínica e cirúrgia odontológica. Revisão. Disponível em: http://www.brazilianapis.com/public/propolisnaclinicarespiratoriaeotorrinolaringologia.pdf. Acesso em 13 de julho de 2012.

[51] Cizmárik J, Matel I. Examination of the chemical composition of propolis I. Isolation and identification of the 3,4-dihydroxycinnamic acid (caffeic acid) from propolis. Experientia. 1970;26(7) 713.

[52] Kadakov, V. P.; Mulearchuk, M. D. Aminoacidos encontrados en el propoleos. Pchelovodstvo 1978; 12: 34.

[53] Endler A L, Oliveira SC, Amorim CA, Carvalho MP, Pileggi M. Teste de Eficácia da Própolis no Combate a Bactérias Patogênicas das Vias Respiratórias. Publicacao UEPG Ciencias Biologicas e Saúde 2003; .9(2)17-20.

[54] Awale S, Shrestha SP, Tezuka Y, Ueda JY, Matsushige K, Kadota S. Neoflavonoids and related constituents from Nepalese propolis and their nitric oxide production inhibitory activity. Journal of Natural Products 2005; 68(6) 858-864.

[55] Funari, C.S.; Ferro, V.O. Análise de própolis. Ciencias e Tecnologia de Alimentos 2006; 26 (1) 171-178.

[56] de Moura SA, Ferreira MA, Andrade SP, Reis ML, Noviello Mde L, Cara DC. Brazilian green propolis inhibits inflammatory angiogenesis in a murine sponge model. Evidence-Based Complementary and Alternative Medicine 2011; 2011:182703. Epub 2011 Mar 9.

[57] Kujumgiev A, Tsvetkova I, Serkedjieva Yu, Bankova V, Christov R, Popov S. Antibacterial, antifungal and antiviral activity of propolis of different geographic origin. Journal of Ethnopharmacology 1999; 64 (3) 235–240.

[58] Paula AMB, Gomes RT, Santiago WK, Dias RS, Cortés ME, Santos VR. Susceptibility of oral pathogenic bacteria and fungi to brazilian green propolis extract. Pharmacologyonline 2006;. 3: 467-473.

[59] Fischer G, Conceição FR, Leite FPL, Dummer LA, Vargas GD, Hübner SO, Dellagostin OA, Paulino N, Paulino AS, Vidor T: Immunomodulaation produced by green propolis extract on humoral and cellular responses in mice immunized with SuHV-1. Vaccine 2007; 25 (1) 1250-1256.

[60] Chan GC, Cheung KW, Sze DM. The Immunomodulatory and Anticancer Properties of Propolis. Clinical Review Allergy Immunology 2012; Jun 17 [Epub ahead of print] PMID: 22707327 [PubMed - as supplied by publisher]

[61] Ozan F, Sümer Z, Polat ZA, Er K, Ozan U, Deger O. Effect of mouthrinse containing propolis on oral microorganisms and human gingival fibroblasts. European Journal Dental 2007; 1(4)195-201.

[62] Tani H, Hasumi K, Tatefuji T, Hashimoto K, Koshino H, Takahashi S. Inhibitory activity of Brazilian green propolis components and their derivatives on the release of cys-leukotrienes. Bioorganic Medicine Chemistry 2010; 18(1) 151-157.

[63] Borrelli, F, Maffia P, Pinto L, Ianaro A, Russo A, Capasso F, Ialenti A. Phytochemical compounds involved in the antiinflamatory effect of propolis extract. Fitoterapia 2002; 73(suppl. 1). S53-S63.

[64] Barros MP, Sousa JP, Bastos JK, de Andrade SF. Effect of Brazilian green propolis on experimental gastric ulcers in rats. Journal of Ethnopharmacology 2007; 110(3) 567-71.

[65] Juman S, Yasui N, Okuda H, Ueda A, Negishi H, Miki T, Ikeda K. Caffeic acid phenethyl ester suppresses the production of adipocytokines, leptin, tumor necrosis factor -alpha and resistin, during differentiation to adipocytes in 3T3-L1 cells. Biological Pharmaceutical Bulletin 2011; 34(4):490-4.

[66] Teerasripreecha D, Phuwapraisirisan P, Puthong S, Kimura K, Okuyama M, Mori H, Kimura A, Chanchao C . In vitro antiproliferative/cytotoxic activity on cancer cell lines of a cardanol and a cardol enriched from Thai Apis mellifera propolis. BMC Complementary and Alternative Medicine 2012; 2:27.

[67] Park YK, Koo, MH, Abreu JA. Antimicrobial activity of propolis on oral microrganisms. Currents Microbiology 1998; 36 (1) 24-28.

[68] Bera A, Muradian LBA. Propriedades físico-químicas de amostras comerciais de mel com própolis do Estado de São Paulo. Ciência e Tecnologia de Alimentos- Campinas 2007; 27(1) 49-52.

[69] Santos VR, Gomes RT, Teixeira KIR, Cortés ME. Antimicrobial activity of a propolis adhesive formulation on different oral pathogens. Brazilian Journal of Oral Sciences 2007; 6 (22) 1387-1391.

[70] Júnior AF, Lopes MMR, Colombari V, Monteiro ACM, Vieira EP. Atividade antimicrobiana de própolis de Apis mellifera obtidas em três regiões do Brasil. Ciência Rural-Santa Maria 2006; 36: 294-297.

[71] Vargas, A. C.; Loguercio, A. P.; Witt, N. M.; Da Costa, M. M.; Sá E Silva, M.; Viana, L. R. Atividade antimicrobiana "in vitro" de extrato alcoólico de própolis. Ciência Rural 2004; 34: 159-163.

[72] Tosi B, Donini A, Romagnoli C, Bruni A. Antimicrobial activity of some commercial extracts of propolis prepared with different solvents. Phytotherapy Research 1996; 10(4) 335-336.

[73] Stepanović S, Antić N, Dakić I, Svabić-Vlahović M. *In vitro* antimicrobial activity of propolis and synergism between propolis and antimicrobial drugs. Microbiological Research 2003; 158(4) 353-357.

[74] Onlen Y, Duran N, Atik E, Savas L, Altug E, Yakan S, Aslantas O. Antibacterial activity of propolis against MRSA and synergism with topical mupirocin. Journal of Alternative and Complementary Medicine 2007; 13(7) 713-718.

[75] Santos VR, Gomes RT, Mesquita RA, De Moura MDG, França EC, Aguiar EG, Naves MD, Abreu JAS, Abreu SRL. Efficacy of Brazilian Propolis Gel for the Management of Denture Stomatitis: a Pilot Study. Phytotherapy Research 2008; 22(11) 1544–1547.

[76] Mello AM, Gomes RT, Lara SR, Silva LG, Alves JB, Cortés ME, Abreu SL, Santos VR. 2006. The effect of Brazilian propolis on the germ tube formation and cell wall of Candida albicans. Pharmacologyonline 2006; 3: 352–358.

[77] De Nollin S, Borgers M. The effects of miconazole on the ultrastructure of Candida albicans. Proceedings of Royal Society of Medicine 1977; 70(Suppl 1) 9-12.

[78] Tajima, H.; Kimoto, H.; Taketo, Y.; Taketo, A. Effects of synthetic hydroxyisothiocinates on microbial systems. Biosciences Biotechnology and Biochemistry 1998; 62: 491-495.

[79] Siqueira AB, Gomes BS, Cambuim I, Maia R, Abreu S, Souza-Motta CM, de Queiroz LA, Porto AL. *Trichophyton* species susceptibility to green and red propolis from Brazil. Letters Applied Microbiology 2009; 48(1) 90-96.

[80] Ota C, Unterkircher C, Fantimato V, Shimizu MT. Antifungal activity of própolis on different species of Candida. Mycoses 2001, 44(9-10) 375-378.

[81] Popova MP, Chinou IB, Marekov IN, Bankova VS. Terpenes with antimicrobial activity from Cretan propolis. Phytochemistry. 2009; 70(10) 1262-1271.

[82] Silva JC, Rodrigues S, Feás X, Estevinho LM. Antimicrobial activity, phenolic profile and role in the inflammation of propolis. Food Chemistry Toxicology 2012; 50(5) 1790-1795.

[83] Havsteen BII. The biochemistry and medical significance of the flavonoids. Pharmacology & Therapeutics 2002; 96(2-3) 67-202.

[84] Marquele FD, Stracieri KM, Fonseca MJ, Freitas LA. Spray-dried propolis extract. I: physicochemical and antioxidant properties. Pharmazie 2006; 61(4) 325-330.

[85] Guo X, Chen B, Luo L, Zhang X, Dai X, Gong S. Chemical compositions and antioxidant activities of water extracts of Chinese propolis. Journal of Agricultural Food Chemistry 2011; 59(23) 12610-12616.

[86] Messerli SM, Ahn MR, Kunimasa K, Yanagihara M, Tatefuji T, Hashimoto K, Mautner V, Uto Y, Hori H, Kumazawa S, Kaji K, Ohta T, Maruta H. Artepillin C (ARC) in Brazilian green propolis selectively blocks oncogenic PAK1 signaling and suppresses the growth of NF tumors in mice. Phytotherapy Research 2009; 23(3) 423-427.

[87] Sud'ina GF, Mirzoeva OK, Pushkareva MA, Korshunova GA, Sumbatyan NV, Varfolomeev SD. Caffeic acid phenethyl ester as a lipoxygenase inhibitor with antioxidant properties. FEBS 1993; 329(1-2) 21-24.

[88] Mani F, Damasceno HC, Novelli EL, Martins EA, Sforcin JM. Propolis: Effect of different concentrations, extracts and intake period on seric biochemical variables. Journal of Ethnopharmacology 2006; 05(1-2):95-98.

[89] Vicentino, A. R. R.; Menezes, F. S. Atividade antioxidante de tinturas vegetais, vendidas em farmácias com manipulação e indicadas para diversos tipos de doenças pela metodologia do DPPH. Revista Brasileira de Farmacognosia 2007; 17(1) 384- 387.

[90] Sulaiman GM, Al Sammarrae KW, Ad'hiah AH, Zucchetti M, Frapolli R, Bello E, Erba E, D'Incalci M, Bagnati R. Chemical characterization of Iraqi propolis samples and assessing their antioxidant potentials. Food Chemistry Toxicology 2011; 49(9) 2415-2421.

[91] Russo A, Longo R, Vanella A. Antioxidant activity of própolis: role of caffeic acid phenethyl ester and galangin. Fitoterapia 2002; 73(suppl. 1) S21-S29.

[92] Cigut T, Polak T, Gašperlin L, Raspor P, Jamnik P. Antioxidative activity of propolis extract in yeast cells. Journal Agricultural Food Chemistry 2011; 59(21) 11449-11455.

[93] Guimarães NS, Mello JC, Paiva JS, Bueno PC, Berretta AA, Torquato RJ, Nantes IL, Rodrigues T. Baccharis dracunculifolia, the main source of green propolis, exhibits potent antioxidant activity and prevents oxidative mitochondrial damage. Food Chemistry Toxicology 2012; 50 (3-4) 1091-1097.

[94] Gong P, Chen F, Liu X, Gong X, Wang J, Ma Y. Protective effect of caffeic acid phenethyl ester against cadmium-induced renal damage in mice. Journal of Toxicology Science 2012; 37(2) 415-25.

[95] Nakamura T, Ohta Y, Ohashi K, Ikeno K, Watanabe R, Tokunaga K, Harada N. Protective Effect of Brazilian Propolis Against Hepatic Oxidative Damage in Rats with Water-immersion Restraint Stress. Phytotherapy Research 2012, Feb 1. doi: 10.1002/ptr. 4601. [Epub ahead of print]

[96] Vynograd N, Vynograd I, Sosnowski Z. A comparative multi-centre study of the efficacy of propolis, acyclovir and placebo in the treatment of genital herpes (HSV). Phytomedicine 2000; 7(1):1-6.

[97] Nolkemper S, Reichling J, Sensch KH, Schnitzler PMechanism of Herpes simplex virus type 2 suppression by propolis extracts. Phytomedicine 2010; 17(2) 132-138.

[98] Huleihel M, Isanu V. Anti-herpes simplex virus effect of an aqueous extract of propolis. Isr Medicine Association Journal. 2002; 4(11 Suppl) 923-927.

[99] Gekker G, Hu S, Spivak M, Lokensgard JR, Peterson PK. Anti-HIV-1 activity of propolis in CD4(+) lymphocyte and microglial cell cultures. Journal of Ethnopharmacology 2005; 102(2) 158-63.

[100] Drago L, De Vecchi E, Nicola L, Gismondo MR. In vitro antimicrobial activity of a novel propolis formulation (Actichelated propolis). Journal of Applied Microbiology 2007; 103(5) 1914-1921.

[101] Schnitzler P, Neuner A, Nolkemper S, Zundel C, Nowack H, Sensch KH, Reichling J. Antiviral activity and mode of action of propolis extracts and selected compounds. Phytotherapy Research 2010; 24(Suppl 1) S20-S28. Erratum in: Phytotherapy Research 2010; 24(4) 632.

[102] Sartori G, Pesarico AP, Pinton S, Dobrachinski F, Roman SS, Pauletto F, Junior LC, Prigol M. Protective effect of brown Brazilian propolis against acute vaginal lesions caused by herpes simplex virus type 2 in mice: involvement of antioxidant and anti-inflammatory mechanisms. Cell Biochem Funct. 2011 Oct 24. doi: 10.1002/cbf.1810. [Epub ahead of print]

[103] Rao CV, Desai D, Rivenson A, Simi B, Amin S, Reddy BS. Chemoprevention of colon carcinogenesis by phenylethyl-3-methylcaffeate. Cancer Research 1995; 55(11) 2310-2315.

[104] Huang MT, Ma W, Yen P, Xie JG, Han J, Frenkel K, Grunberger D, Conney AH. Inhibitory effects of caffeic acid phenethyl ester (CAPE) on 12-O-tetradecanoylphorbol-13-acetate-induced tumor promotion in mouse skin and the synthesis of DNA, RNA and protein in HeLa cells. Carcinogenesis 1996; 17(4) 761-765.

[105] Orsolić N, Basić I Antitumor, hematostimulative and radioprotective action of water-soluble derivative of propolis (WSDP). Biomedicine and Pharmacotherapy 2005; 59(10) 561-570.

[106] Szliszka E, Czuba ZP, Domino M, Mazur B, Zydowicz G, Krol W. Ethanolic extract of propolis (EEP) enhances the apoptosis- inducing potential of TRAIL in cancer cells. Molecules 2009; 14(2) 738-754.

[107] Endo S, Matsunaga T, Kanamori A, Otsuji Y, Nagai H, Sundaram K, El-Kabbani O, Toyooka N, Ohta S, Hara. A selective inhibition of human type-5 17β-hydroxysteroid dehydrogenase (AKR1C3) by baccharin, a component of Brazilian propolis. Journal of Natural Products 2012; 75(4) 716-21.

[108] Akao Y, Maruyama H, Matsumoto K, Ohguchi K, Nishizawa K, Sakamoto T, Araki Y, Mishima S, Nozawa Y. Cell Growth inhibitory effect of cinnamic acid derivatives from própolis on human tumor cell lines. Biological and Pharmaceutical Bulletin 2003; 26(7) 1057-1059.

[109] Awale S, Li F, Onozuka H, Esumi H, Tezuka Y, Kadota S. Constituents of Brazilian red propolis and their preferential cytotoxic activity against human pancreatic PANC-1 cancer cell line in nutrient-deprived condition. Bioorganic Medical Chemistry 2008; 16(1)181-189.

[110] Li F, Awale S, Tezuka Y, Kadota SCytotoxicity of constituents from Mexican propolis against a panel of six different cancer cell lines. Natural Products Communication 2010; 5(10) 1601-1606.

[111] Seda Vatansever H, Sorkun K, Ismet Deliloğlu Gurhan S, Ozdal-Kurt F, Turkoz E, Gencay O, Salih B. Propolis from Turkey induces apoptosis through activating caspases in human breast carcinoma cell lines. Acta Histochemica 2010; 112(6) 546-556.

[112] Sobočanec S, Balog T, Šariċ A, Mačak-Šafranko Ž, Štroser M, Žarković K, Žarković N, Stojković R, Ivanković S, Marotti T. Antitumor effect of Croatian propolis as a consequence of diverse sex-related dihydropyrimidine dehydrogenase (DPD) protein expression. Phytomedicine 2011; 18(10) 852-858.

[113] Badr MO, Edrees NM, Abdallah AA, El-Deen NA, Neamat-Allah AN, Ismail HT. Antitumour effects of Egyptian propolis on Ehrlich ascites carcinoma. Veterinaria Italiana 2011; 47(3) 341-350.

[114] Benkovic V, Kopjar N, Knezevic AH, Dikiv D, Basic I, Ramic S, Viculin T, Knezevic F, Orsolic N. Evaluation of Radioprotective Effects of Propolis and Quercetin on Human White Blood Cells in Vitro. Biological. Pharmaceutical Bulletin 2008; 31(9) 1778-1785.

[115] Búfalo MC, Candeias JM, Sousa JP, Bastos JK, Sforcin JM. In vitro cytotoxic activity of *Baccharis dracunculifolia* and propolis against HEp-2 cells. Natural Product Research 2010; 24(18) 1710-1718.

[116] Tanaka M, Okamoto Y, Fukui T, Masuzawa T. Suppression of interleukin 17 production by Brazilian propolis in mice with collagen-induced arthritis. Inflammopharmacology 2012; 20(1)19-26.

[117] Bachiega TF, Orsatti CL, Pagliarone AC, Sforcin JM The Effects of Propolis and its Isolated Compounds on Cytokine Production by Murine Macrophages. Phytotherapy Research 2012; doi: 10.1002/ptr.3731.

[118] Okamoto Y, Tanaka M, Fukui T, Masuzawa T.Brazilian propolis inhibits the differentiation of Th17 cells by inhibition of interleukin-6-induced phosphorylation of signal

transducer and activator of transcription 3. Immunopharmacology and Immunotoxicology 2012; Feb 9. [Epub ahead of print] PMID: 22316079 [PubMed

[119] Dimov V, Ivanovska N, Bankova V, Popov S. Immunomodulatory action of propolis: IV. Prophylactic activity against Gram-negative infections and adjuvant effect of the water-soluble derivate. Vaccine 1992; 10(12) 817-823.

[120] Nunes A, Faccioli LH, Sforcin JM. Propolis: lymphocyte proliferation and IFN-g production. Journal of Ethnopharmacology 2003; 87(1)93-97.

[121] You KM, Son KH, Chang HW, Kang SS, Kim HP. Vitexicarpin, a flavonoid from the fruits of Vitex rotundifolia, inhibits mouse lymphocyte proliferation and growth of cell lines in vitro. Planta Medica 1998; 64(1) 546–550.

[122] Orsolic N, Sver L, Terzié S, Tadie Z, Basic I. Inhibitory effect of water-soluble derivative of propolis and its polyphenolic compounds on tumor growth and metastasizing ability: a possible mode of antitumor action. Nutrition and Câncer 2003; 47(2) 156-163.

[123] Orsolic N, Benkovic V, Knezevic AH, Kopjar N, Kosalec I, Bakmaz M, Mihaljevic Z, Bendelja K, Basic I. Assessment by Survival Analysis of the Radioprotective Properties of Propolis and Its Polyphenolic Compounds. Biological Pharmaceutical Bulletin 2007; 30(5) 946-951.

[124] Kimoto T, Arai S, Kohguchi M, Aga M, Nomura Y, Micallef MJ, Kurimoto M, Mito K. Apoptosis and suppression of tumor growth by artepillin C extracted from Brazilian propolis. Cancer Detect Prevention 1998; 22(6) 506-15.

[125] Missima F, Pagliarone AC, Orsatti CL, Araújo JP Jr, Sforcin JM. The Effect of propolis on Th1/Th2 cytokine expression and production by melanoma-bearing mice submitted to stress. Phytotherapy Research 2010; 24(10)1501-1507.

[126] Orsatti CL, Sforcin JM. Propolis immunomodulatory activity on TLR-2 and TLR-4 expression by chronically stressed mice. Natural Product Research 2012; 26(5) 446-453.

[127] Zedan H, Hofny ER, Ismail SA. Propolis as an alternative treatment for cutaneous warts. International Journal of Dermatology 2009; 48(11) 1246-1249.

[128] de Sousa JP, Bueno PC, Gregório LE, da Silva Filho AA, Furtado NA, de Sousa ML, Bastos JK. A reliable quantitative method for the analysis of phenolic compounds in Brazilian propolis by reverse phase high performance liquid chromatography. Journal of Separation Science 2007; 30(16) 2656-2665.

[129] Ramanauskiene K, Savickas A, Inkeniene A, Vitkevicius K, Kasparaviciene G, Briedis V, Amsiejus A. Analysis of content of phenolic acids in Lithuanian propolis using high-performance liquid chromatography technique. Medicina (Kaunas) 2009; 45(9) 712-717.

[130] Volpi N, Bergonzini G. Analysis of flavonoids from propolis by on-line HPLC-electrospray mass spectrometry. Journal of Pharmacy and Biomedical Analysis 2006; 42(3) 354-361.

[131] Gómez-Caravaca AM, Gómez-Romero M, Arráez-Román D, Segura-Carretero A, Fernández-Gutiérrez A. Advances in the analysis of phenolic compounds in products derived from bees. Journal of Pharmacology and Biomedicine Analysis 2006; 41(4) 1220-34.

[132] Watson DG, Peyfoon E, Zheng L, Lu D, Seidel V, Johnston B, Parkinson JA, Fearnley J. Application of principal components analysis to 1H-NMR data obtained from propolis samples of different geographical origin. Phytochemical Analysis 2006; 17(5) 323-331.

[133] Mutinelli F. The spread of pathogens through trade in honey bees and their products (including queen bees and semen): overview and recent developments. Revue Scientifique et Technique 2011; 30(1) 257-271.

[134] Ceschel GC, Maffei P, Sforzini A, Lombardi Borgia S, Yasin A, Ronchi C. In vitro permeation through porcine buccal mucosa of caffeic acid phenetyl ester (CAPE) from a topical mucoadhesive gel containing propolis. Fitoterapia. 2002; 73 (Suppl 1) S44- S52.

[135] Iyyam Pillai S, Palsamy P, Subramanian S, Kandaswamy M. Wound healing properties of Indian propolis studied on excision wound-induced rats. Pharmaceutical Biology 2010; 48(11):1198-1206.

[136] Dodwad V, Kukreja BJ. Propolis mouthwash: A new beginning. Journal of Indian Society of Periodontology 2011; 15(2) 121-125.

[137] Eley BM. Antibacterial agents in the control of supragingival plaque: a review. British Dental Journal 1999; 186(6) 286-296.

[138] Vervelle A, Mouhyi J, Del Corso M, Hippolyte MP, Sammartino G, Dohan Ehrenfest DM. Mouthwash solutions with microencapsuled natural extracts: Efficiency for dental plaque and gingivitis. Revue de Stomatologie et Chirurgie Maxillofacialle 2010; 111(3)148-151.

[139] Koo H, Cury JA, Rosalen PL, Ambrosano GM, Ikegaki M, Park YK Effect of a mouthrinse containing selected propolis on 3-day dental plaque accumulation and polysaccharide formation. Caries Research 2002; 36(6):445-448.

[140] Cairo do Amaral R, Gomes RT, Rocha WMS, Abreu SLR, Santos VR. Periodontitis treatment with brazilian green própolis gel. Pharmacologyonline. 2006; 3(3) 336-341.

[141] Martins RS, Péreira ES Jr, Lima SM, Senna MI, Mesquita RA, Santos VR Effect of commercial ethanol propolis extract on the in vitro growth of *Candida albicans* collected from HIV-seropositive and HIV-seronegative Brazilian patients with oral candidiasis. Journal of Oral Sciences 2002; 44(1) 41-48.

[142] Jeon JG, Rosalen PL, Falsetta ML, Koo H. Natural products in caries research: current (limited) knowledge, challenges, and future perspective. Caries Research 2011; 45(3) 243-263.

[143] Samet N, Laurent C, Susarla SM, Samet-Rubinsteen N. The effect of bee propolis on recurrent aphthous stomatitis: a pilot study. Clinical Oral Investigation 2007; 11(2)143-147.

[144] Santos VR, Pimenta FJ, Aguiar MC, do Carmo MA, Naves MD, Mesquita RA. Oral candidiasis treatment with Brazilian ethanol propolis extract. Phytotherapy Research 2005; 19(7) 652-654.

[145] Kalogeropoulos N, Konteles S, Mourtzinos I, Troullidou E, Chiou A, Karathanos VT. Encapsulation of complex extracts in beta-cyclodextrin: an application to propolis ethanolic extract. Journal of Microencapsulations 2009; 26(7) 603-613.

[146] Koru O, Toksoy F, Acikel CH, Tunca YM, Baysallar M, Uskudar Guclu A, Akca E, Ozkok Tuylu A, Sorkun K, Tanyuksel M, Salih B. *In vitro* antimicrobial activity of propolis samples from different geographical origins against certain oral pathogens. Anaerobe 2007; 13(3-4) 140-145.

[147] De Luca MP. Verniz a base de quitosana contendo própolis verde brasileira: avaliação da atividade antimicrobiana, citotoxicidade e perfil de liberação. Thesis. Universidade Federal de Minas Gerais; 2011.

[148] da Silva WJ, Rached RN, Rosalen PL, Del bel Cury AA. Effects of nystatin, fluconazole and propolis on poly(methyl methacrylate) resin surface. Brazilian Dent Journal 2008; 19(3)190-196.

[149] Sforcin JM, Bankova V. Propolis: is there a potential for the development of new drugs? Journal of Ethnopharmacology 2010; 133(2) 253-260.

[150] Chan GC, Cheung KW, Sze DM. The Immunomodulatory and Anticancer Properties of Propolis. Clinical Review of Allergy and Immunology 2012 Jun 17. [Epub ahead of print] PMID: 22707327 [PubMed - as supplied by publisher]

[151] Chang FR, Hsieh YC, Chang YF, Lee KH, Wu YC, Chang LK. Inhibition of the Epstein-Barr virus lytic cycle by moronic acid. Antiviral Research 2010; 85(3) 490-495.

[152] Iio A, Ohguchi K, Inoue H, Maruyama H, Araki Y, Nozawa Y, Ito M Ethanolic extracts of Brazilian red propolis promote adipocyte differentiation through PPARγ activation. Phytomedicine. 2010; 17(12) 974-9.

[153] Chuu CP, Lin HP, Ciaccio MF, Kokontis JM, Hause RJ Jr, Hiipakka RA, Liao S, Jones RB. Caffeic acid phenethyl ester suppresses the proliferation of human prostate cancer cells through inhibition of p70S6K and Akt signaling networks. Cancer Prevention Research (Philadephia) 2012; 5(5) 788-797.

[154] Gjertsen AW, Stothz KA, Neiva KG, Pileggi R. Effect of propolis on proliferation and apoptosis of periodontal ligament fibroblasts. Oral Surgery Oral Medicine Oral Pathology Oral Radiology and Endodontics 2011; 112(6) 843-848.

[155] Choudhari MK, Punekar SA, Ranade RV, Paknikar KM. Antimicrobial activity of stingless bee (Trigona sp.) propolis used in the folk medicine of Western Maharashtra, India. Journal of Ethnopharmacology 2012; 141(1) 363-367.

[156] Ha SK, Moon E, Kim SY. Chrysin suppresses LPS-stimulated proinflammatory responses by blocking NF-κB and JNK activations in microglia cells. Neuroscience Letters 2010; 485(3) 143-147.

[157] Watanabe MA, Amarante MK, Conti BJ, Sforcin JM. Cytotoxic constituents of propolis inducing anticancer effects: a review.Journal of Pharmacy and Pharmacology 2011; 63(11) 1378-1386.

[158] Salomão K, Pereira PR, Campos LC, Borba CM, Cabello PH, Marcucci MC, de Castro SL. Brazilian propolis: correlation between chemical composition and antimicrobial activity. Evidence Based Complementary and Alternative Medicine 2008; 5(3) 317-324.

[159] Salomão K, de Souza EM, Henriques-Pons A, Barbosa HS, de Castro SL. Brazilian Green Propolis: Effects In Vitro and In Vivo on Trypanosoma cruzi. Evidence Based Complementary and Alternative Medicine. 2011;2011:185918. Epub 2011 Feb 13. PMID: 19213854 [PubMed]

[160] Dias LG, Pereira AP, Estevinho LM. Comparative study of different Portuguese samples of propolis: Pollinic, sensorial, physicochemical, microbiological characterization and antibacterial activity. Food Chemistry Toxicology. 2012 Sep 5. pii: S0278-6915(12)00640-0. doi: 10.1016/j.fct.2012.08.056. [Epub ahead of print] PMID: 22981908 [PubMed - as supplied by publisher]

[161] Mattigatti S, Ratnakar P, Moturi S, Varma S, Rairam S. Antimicrobial Effect of Conventional Root Canal Medicaments vs Propolis against *Enterococcus faecalis, Staphylococcus aureus* and *Candida albicans*. Journal of Contemporary Dental Practice. 2012;13(3)305-309.

Chapter 8

Functional Evaluation of Sasa Makino et Shibata Leaf Extract as Group III OTC Drug

Hiroshi Sakagami, Tomohiko Matsuta,
Toshikazu Yasui, Oguchi Katsuji, Madoka Kitajima,
Tomoko Sugiura, Hiroshi Oizumi and
Takaaki Oizumi

Additional information is available at the end of the chapter

http://dx.doi.org/10.5772/52187

1. Introduction

Over the counter (OTC) drugs in Japan are classified into three groups (I, II and III), based on the safety [1]. Group I drugs have the highest risk of exerting the adverse effects on our health. The intensity of such side effects declines in the order of Group I, II and III. Only Group III drugs with the least side effects can be purchased through the internet.

	Safety	
Group I	+	
Group II	++	Kampo medicine, herb extracts
Group III	+++	herb extracts, SE

Table 1. Classification of OTC drugs in Japan, based on the safety.

Kampo Medicines, classified as Group II, are usually available as hot water extracts of more than two different plant species. Recently, the presentation of the detailed compositional analysis by HPLC has become mandatory for the publication of the biological activity of Kampo Medicines. However, we often experience the loss of biological activity of Kampo medicines during the purification steps, thus making it difficult to assign the active principles. Herb extracts are classified into Group II and Group III. Three major products of bamboo leaf extract (products A, B, C) are classified into Group III (Table 2), and other drugs are classified into Group I.

Three major products of bamboo leaf extract		
Product A (=SE)	Fe (II)-chlorophyllin	Pure *Sasa senanensis* Rehder extract
Product B	Cu (II)-chlorophyllin	LCC was removed
Product C	Cu (II)-chlorophyllin	Supplemented with ginseng and pine (*Pinus densiflora*) leaf extracts.

Table 2. Three major products of Bamboo leaf extract available in the drug store in Japan.

Two bamboos, "Take" and "Sasa" (Japanese names) belong to grasses, but are not strictly distinguished each other botanically. There are 70 genera of bamboos in the world and 14 genera (approximately 600 species) in Japan. Sasa culms are 1-2 m high, 5-8 mm in diameter, robust, ramose at lower portions. Leaf-blades are oblong-lanceolate, 20-25 cm long and 4-5 cm broad (Figure 1A, B). They are distributed into Saghalien, the Kuriles, Hokkaido, Honshu, Shikoku and Kyushu in Japan. Product A (Sasa Health®, referred to as "SE") (Figure 1C) is a pure alkaline extract of the leaves of *Sasa senanensis* Rehder (dry weight: 58.8 mg/ml [2-4]) that contains Fe (II)-chlorophyllin, in which Mg (II) is replaced by Fe (II) by adding $FeCl_2$. SE-10 (Figure 1D) is a granulated powder of SE supplemented with lactose, lactitol, trehalose and tea extract, and sold as dried and packaged powder in drug stores.

Products B (Sunchlon®, referred to as "BLE") is an alkaline extract of Sasa Makino et Shibata (dry weight 77.6 mg/ml [4]) that contains Cu (II)-chlorophyllin, but approximately 80% of lignin-carbohydrate complex (LCC) has been removed as precipitate [5].

Product C (Shojusen®, referred to as "KS) is a hot water extract of the leaves of *Sasa krilensis Makino* et Sibata (27.0 mg/ml), supplemented with ethanol extract of the leaves of *Pinus densiflora* Sieb et Zucc. (1.2 mg/ml), ethanol extract of the roots of *Panax ginseng* C.A. Meyer (0.92 mg/ml) and paraben as a preservative [6] (Table 2).

These bamboo leaf products is recognized as being effective in treating various malaises including fatigue, low appetite, halitosis, body odor and stomatitis [7-10]. However, there is no scientific evidence that demonstrates their efficacy due to the lack of appropriate biomarkers, although their *in vitro* antiseptic [11], membrane stabilizing [12], anti-inflammatory [13-16], phagocytic [17], radical scavenging [2, 4, 18, 19], anti-oxidant [20-23], antibacterial [2, 9], anti-viral [2, 4, 18, 19, 24] and antitumor activities [2, 25, 26] have been reported. SE showed several common biological properties with LCCs, that is, the prominent anti-HIV, anti-UV and synergistic activity with vitamin C [27, 28].

Lignins are major class of natural products present in the natural kingdom, and are formed through phenolic oxidative coupling processes in the plant [29]. Lignins are formed by the dehydrogenative polymerization of three monolignols: *p*-coumaryl, *p*-coniferyl and sinapyl alcohols [29]. These monolignols were produced from $_L$-phenylalanine by general phenyl-

http://dx.doi.org/10.5772/52187

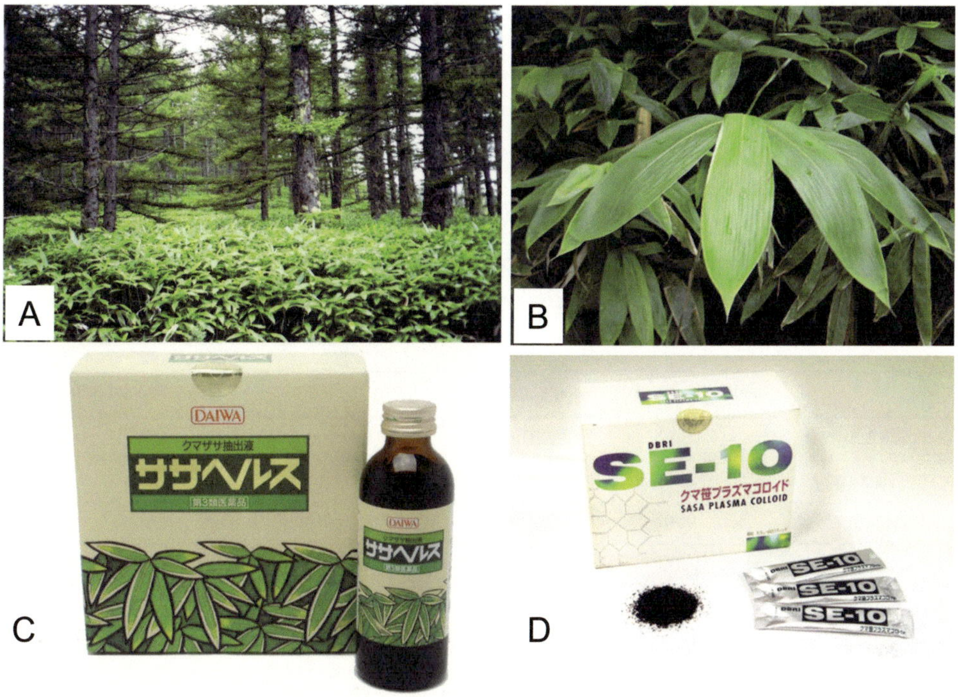

Figure 1. The primeval forest of *Sasa senanensis* Rehder (A), its leaves (B), SE (C) and SE-10 (D).

propanoid pathway [30]. Some polysaccharides in the cell walls of lignified plants are linked to lignin to form lignin-carbohydrate complexes (LCCs). Considering that both of SE and LCC are prepared by extraction with alkaline solution, it is not surprising that they display common biological activities with each other. Furthermore, we have recently identified the anti-UV substances of SE as *p*-coumaric acid derivative(s), one of lignin precursors [31]. Alkaline extraction step that is necessary for the preparation of SE provides higher amounts of LCC as compared with hot-water extracted Kampo medicines. One or two-order higher anti-HIV activity of both SE and LCC over tannins and flavonoids suggest their possible applicability towards virally-induced diseases.

However, there is a possibility that the components from SE and other plants are associated with each other, thus modify their biological activities. Also, SE components may inhibit the activity of CYP3A4, the most abundant drug-metabolizing enzyme, so as to increase the bioavailability of co-administered drugs (especially, CYP3A4 substrates). Lastly, the clinical evidences that demonstrate how the treatment of SE products improves the patient's conditions are limited.

Based on these circumstances, we review the functional analysis of SE products as alternative medicines, citing the literatures of other groups and ours, focusing on the following points: (i) component analysis, (ii) spectrum of reported biological activities in comparison with those of Kampo medicines, (iii) possibility of complex formation between the components, (iv) inhibition of CYP3A4 activity and (v) the clinical application for the treatment of oral diseases.

2. Component analysis

Components of SE are listed in Table 3. Dietary fibre was the major component of SE. Water-soluble and water-insoluble dietary fibres are present approximately at the 1: 2 ratio.

	mg/100 ml	mg/100 g*		mg/100 ml	mg/100 g*
Protein	1500	22700	Glycine		
Lipid	200	3030	Proline	84	1270
Ash content	900	13600	Glutamic acid	186	2800
Sugar	1200	18200	Serine	21	320
Glucose	90	1360	Threonine	13	200
Arabinose	380	5700	Aspartic acid	159	2400
Xylose	1060	16000	Tryptophan	28	420
Galactose	180	2700			
Dietary fibre	2100	31800	Folic acid	0.008	0.12
Water-soluble	1400	21200	Lutein	0.3	4.5
Water-insoluble	700	10600			
			Sodium	395	5980
Arginine	19	290	Iron	1.02	15
Lysine	59	890	Calcium	1.0	15
Histidine	23	350	Potassium	4.9	74
Phenylalanine	86	1300	Magnesium	0.5	8
Tyrosine	63	950	Zinc	0.08	1.2
Leucine	135	2040			
Isoleucine	53	800	Vitamin A	0.003	0.05
Methionine	32	480	β-Carotene	0.032	0.5
Valine	95	1440	Vitamin K1	0.006	0.09
Alanine	105	1590	Glycine	99	1500

Table 3. Composition of SE. *corrected, assuming that 1 ml contains 66.1 mg SE. Cited from [19], with permission.

According to this information, we have fractionated the LCC into the following three fractions Fr I, II and III by repeated acid precipitation and solubization with $NaHCO_3$ or NaOH

http://dx.doi.org/10.5772/52187

solution, and polysaccharide fraction was recovered as Fr. IV by addition of equal volume of ethanol in Figure 2.

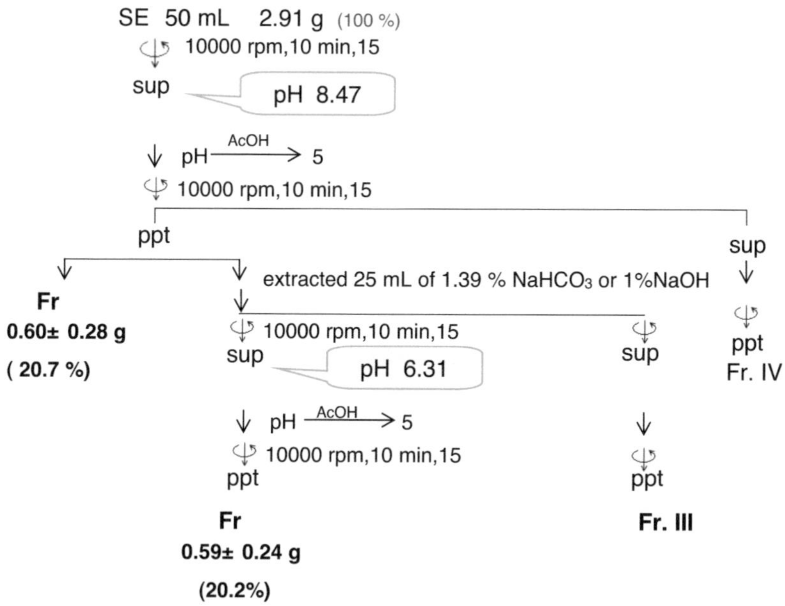

Figure 2. Fractionation of lignin-carbohydrate complex (LCC) fractions Fr I-III and polysaccharide fraction Fr IV. *Yield of Frs. I and II represents mean±S.D. from three independent experiments.* Cited from [18], with permission

Luteolin glycosdes are isolated from the leaves of *Sasa senanensis* Rehder and their structures were identified as decribed below (Figure 3) [32]. Luteolin 6-*C*-β-D-glucoside [compound 1]: yellow amorphous powder, $[\alpha]^{25}_{D}$ +30.7° (*c*=0.12, CH_3OH), mp 232° (dec.), ultraviolet (UV) λmax (MeOH) nm (ε): 348 (22,200), 270 (17,600) and 258 (17,400). Electrospray ionization time of flight mass spectra (ESI-TOF-MS) *m/z*: 448 ($[M+H]^+$), high-resolution mass spectra (HR-MS) *m/z*: 449.1094 (calcd. for $C_{21}H_{21}O_{11}$, 449.1084).

Luteolin 7-*O*-β-D-glucoside [compound 2]:yellow amorphous powder, $[\alpha]^{25}_{D}$ -81.1° (*c*=0.10, CH_3OH), mp 261° (dec.), UV λmax (MeOH) nm (ε): 346 (20,500) and 270 (18,400). ESI-TOF-MS *m/z*: 448 ($[M+H]^+$), 287 ($[aglycon+H]^+$), HR-MS *m/z*: 449.0976 (calcd. for $C_{21}H_{21}O_{11}$, 449.1084).

Luteolin 6-*C*-α-L-arabinoside [compound 3]:yellow amorphous powder, $[\alpha]^{25}_{D}$ +66.0° (*c*=0.11, CH_3OH), mp > 300° (dec.), UV λmax (MeOH) nm (ε): 348 (22,100), 270 (17,600) and 258 (17,400). ESI-TOF-MS *m/z*: 419 ($[M+H]^+$), HR-MS *m/z*: 419.1027 (calcd. for $C_{20}H_{19}O_{10}$, 419.0978).

Tricin [compound 4]: yellow amorphous powder, UVλmax (MeOH) nm (ε): 349 (41,000) and 269 (27,200). ESI-TOF-MS *m/z*: 331 ($[M+H]^+$): HR-MS *m/z*: 331.0837 (Calcd. for $C_{17}H_{15}O_7$, 331.0818).

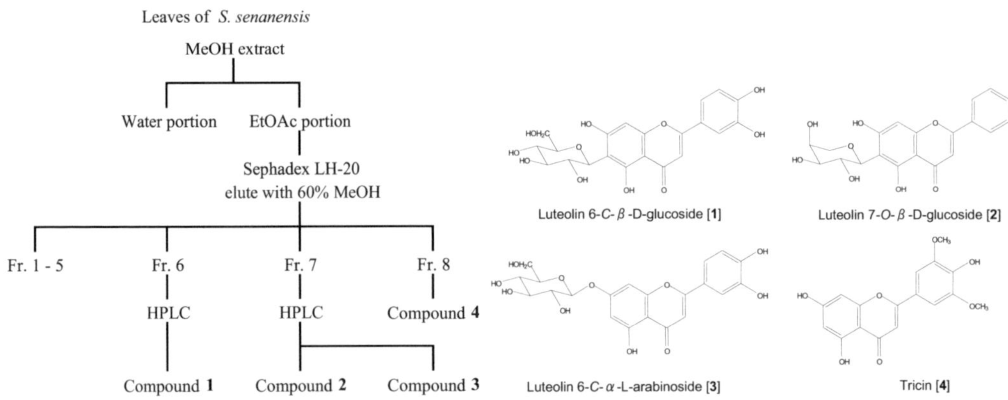

Figure 3. Purification of luteolin 6-*C*-β-$_D$-glucoside [compound 1], luteolin 7-*O*-β-D-glucoside [compound 2], luteolin 6-*C*-α-$_L$-arabinoside [compound 3] and tricin [compound 4] from the leaves of *Sasa senanensis* Rehder. Cited from [32], with permission.

We also isolated substances (SEE-1) that protected the cells from the UV-induced cytotoxicity, by ethanol extraction, Wakosil 40C18 chromatography (H_2O elution) and preparative HPLC (Shimadzu LC-10AD pump, Shimadzu SPD-M10AVP photodiode array detector, separation column: Inatsil ODS-3, eluted with H_2O : acetonitrile : formic acid (90:10:0.1), and proposed the putative structures as *p*-coumaric acid derivative(s) (Figure 4) [31].

A

B

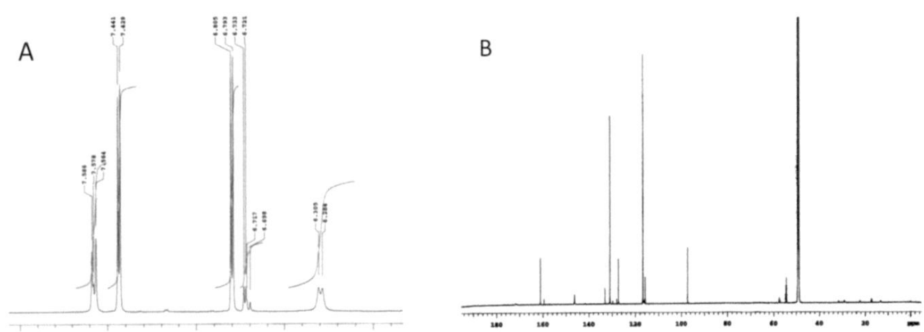

C

	^{13}C	^{1}H
1	127.4	
2,6	131.0	7.44(d, *J*=8.6Hz)
3,5	116.8	6.80(d, *J*=8.6Hz)
4	161.0	
7	146.2	7.58(d, *J*=15.5Hz)
8	115.8	6.29(br.d, *J*=14.7Hz)
9	159.5	

D

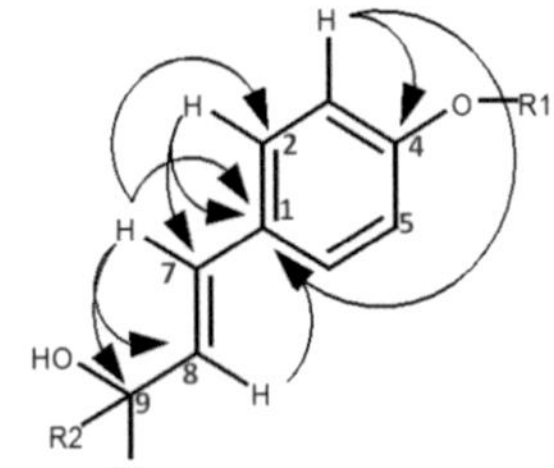

Figure 4. Identification of anti-UV substance(s) as *p*-coumaric acid derivative(s). Cited from [31] with permission.

3. Biological activities

3.1. Antiviral activity

Anti-human immunodeficiency virus (HIV) activity was assessed quantitatively by a selectivity index ($SI=CC_{50}/EC_{50}$, where CC_{50} is the 50% cytotoxic concentration against mock-infected MT-4 cells, and EC_{50} is the 50% effective concentration against HIV-infected cells). Products A, B and C all effectively and dose-dependently reduced the cytopathic effect of HIV infection (closed symbols in Figure 5), although their anti-HIV activity was much lower than that of positive controls [dextran sulfate (SI=1378), curdlan sulfate (SI=5606), azidothymidine (SI=17746), 2′,3′-dideoxycytidine (SI=5123)] (Table 4). The potency of anti-HIV activity was in the order of product A (Sasa-Health®, SE) (SI=607) > product C (SI=117) > product B (SI=111) (Exp. I, Table 4) [4]. A granulated powder of *Sasa senanensis* Rehder leaf extract (SE-10) (Figure 1D) (SI=54) showed slightly higher anti-HIV activity than SE (SI=45) (Exp. 2, Table 4) [19]. Among the components of SE, LCC fractions prepared as described in Figure 3 (SI=37~62) showed comparable or slightly higher activity anti-HIV activity than unfractionated SE (SI=36) (Exp. 3, Table 4) [28]. Luteolin glycosides, luteolin 6-*C*-β-D-glucoside, luteolin 7-*O*-β-D-glucoside, luteolin 6-*C*-α-L-arabinoside and tricin from *Sasa senanensis* Rehder leaf extract showed somewhat lower anti-HIV activity (SI=2~24) (Exp. 4, Table 4) [32]. The anti-HIV activity of LCCs isolated from SE was comparable with that of LCCs from pine cone, catuaba bark [33], cacao husk [34], cacao mass [35], cultured extract of *Lentinus edodes* mycelia extract [36] and mulberry juice [37, 38], and synthetic lignin (dehydrogenation polymers of phenylpropanoids) [39], and was generally higher than that of tannins [40], flavonoids [41], gallic acid, (-)-epigallocatechin 3-*O*-gallate (EGCG), curcumin, and chemically modified glucans [42] (Exp. 5, Table 4) and Kampo medicines and its constituent plant extracts [43] (Exp. 6, Table 4).

SE also protected the MDCK cells from the cytopathic effect of influenza virus infection (CC_{50}=0.67%, EC_{50}=0.060%, SI=11) (Figure 6). Tricin showed potent anti-human cytomegalovirus activity [24].

3.2. Anti-bacterial activity

Product B (BLE) significantly reduced the bacterial growth and lactate production *in vitro* in the total saliva [9].

Product A (SE) showed a bacteriostatic, but not a bactericidal effect on *Fusobacterium nucleatum* and *Prevotella intermedia* (Figure 7A, 7B). The MIC_{50} for the *Fusobacterium nucleatum* and *Prevotella intermedia* was calculated to be 0.63 and 1.25%, respectively, and at the highest concentration (2.5%), 12.0 and 17.2% of the bacteria remained viable, respectively.

Gas chromatography demonstrated that these bacteria produced H_2S and CH_3SH, but not $(CH_3)_2H$. SE more efficiently reduced the production of H_2S in *Fusobacterium nucleatum*, with a 50% inhibitory concentration (IC_{50}) of 0.04% (Figure 7C). On the other hand, SE more efficiently reduced the production of CH_3SH in *Prevotella intermedia*, with an IC_{50} of 0.16% (Figure 7D). A higher concentration of SE (2.5%) completely eliminated both H_2S and CH_3SH [2].

	S I		SI
Exp. 1 (Alkaline extract)		**Exp. 5 (other plant extracts)**	
Product A (SE)	607	LCC from pine trees (n=2)	27
Product B	111	LCC from pine seed shell	12
Product C	117	LCC from catuaba bark	43
Dextran sulfate	1378	LCC from cacao husk	311
Curdlan sulfate	5606	LCC from cacao mass	46
AZT	17746	LCC from cultured LEM	94
ddC	5123	LCC from mulberry juice	7
Exp. 2 (SE product)		Phenylpropenoid polymers (n=23)	105
SE	45		
SE-10	54	Neutral polysaccharide from pine cone	1
Dextran sulfate	160	*N,N*-dimethylaminoethyl paramylon	<1
Curdlan sulfate	781	*N,N*-diethylaminoethyl paramylon	<1
AZT	6931	*N,N*-dimethylaminoethyl curdlan	<1
ddC	905	Hydrolyzable tannins monomer (n=21)	<1
		Hydrolyzable tannins dimer (n=39)	<1
Exp. 3 (SE component)		Hydrolyzable tannins trimer (n=4)	3
SE	36	Hydrolyzable tannins tetramer (n=3)	11
LCC Fr I (acid precipitation)	37	Condensed tannins (n=8)	<1
LCC Fr II (acid precipitation ×2))	58		
LCC Fr III (acid precipitation × 2)	62	Flavonoids (n=160)	<1
Polysaccharide fraction Fr IV	><1	Gallic acid	<1
Butanol extract	<1	(-)-Epigallocatechin 3-*O*-gallate	<1
		Curcumin	<1
Exp. 4 (SE component)		Chlorophyllin	5
SE	40		
Luteolin 6-*C*-β-D-glucoside [**1**]	>2	**Exp. 6 (Plant extracts)**	
Luteolin 7-*O*-β-D-glucoside [**2**]	7	Kampo medicines (n=10)	<1.0
Luteolin 6-C-α-L-arabinoside [**3**]	>7	Constituent plant extracts (n=25)	1.3
Tricin [**4**]	24	AZT	17850

Table 4. Anti-HIV activity of polyphenols.

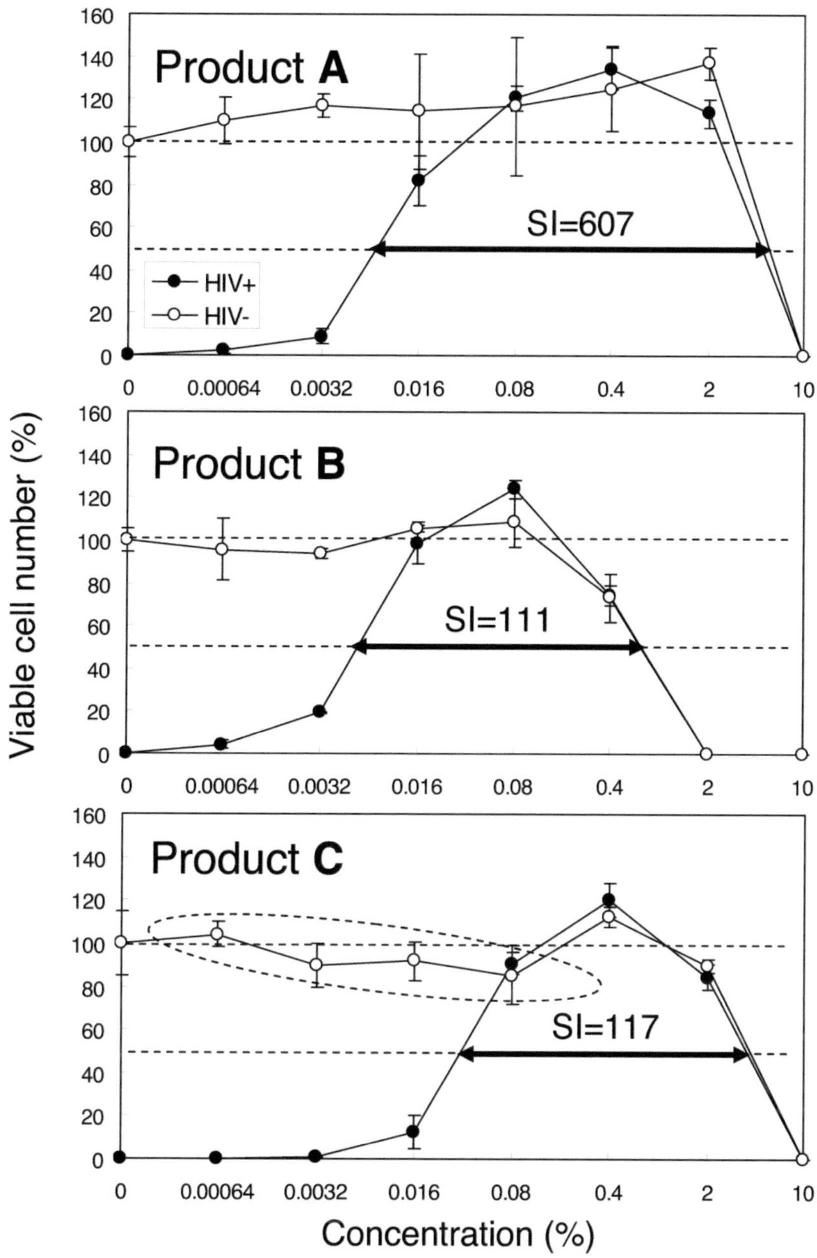

Figure 5. Figure 1. Anti-HIV activity of three commercial products of *Sasa senanensis* Rehder extract. HIV-1_{IIIB}-infected (HIV+) and mock-infected (HIV–) MT-4 cells were incubated for 5 days with the indicated concentrations of products A (upper panel), B (center panel) and C (lower panel) and the viable cell number was determined by the MTT assay and expressed as a percentage that of the control. Data represent the mean±standard deviation from triplicate assays. It should be noted that product C exhibited a weak cytostatic effect at lower concentrations (indicated by dotted circle). Cited from [4], with permission.

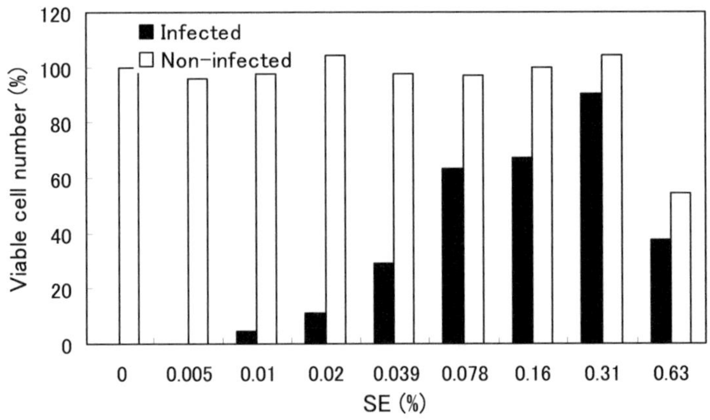

Figure 6. Anti-influenza virus activity of SE. Influenza virus-infected or mock-infected MDCK cells were incubated for 3 days with the indicated concentrations of SE, and the viable cell number was determined by MTT method. Each value represents a mean from triplicate assays. Cited from [2] with permission.

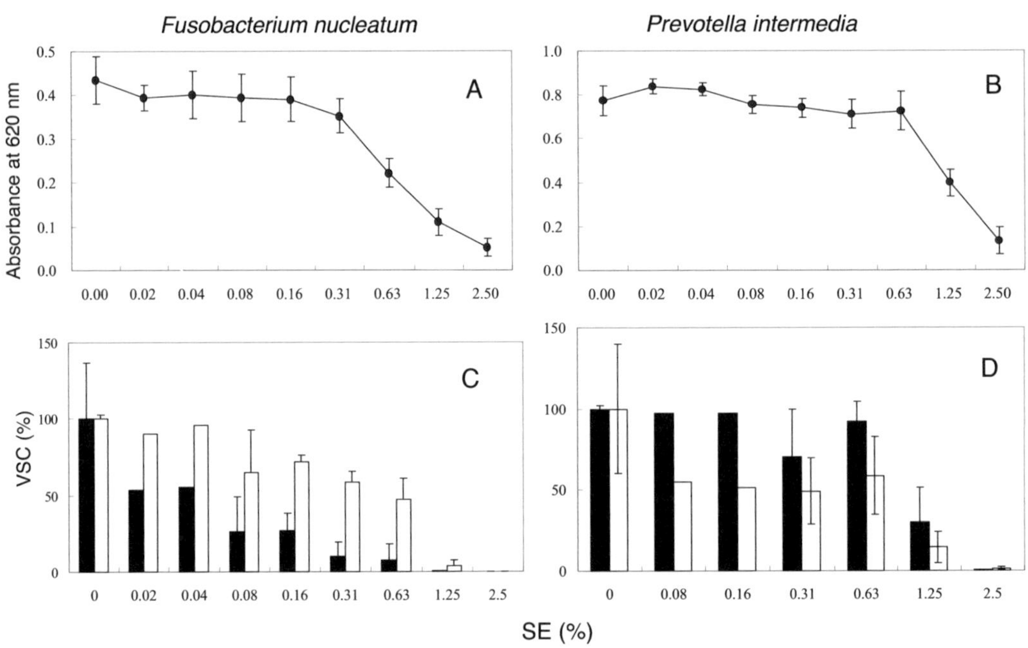

Figure 7. Antibacterial activity of SE. *Fusobacterium nucleatum* (A, C) and *Prevotella intermedia* (B, D) were cultured anaerobically for 24 hours at 37°C with the indicated concentrations of SE in capped 15-cm centrifugation tubes. The VSC released into the culture medium (black bar: H_2S, white bar, CH_3SH) was quantified by gas chromatography (C, D). Bacterial growth was measured by recording the absorbance at 620 nm, using a microplate reader (A, B). (A, B) Bacteriostatic activity of SE. Each point represents mean ±S.D. from triplicate assays. (C, D) Effect on VSC. Each bar represents mean ±S.D. from triplicate assays. Without bar (0.02 and 0.04%SE (C), and 0.08 and 0.16% SE (D)) means the value from a single assay. Cited from [2] with permission.

3.3. Antitumor activity

Oral administration of SE (*ad lib.*) significantly delayed the development and growth of mammary tumors in a mammary tumor strain of virgin SHN mice [25]. Oral administration of SE (*ad lib.*) significantly inhibited spontaneous mammary tumorigenesis, reduced tumor multiplicity, inhibited the mammary duct branching, side bud development and angiogenesis in another mouse model of human breast cancer, transgenic FVB-Her2/NeuN mouse model [26].

SE showed slightly higher cytotoxicity against the human squamous cell carcinoma cell lines (HSC-2, HSC-3, HSC-4, Ca9-22, NA) (mean CC_{50}=6.22%, 3.62 mg/mL) and the human glioblastoma cell lines (T98G, U-87MG) (mean CC_{50}=5.43%, 3.16 mg/mL), as compared with the human oral normal cells [gingival fibroblast (HGF), pulp cell (HPC), periodontal ligament fibroblast (HPLF)] (mean CC_{50}=6.90%, 4.01 mg/mL), and was more cytotoxic to the human myelogenous leukemic cell lines (HL-60, ML-1, KG-1) (CC_{50}=1.18%, 0.68 mg/mL) and the human T-cell leukemia cell line (MT-4) (CC_{50}=1.41%, 0.82 mg/mL), with an approximate tumor specificity index of 1.62 (Table 5). Although SE did not show high tumor-specific cytotoxicity, it was highly cytotoxic to three human myelogenous leukemic cell lines (HL-60, ML-1, KG-1) and one T-cell leukemic cell line (MT-4). The type of cell death induced by SE remains to be investigated [2].

3.4. Membrane stabilizing activity

In order to investigate whether SE contains membrane -stabilizing activity, SE was defatted with hexane, and fractionated on Silica gel chromatography, according to the polarity, into Fr. 1 (eluted with *n*-hexane: CH_2Cl_2), Fr. 2 (CH_2Cl_2), Fr. 3 (acetone), Frs 4 and 5 (methanol) and Fr. 6 (residue). SE inhibited the hemolysis of rat red blood cells in hypotinic buffer by 13%. Frs. 3, 4 and 5 ihibited the homolysis approximately 35, 20 and 35%, respectively [12], suggesting the membrane-stabilization activity of SE and its fractions.

Membrane stability can be evaluated by the extracellular leakage of glutamic-oxaloacetic transaminase (GOT) and glutamic-pyruvic transamiase (GPT) from the hepatocytes. Control hepatocytes released 85.1± 5.4 (mean±SD) K.U./ml GOT into the culture medium. SE (1~5 μi=60~300 μg/ml) significantly inhibited the release of GOT. Among the SE fractions, Frs. 1, 4 and 6 showed the inhibitory effects (Figure 8A). Control hepatocytes released 37.0 ± 3.6K.U./ml GPT inoto the culture medium. SE (1~2 μl=60, 120 μg/ml) significantly inhibited the GTP release (Figure 8B) [13].

SE, Fr. 3 and Fr. 5 showed the surfactant action by reducing the surface tension. These substances did not significantly affect the phase-transtion temperature of dipalmitoyl phosphatidylcholine (DPPC)-liposome bilayer nor the membrane-fluidity. These data suggest that the membrane-stabilizing activity of SE may be generated by polysaccharide, lignin, or chlorophyll present in Fr. 3, 4 and 5.

	CC_{50}	
	% (v/v)	mg/mL
Human normal cells		
Gingival fibroblast (HGF)	6.96	4.05
Pulp cell (HPC)	7.54	4.38
Periodontal ligament fibroblast (HPLF)	6.19	3.60
(mean)	6.90	4.01
Human oral squamous cell carcinoma cell lines		
HSC-2	8.49	4.94
HSC-3	5.99	3.49
HSC-4	5.69	3.31
Ca9-22	4.20	2.44
NA	6.71	3.91
(mean)	6.22	3.62
Human glioblastoma cell lines		
T98G	6.92	4.03
U87MG	3.94	2.29
(mean)	5.43	3.16
Human myelogenous leukemia cell lines		
HL-60	1.14	0.66
ML-1	0.39	0.23
KG-1	2.00	1.16
(mean)	1.18	0.68
Human T-cell leukemia cell line		
MT-4	1.41	0.82
TS value	1.62	

The tumor-specificity index (TS) was measured by the following equation: TS= [CC_{50} (HGF) + CC_{50} (HPC) + CC_{50} (HPLF)] / [CC_{50} (HSC-2) + CC_{50} (HSC-3) + CC_{50} (HSC-4) + CC_{50} (Ca9-22) + CC_{50} (NA) + CC_{50} (T98G) + CC_{50} (U87MG) + CC_{50} (HL-60) + CC_{50} (ML-1) + CC_{50} (KG-1) + CC_{50} (MT-4)] x (11/3). Cited from [2] with permission.

Table 5. Cytotoxic activity of SE against human normal and tumor cells.

http://dx.doi.org/10.5772/52187

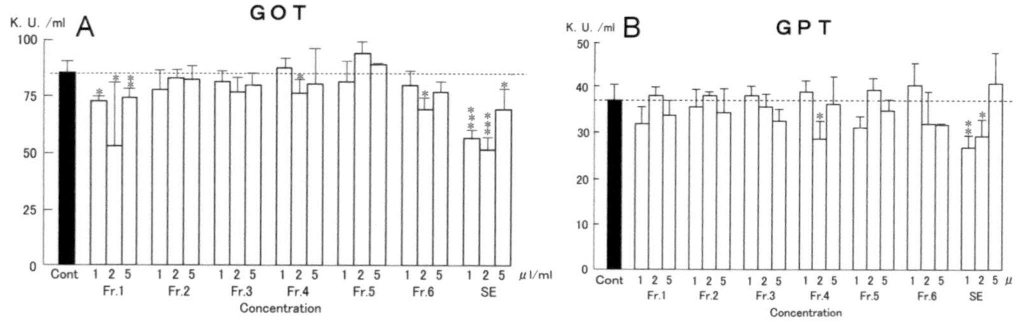

Figure 8. Effect of SE and each fraction on the leakage of GOT (A) and GPT (B) from rat cultured hepatocytes. Hepatocytes were suspended in Williams' E medium for 24 h at 37°C and culture was continued in the same medium with SE or each fraction for 24 h at 37°C. Each value was mean±S.D. of five experiments, and expressed as Karmen Units/ml of medium. Values are significant: *p<0.05, **p<0.01, ***p<0.001; control *vs* experiments (students *t*-test). Cited from [13] with permission.

We next compared the hepatocyte protective effect of SE, other Herbal extracts and tinctures (Aloe, Gambir, Swertiae, Plantaginis, Geranii, Houttuyniae extracts). Aloe extract rather enhanced the leakage of liver enzymes, whereas SE and Gambir extract were inhibitory. SE more significantly inhibited the enzyme leakage, as compared with other herbal extracts and tinctures, suggesting that the hepatocyte protective activity of SE may be more potent that other herbal extracts [13].

3.5. Anti-inflammatory activity

Oral administration of hot water extract of leaves of bamboo of genus *Sasa* spp (HSBE) inhibited the carrageenan-induced edema and 12-*O*-tetradecanoylphorbol-13-acetate-induced ear swelling in mice, possibly by inhibiting the production of proinflammatory substances [prostaglandin E_2 (PGE_2), serotonin) and expression of 5-lipoxygenase, cycooxygenase-2 (COX-2), tumor necrosis factor-α (TNF-α), interleukin-6 (IL-6) and IL-10. Although the anti-inflammatory activity of HSBE was much less than that of dexamethasone, the major activity was concentrated into lower molecular weight, dialyzable and methanol eluted fraction [16].

Single oral administration of SE (10~20 ml =0.6~1.2 mg/kg) slightly reduced the vasopermeability in ddY male mice (assessed by Whittle method). Single oral administration of SE (5 ml=0.3 mg/kg) slightly inhibited the formation of carrageenin-induced edema in SD male rats at 1 h, but rather enhanced the formation of edema at 3 h and thereafter (Figure 9A). Single oral administration of SE (5 ml=0.3 mg/kg) inhibited the formation of formalin-induced edema at 3 h (Figure 9B). Repeated oral administration of SE (1, 5, 10 ml/kg/day×7 or 9days) stimulated the growth of fibroblasts and neovascularization, in contrast to the enhanced formation of collagen fiber. This suggests that SE may stimulate the regeneration of normal tissue during the restoration process of inflammatory tissues [12].

Oral administration of SE slightly increased the phagocytic index (assessed by carbon clearance method) after 3~5 h, but did not affect the phagocytic index at 7 days, suggesting that SE does not reduce the function of reticuloendothelial system.

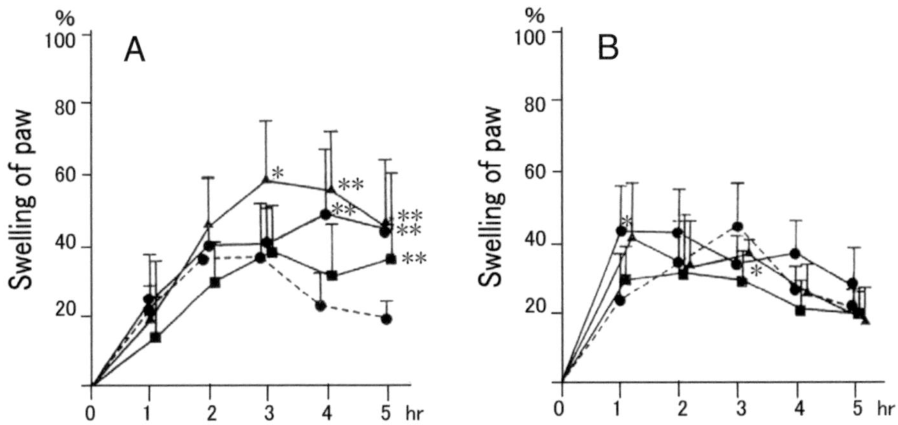

Figure 9. Effect of SE on carrageenin (A) and formalin (B)-induced hind paw edema in rats.Each point represents the mean of eight rats with S.D. ●---● : control, ●———● : SE 1ml/kg, ■———■ : SE 5 ml/kg,▲———▲ : SE 10 ml/kg,. *,** : significantly different from the control value with $p<0.05$, $p<0.01$ (Student's t-test). Cited from [12] with permission.

SE also inhibited the production of nitric oxide (NO) and prostaglandin E_2 (PGE_2) from the LPS-activated mouse macrophage-like cells RAW264.7 *via* inhibition of the expression of iNOS and COX-2 at protein and mRNA levels [14].

IL-1β induced one to two order higher production of proinflammatory substances (PGE_2, IL-6, IL-8, MCP-1), but not NO and TNFα by human gingival fibroblast (HGF). SE also inhibited the production of IL-8 production by IL-1β-stimulated human gingival fibroblast (Figure 10)[15].

3.6. Radical scavenging activity

ESR spectroscopy showed that SE (50%=29.1 mg/mL) did not produce any detectable ESR signal at pH 7.4 (radical intensity (RI)<0.089) and pH 10.0 (RI<0.11). At pH 13.0, a weak broad peak, similar to that of typical lignin [28], appeared (RI=0.14) [2].

Products A, B and C dose-dependently reduced the intensity of superoxide anion (O_2^-) (detected as DMPO-OOH) generated by hypoxanthine and xanthine oxidase reaction. The potency of O_2^- scavenging activity of the three products was comparable: product A (IC_{50}=0.46 mg/ml), product B (IC_{50}=0.52 mg/ml) and product C (IC_{50}=0.54 mg/ml) (Table 6) [4].

Products A, B and C dose-dependently reduced the intensity of hydroxyl radical (OH) (detected as DMPO-OH) generated by the Fenton reaction. The potency of products A and C was comparable with each other (IC_{50}=2.1 and 1.9 mg/ml, respectively), but 4-fold higher than that of product B (IC_{50}=8.0 mg/ml) (Table 6) [4].

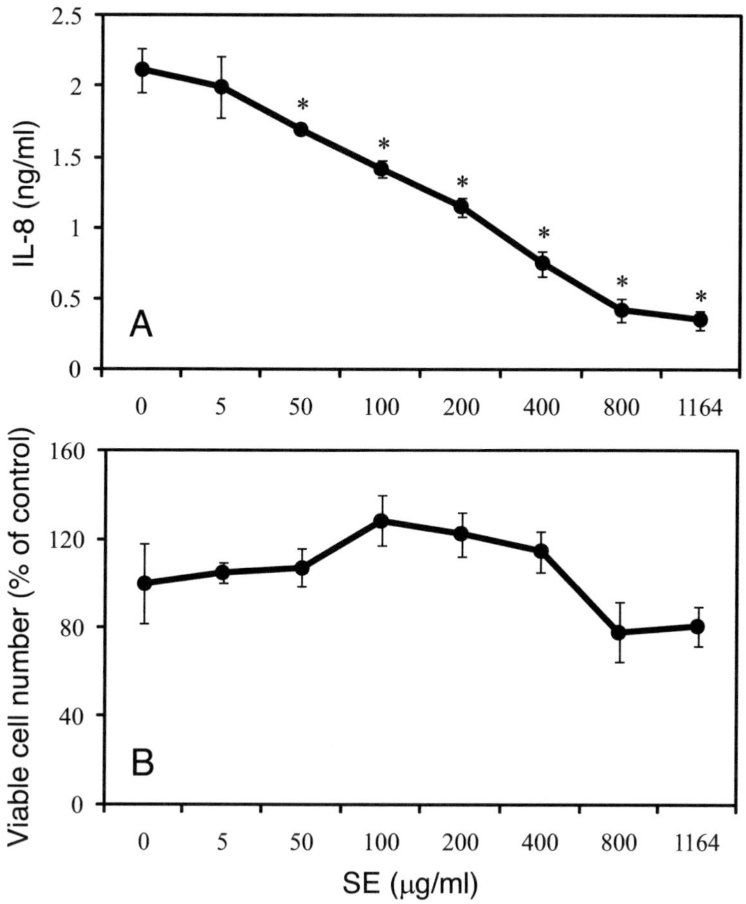

Figure 10. SE inhibited the IL-1β-stimulated IL-8 production by HGF cells. HGF cells were incubated for 48 h with the indicated concentrations of SE in the presence of IL-1β (1 ng/ml), and the extracellular IL-8 concentration (A) and viable cell number (B) were determined. mean± S.D (n=3). *<0.01. Cited from [15] with permission.

	$O_2^{\cdot-}$–Scavenging activity (IC_{50})	·OH–Scavenging activity (IC_{50})
Product **A**	0.69% (0.46 mg/ml)	3.2% (2.1 mg/ml)
Product **B**	0.67% (0.52 mg/ml)	10.3% (8.0 mg/ml)
Product **C**	1.9% (0.54 mg/ml)	6.6% (1.9 mg/ml)

Table 6. Radical scavenging activity of three commercial products of *Sasa senanensis* Rehder extract. Data was cited from [2], with permission.

3.7. Anti-UV activity

UV irradiation (6 J/m^2/min) for 1 min followed by 48 h culture resulted in extensive cell death (closed circles in Figure 11). Popular antioxidants, *N*-acetyl-L-cysteine (NAC) and catalase (enzyme that degrades hydrogen peroxide), could not prevent the UV-induced cellular damage, suggesting that hydrogen peroxide may not be involved in the UV-induced cytotoxicity, but the type of radical species produced by UV irradiation remains to be identified (Exp. 1, Table 7). SE dose-dependently inhibited the UV-induced cytotoxicity in a bell-shaped fashion (Figure 11). The viability of the cells was recovered to 50% by the addition of 0.53 mg/ml SE (=EC_{50}). From the dose-response curve without UV irradiation, CC_{50} of SE was calculated to be 22.24 mg/ml. From these values, selectivity index SI (CC_{50}/EC_{50}) was calculated to be 41.96. Similar experiments were repeated three times to yield the mean value of SI=19.7±15.1 (mean of four independent experiments) (Exp. I, Table 7). The ant-UV activity of SE was slightly less than that of sodium ascorbate (SI=30.2±13.4) (mean of five independent experiments), but higher than that of luteolin 6-*C*-β-$_D$-glucoside [1] (SI>8), luteolin 7-*O*-β-$_D$-glucoside [2] (SI>6), luteolin 6-*C*-α-$_L$-arabinoside [3] (SI>6), Tricin [4] (TS>3), gallic acid (SI=17.1), EGCG (SI=7.7), chlorophyllin (SI=0.53) and chlorophyll a (SI<0.24) (Exp. I, Table 7) [3].

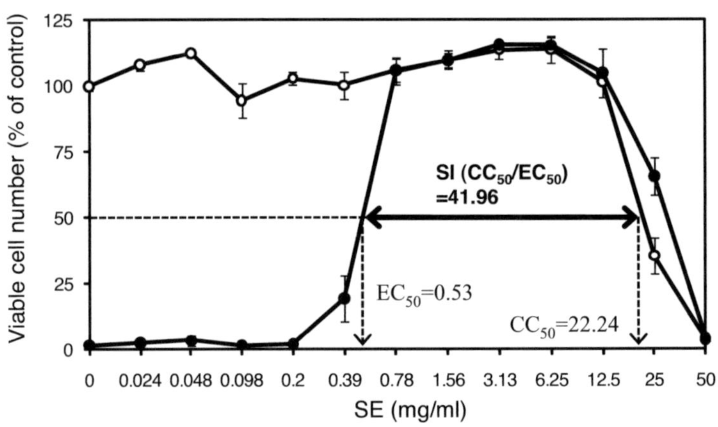

Figure 11. Anti-UV activity of SE. HSC-2 cells were treated without (○) or with UV (●) irradiation (6 J/m^2/min) for 1 min in PBS(−) containing SE. Viable cell number determined by MTT method 48 h after irradiation, and expressed as percent of control (without UV irradiation). EC_{50}: 50% effective concentration, CC_{50}: 50% cytotoxic concentration.Mean ± S.D. of triplicate determinations. Cited from [3] with permission.

SE (product A) showed higher anti-UV activity (SI=20) than other *Sasa senanensis* Rehder leaf products B (SI=4) (that has lower amounts of LCC) and C (SI=13) (that contains ginseng extract and pine (*Pinus densiflora*) leaf extract) [4], suggesting the importance of LCC for the anti-UV activity. A granulated powder of *Sasa senanensis* Rehder leaf extract (SE-10) (SI=129) showed approximately three-fold higher anti-UV activity than SE (Exp. 2, Table 7)[19], suggesting some synergistic effect of SE and other components present in SE-10.

LCCs from pine cones, pine seed and cultured LEM (SI=26-42) showed comparable anti-UV activity with SE (SI=39). Lignin precursor, vanillin, showed higher anti-UV activity comparable with that of sodium ascorbate (SI=64) (Exp. 3, Table 7) [44, 45]. On the other hand, chemically-modified glucans, such as *N,N*-dimethylaminoethyllaminarin, *N,N*-dimethylaminoethylpullulan, *N,N*-dimethylaminoethyldextran and paramylon sulfate (SI<1) [45] (Exp. 4, Table 7), hot water extract (Kampo medicines and constituent plant extracts) [43] (SI=1~2) (Exp. 5, Table 7) and tea extracts (green tea, black tea, oolong tea, burley tea, Jasmine tea) [44] (Exp. 6, Table 7) were also inactive (SI=1~2). These data suggests the alkaline extracts (such as SE and LCCs) show higher anti-UV activity than hot-water extracts (such as Kampo medicines, tea extracts).

	S I		**SI**
Exp. 1		Exp. 3 (LCCs)	
SE	20	LCC from pine cones (n=3)	33
Luteolin 6-*C*-β-$_D$-glucoside [**1**]	>8	LCC from pine seed	26
Luteolin 7-*O*-β-$_D$-glucoside [**2**]	>6	LCC from cultured LEM	42
Luteolin 6-*C*-α-$_L$-arabinoside [**3**]	>6	SE	39
Tricin [**4**]	>3	Vanilline	64
Chlorophyllin	<1	Sulfated lignin (n=2)	>8
Chlorophyl a	<1	Sodium acorbate	64
Sodium ascorbate	30	Exp. 4 (polysaccharides)	
Gallic acid	17	*N,N*-Dimethylaminoethyllaminarin	<1
EGCG	8	*N,N*-Dimethylaminoethylpullulan	<1
Curcumin	<1	*N,N*-Dimethylaminoethyldextran	<1
Ar-turmerone	<1	Paramylon sulfate	<1
		Sodium ascorbate	89
N-Acetyl-L-cysteine	<1		
Catalase	<1	Exp. 5 (Plant extracts)	
		Kampo medicines (n=10)	2
Exp. 2 (SE products)		Constituent plant extracts (n=25)	1
Product A (SE)	20		
Product B (BLE)	4	Exp. 6 (Tea extract)	
Product C (KS)	13	Green tea	3
Sodium acorbate	33	Black tea	<1
		Oolong tea	<1
SE	39	Burley tea	<1
SE-10	129	Jasmine tea	<1
Sodium ascorbate	90	Sodium ascorbate	30

Table 7. Anti-UV activity of various natural products.

3.8. Synergistic action with vitamin C

Vitamin C exhibited either antioxidant or prooxidant activity, depending on the concentration [46]. We have reported that ascorbate derivatives that produced the doublet signal of ascorbate radical (sodium-L-ascorbate, L-ascorbic acid, D-isoascorbic acid, 6-β-D-galactosyl-L-ascorbate, sodium 5,6-benzylidene-L-ascorbate) induced apoptosis (characterized by internucleosomal DNA fragmentation and an increase in the intracellular Ca^{2+} concentration) in HL-60 cells. On the other hand, ascorbate derivatives that did not produce radicals (L-ascorbic acid-2-phosphate magnesium salt, L-ascorbic acid 2-sulfate and dehydroascorbic acid) did not induce apoptosis [47, 48]. This suggests the possible involvement of the ascorbate radical in apoptosis-induction by ascorbic acid-related compounds.

We accidentally found that LCCs from the pine cone of *Pinus parviflola* Sieb et Zucc, pine cone of *Pinus elliottii* var. Elliotti, leaf of *Ceriops decandra* (Griff.) Ding Hou and, thorn apple of *Crataegu Cuneata* Sieb. et Zucc modulated the radical intensity of ascorbate bi-phasically, depending on the concentrations. At higher concentration, LCCs strongly enhanced the radical intensity of sodium ascorbate, which rapidly decayed, possibly due to the breakdown of ascorbic acid or to the consumption of ascorbyl radical. LCCs, not only from pine cones (Fr. VI), but also from Catuaba bark, pine seed shell, *A. nikoense* Maxim. and *C. Cuneata Sieb.* et Zucc. enhanced the radical intensity and cytotoxic activity of sodium ascorbate [27]. On the other hand, tannins such as gallic acid, EGCG, and tannic acid counteracted the radical intensity and cytotoxic activity of sodium ascorbate [49].

Sodium ascorbate rapidly reduced the oxygen concentration in the culture medium, possibly due to oxygen consumption *via* its pro-oxidation action. Simultaneous addition of LCCs further enhanced the ascorbate-stimulated consumption of oxygen [50]. These data suggest that the synergistic enhancement of the cytotoxic activity of LCCs and ascorbate might be due at least in part to the stimulated induction of hypoxia.

Lower concentration of LCC (pine cone Fr. VI) and sodium ascorbate showed radical scavenging activity. LCC further stimulated the superoxide anion (O_2^-) and 1,1-diphenyl-2-picrylhydrazyl (DPPH) radical scavenging activity of sodium ascorbate. LCCs from *Ceriops decandra* (Griff.) Ding Hou. and cacao husk scavenged O_2^- and hydroxyl radical, and synergistically enhanced the radical scavenging activity of sodium ascorbate [27, 34].

Similarly, SE and vitamin C synergistically enhanced the activity that scavenging superoxide anion radical (determined by the intensity of DMPO-OOH) and hydroxyl radical (determined by the intensity of DMPO-OH radical) (Table 8) [2].

	DMPO-OOH radical intensity (% of control)		**DMPO-OH radical intensity (% of control)**	
	0.5% VC	0.25% + 5 μM VC	1% VC	0.5% + 5 μM VC
SE	48.3	47.1 < 60.4 [(48.3+72.4)/2]	65.4	75.5 < 87.3 [(65.4+109.1)/2]
10 μM vitamin C	72.4		109.1	

Table 8. Synergistic radical scavenging activity of SE and vitamin C. Cited from [2] with permission.

http://dx.doi.org/10.5772/52187

3.9. Inhibition of CYP3A4 activity

CYP3A4 activity was measured by β-hydroxylation of testosterone in human recombinant CYP3A4. Products A, B and C dose-dependently inhibited the β-hydroxylation of testosterone, generally used for the assay of CYP3A4 activity. Product C exhibited the highest CYP3A4–inhibitory activity (IC_{50}=58 μg/ml), followed by product B (IC_{50}=124 μg/ml) and then product A (IC_{50}=403 μg/ml). Product B inhibited the CYP3A4 to an extent similar to that attained by Cu (II)- chlorophyllin; product A inhibited CYP3A4 to lower extent than that achieved by grapefruit juice (Figure 12) [4].

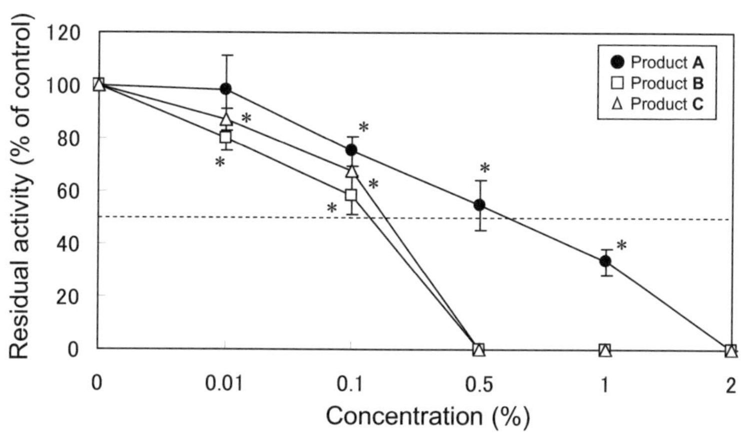

Figure 12. CYP3A4 inhibitory activity of products **A**, **B** and **C**. One millilitre of products **A**, **B** and **C** was freeze dried to produce the powder (66.1, 77.6 and 28.5 mg, respectively).Each value represents the mean ± S.D. (n=3). *p<0.05 relative to the control (0%). Cited from [4] with permission.

SE-10 and SE dose-dependently inhibited the β-hydroxylation of testosterone, generally used for the assay of CYP3A4 activity. SE-10 (IC_{50}= 0.516 μg SE equivalent/ml) had an approximately 16% lower CYP3A4-inhibitory activity (IC_{50}= 0.445 μg/ml) [19].Combined with our recent report [4], CYP3A4 inhibitory activity increases in the following order (from lower to higher): SE-10 < SE < products B and C. SE-10 and SE seem likely to be safer drugs as compared with products B and C, since the latter are expected to enhance the side-effects of CYP3A4-metabolizable drugs more potently.

3.10. Possibility of complex formation between the components

Solvent fractionation of SE demonstrated that the majority of chlorophyllin and the activity that inhibited the NO production by macrophages were recovered from the water layer that contains majority of compounds (more than 81%) [18]. This suggests the possibility that chlorophyllin in SE may be associated with hydrophilic substances, especially LCC in the native state or after extraction with alkaline solution, since the preparative method of SE is the same with that of LCC. This was supported by the observation that LCC isolated from SE has greenish color (absorption peak = 655 nm), characteristic to chlorophyllin (absorption peak = 629 nm), expected to contain 1.7-2.6% chlorophyllin in the molecule, and that 68.5% of SE eluted as a single peak at the retention time of 22.175 min in HPLC [18]. Upon binding to chlorophyllin, LCC may obtain the activity of inhibiting the NO production by activated macrophages.

3.11. Clinical application for the treatment of oral diseases

Oral intake of product B (BLE) slightly but significantly reduced the gingival crevicular fluid (determined by Periometer®), and tended to reduce gingival index in the experimentally induced gingivitis patients [9].

Lichen planus is a chronic mucocutaneous disease that affects the skin, tongue, and oral mucosa. The most common presentation of oral lichen planus is the reticular form that manifests as white lacy streaks on the mucosa (known as Wickham's striae) or as smaller papules (small raised areas). The cause of lichen planus is not known. Some lichen planus-type rashes occur as allergic reactions to medications and a complication of chronic hepatitis C virus infection [51]. Hepatitis C virus has been reported to occasionally replicate in oral lichen tissue and contribute to mucosal damage [52, 53]. It has been reported that the Epstein-Barr virus is more frequently detected in oral lesions such as oral lichen planus and oral squamous cell carcinoma in comparison with healthy oral epithelium [54].

Potent antiviral, antibacterial, and anti-inflammatory activity of SE prompted us to investigate whether SE is effective on oral lichenoid dysplasia and osteoclastogenesis. A male patient with white lacy streaks in the oral mucosa was orally administered SE three times a day for ten months. Long-term treatment cycle of SE progressively reduced both the area of white steaks (Figure 13) and the base-line levels of salivary interleukin-6 and 8 (Figure 14) [55]. IL-8 concentration after SE treatment was below the initial level throughout the experimental period. This was accompanied by the improvement of patient's symptoms. Before the SE treatment, the patient felt that the mucosa is uneven, rough and cut by touching with his tongue. Three weeks after the treatment, such feeling reduced and the mucosa became much smooth. At four weeks, the rough mucosa was narrowed into smaller area, and the patient could eat without pungent feeling on the oral mucosa. Oral intake of SE also improved the patient's symptom of pollen allergy, and loose teeth, giving an impression that the oral mucosa became much tighter. SE significantly inhibited the RANKL-induced differentiation of mouse macrophage-like RAW264.7 cells towards osteoclasts (evaluated by TRAP-positive multinuclear cell formation). These pilot clinical study suggests the therapeutic potentiality of SE against oral diseases [55].

4. Conclusion

SE (Sasa Health®), alkaline extract of *Sasa senanensis* Rehder extract has shown diverse biological activities including membrane stabilizing, anti-leukemia, anti-inflammatory, radical scavenging, anti-UV, bacteriostatic, antiviral, anti-stomatitis, and anti-lichen planus activity

http://dx.doi.org/10.5772/52187

(Figure 15). Among these biological activities, antiviral, anti-UV and synergism with vitamin C are unique properties to SE as well as LCC (Figure 15).

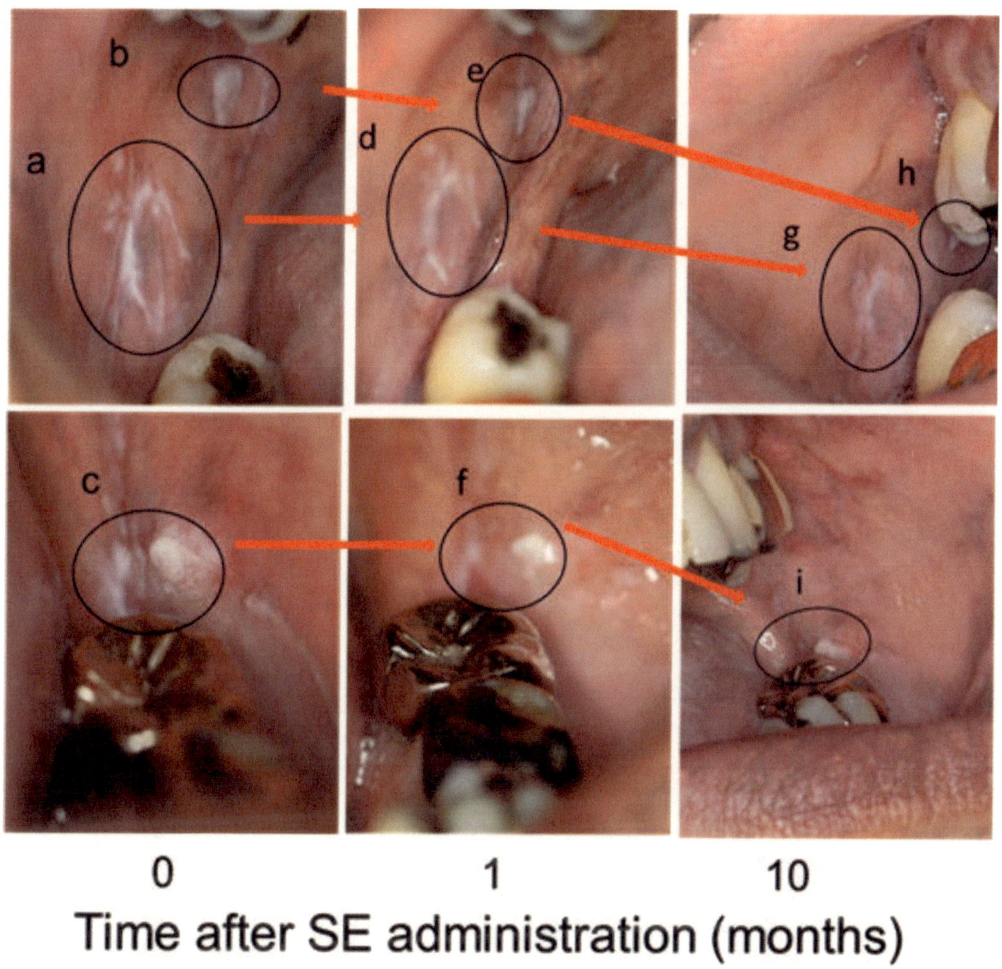

Figure 13. Time-dependent effect of SE on the oral lichenoid dysplasia. One 51 years old male patient with lichenoid dysplasia was treated for 0, 1 or 10 months with 13.3 ml of 50% diluted SE (containing 33 mg dried material/ml) at each meal, 3 times a day. Intraoral photographs in the right side (upper panel) and left side (lower panel) of buccal mucosa were taken. It should be noted that the SE treatment progressively reduced the area of the white streaks (a → d → g, b → e → h in the right side of buccal mucosa and c → f → i in the left side of buccal mucosa). Cited from [55] with permission.

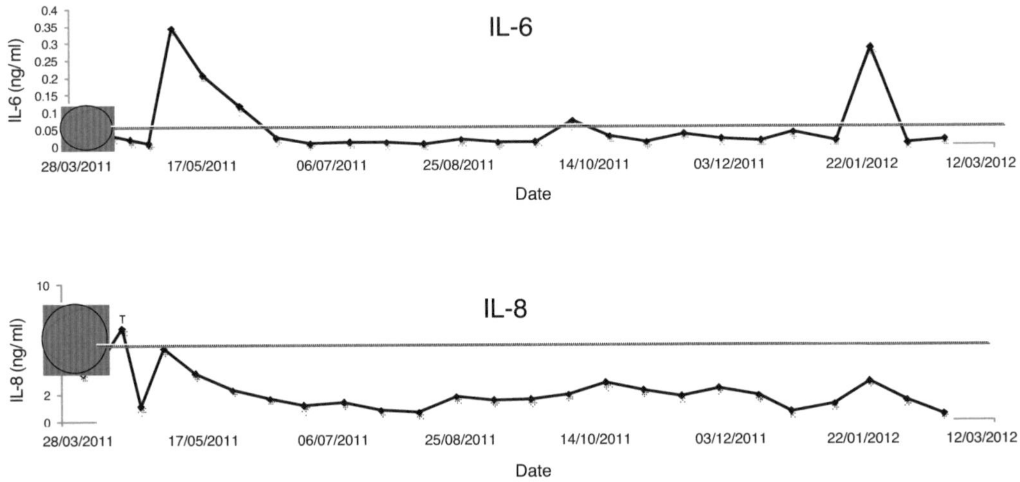

Figure 14. Effect of SE on saliva inflammatory cytokine level. One lichenoid dysplasia patient was treated with SE for the indicated periods, and the salivary IL-6 and IL-8 concentrations were determined by ELISA. Each value represents mean±S.D. of triplicate assays. ○: Control, ●:SE treatment. Cited from [55] with permission.

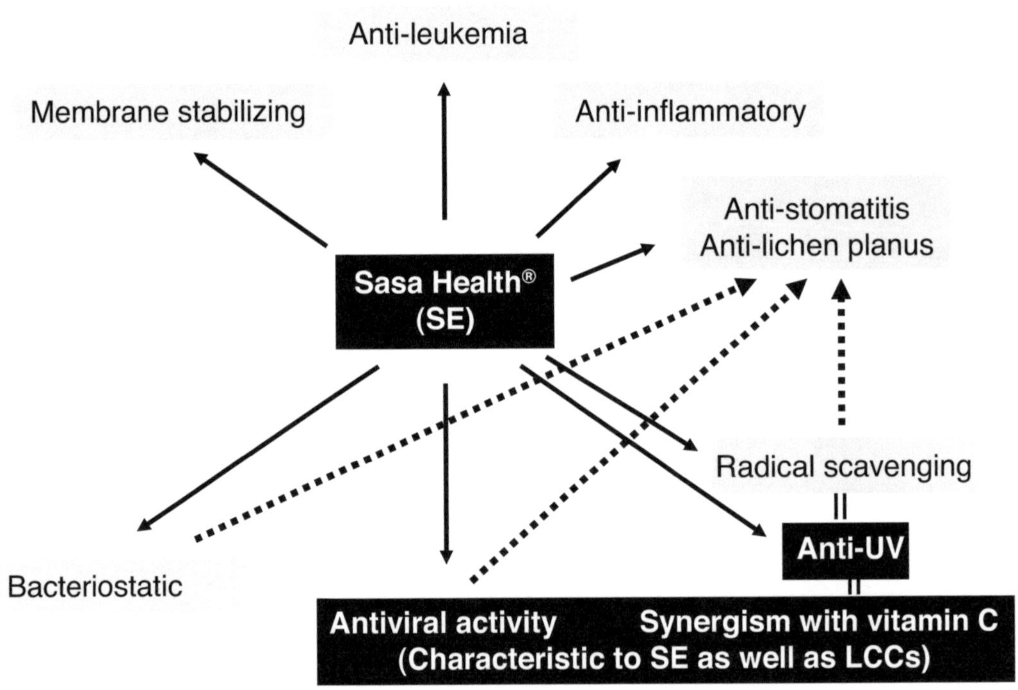

Figure 15. Diverse biological activity of SE..

SE as well as LCCs, which are efficiently extracted with alkaline solution, showed higher anti-HIV and anti-UV activity, as compared with hot water extract of many plant species including Kampo medicines (Figure 16). Antitumor activity of polysaccharide fractions of pine cone extracts against ascites tumor cells transplanted in mice also increased with acidity (binding strength to DEAE-cellulose column) [56], suggesting the potency of alkaline extract against certain types of diseases.

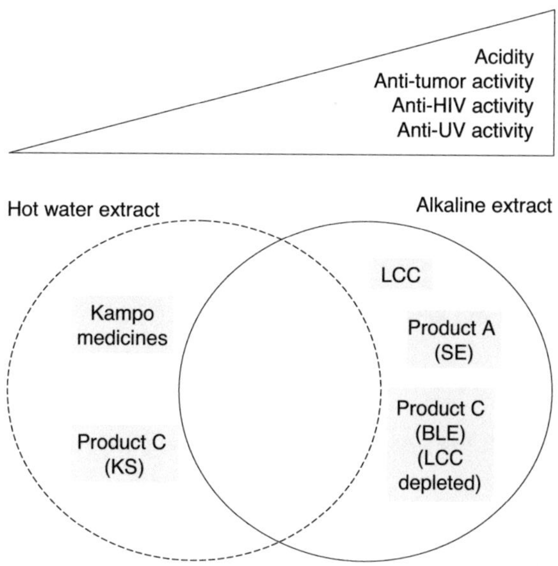

Figure 16. Comparison of several biological activities between hot water and alkaline extracts.

We have reported broad antiviral spectrum of LCC ranging from HIV [57-59], influenza virus [60-62], herpes simplex virus [63-65]. Oral administration of LCC from pine cone extract significantly improved the symptom of HSV-infected patients [66, 67], and lichenoid dysplasia patient [55]. These data suggest the possible application of SE to virally-induced diseases. Considering to low absorption through the intestinal tract [68], the application through the mucosa membrane is recommended. We are now studying the interaction between SE, antibacterial agent and charcoal to optimize the therapeutic potential of SE for the main component of toothpaste.

LCC is composed of two major components: polysaccharide and phenylpropanoide polymer [29, 30, 69, 70]. Limited digestion study demonstrated that anti-viral activity of LCC is generated by its phenylpropanoid portion [58, 61], and immnopotentiation activity possibly by polysaccharide. Using DNA microarray analysis, we have recently reported that treatment of mouse macrophage-like J774.1 cells with LCC fractions isolated from LEM (Fr4) enhanced the expression of dectin-2 (4.2-fold) and toll-like receptor (TLR)-2 (2.5-fold) prominently, but only slightly modified the expression of dectin-1 (0.8-fold), complement receptor 3 (0.9-fold), TLR1, 3, 4, 9 and 13 (0.8- to 1.7-fold), spleen tyrosine kinase (Syk)b, zeta-chain (TCR) associated protein kinase 70kDa (Zap70), Janus tyrosine kinase (Jak)2 (1.0- to 1.2-fold), nuclear factor (Nf)κb1, NFκb2, reticuloendotheliosis viral oncogene homolog (Rel)a, Relb (1.0- to 1.6-fold), Nfκbia, Nfκbib, Nfκbie, Nfκbi12 Nfκbiz (0.8- to 2.3-fold). On the other hand, LPS did not affect the expression of dectin-2 nor TLR-2. These data suggest the significant role of the activation of the dectin-2 signaling pathway in the action of LCC on macrophages [71]. It is generally accepted that dectin- 2 is the receptor for mannan, whereas dectin-1 is that for glucan [72-76]. It remains to be investigated the signaling pathway of LCC via dectin-2.

Author details

Hiroshi Sakagami[1*], Tomohiko Matsuta[1], Toshikazu Yasui[1], Oguchi Katsuji[2], Madoka Kitajima[3], Tomoko Sugiura[3], Hiroshi Oizumi[3] and Takaaki Oizumi[3]

*Address all correspondence to: sakagami@dent.meikai.ac.jp

1 Meikai University School of Dentistry, Sakado, Saitama, Japan

2 School of Medicine, Showa University, Tokyo, Japan

3 Daiwa Biological Research Institute Co., Ltd., Kanagawa, Japan

References

[1] The Pharmaceutical Affairs Law in Japan, Pharmaceuticals and Medical Safety Bureau, Ministry of Health, Labour and Welfare, Tokyo, 2009.

[2] Sakagami H, Amano S, Kikuchi H, Nakamura Y, Kuroshita R, Watanabe S, Satoh K, Hasegawa H, Nomura A, Kanamoto T, Terakubo S, Nakashima H, Taniguchi S, Oizumi T. Antiviral, Antibacterial and vitamin C-synergized radical scavenging activity of *Sasa senanensis Rehder* extract. In Vivo 2008;22(4) 471-476.

[3] Matsuta T, Sakagami H, Kitajima M, Oizumi H and Oizumi T. Anti-UV activity of alkaline extracts of the leaves of *Sasa senanensis* Rehder. In Vivo 2011;25(5) 751-755.

[4] Sakagami H, Iwamoto S, Matsuta T, Satoh K, Shimada C, Kanamoto T, Terakubo S, Nakashima H, Morita Y, Ohkubo A, Tsuda T, Sunaga K, Kitajima M, Oizumi H, Oizumi T. Comparative study of biological activity of three commercial products of bamboo leaf extract. In Vivo 2012;26(2) 259-264.

[5] Kuboyama N, Fujii A, Mizuno S, Tamura T. Studies on the toxicity of drugs (No. 29) – acute and subacutte toxicities of bamboo leaf extracts (BLE). (in Japanese) Japanese Pharmacology & Therapeutics 1982;10(5) 97-111, 1982.

[6] Tomioka H, Kpya S, Satake F, Nakamura T, Kurashige S. The effect of *in vitro* stimulation with Shojusen on the cytokine production of mouse peritoneal macrophages. (in Japanese) The Kitakanto Medical Journal 2000;50(6) 523-528.

[7] Tamura T, Fujii A, Kobayashi T. Studies on clinical pharmacology No. 9 – Antifatigue effect of bamboo leaf extract (BLE) - (in Japanese) Japanese Pharmacology & Therapeutics 1984;12(12) 47-51.

[8] Kuboyama N, Fujii A, Ookuma K, Tamura T. Orexiant activities of bamboo leaf extracts (BLE). Japanese Pharmacology & Therapeutics 1983;11(6) 43-53.

[9] Sato T, Tsuchiya A, Kobayashi, Kimura J, Hayashi H, Kobayashi H, Hobo H, Kamoi K. An application for periodontal therapy on the bamboo leaf extracted solution. (in Japanese) Nihon Shishubyo Gakkai Kaishi 1986;28(2) 752-757.

[10] Ichikawa S, Takigawa, Nara S, Ozawa M, Ito K, Yagihara Y, Seda K, Baba N, Mou M, Matsuo H, Suga H, Kogure M. Clinical effect of herbal extract "Shojusen on malaises. (in Japanese) J New Remedies & Clinics 1998;47(5) 207-215.

[11] Chuyen N V, Kurata T, Kato H. Anti-septic activity of *Sasa senanensis Rehder* extract. (in Japanese). J Antibac Antifung Agents 1983;11, 69-75, 1983.

[12] Ohizumi T, Kodama K, Tsuji M, Okuchi K. The effect of *Sasa senanensis Rehder* extract and crude herb medicine extract on the membrane (in Japanese). Showa Med J 1989;49, 315-321.

[13] Ohizumi T, Shirasaki K, Tabata T, Nakayama S, Okazaki M, Sakamoto K. Pharmacological studies of *Sasa senanensis* Rehder extract on anti-inflammatory effect and phagocytic activity. (in Japanese) Showa Med J 1988;48, 595-600.

[14] Zhou L, Hashimoto K, Satoh K, Yokote Y, Kitajima M, Oizumi T, Oizumi H, Sakagami H. Effect of *Sasa senanensis* Rehder extract on NO and PGE_2 production by activated mouse macrophage-like RAW264.7 cells. *In Vivo* 2009;23(5), 773-778..

[15] Ono M, Kantoh K, Ueki J, Shimada A, Wakabayashi H, Matsuta T, Sakagami H, Kumada H, Hamada N, Kitajima M, Oizumi H, Oizumi T. Quest for anti-inflammatory substances using IL-1β-stimulated gingival fibroblasts. In Vivo 2011;25(5) 763-768.

[16] Akazaki N, Sasaki Y, Takeda, H, Hosokawa T, Takeshita K, Kanamori M, Tsuboi M, Nagumo S. Anti-inflammatory effects of Kumazasa water extract. Pharmacometrics 2011;80, 35-42.

[17] Komatsu M, Hiramatsu M. Free radical scavenging activity of *Sasa Senanensis Rehder* extract. (in Japanese). KISO TO RINSHO 1997;31, 3321-3324.

[18] Sakagami H, Zhou L, Kawano M, Thet MM, Takana S, Machino M, Amano S, Kuroshita R, Watanabe S, Chu Q, Wang QT, Kanamoto T, Terakubo S, Nakashima H, Sekine K, Shirataki Y, Hao ZC, Uesawa Y, Mohri K, Kitajima M, Oizumi H, Oizumi T. Multiple biological complex of alkaline extract of the leaves of *Sasa senanensis* Rehder. In Vivo 2010;24(5) 735-744.

[19] Sakagami H, Matsuta T, Satoh K, Ohtsuki S, Shimada C, Kanamoto T, Terakubo S, Nakashima H, Morita Y, Ohkubo A, Tsuda T, Sunaga K, Maki J, Sugiura T, Kitajima M, Oizumi H, Oizumi T. Biological Activity of SE-10, a granulated powder of *Sasa senanensis* Rehder leaf extract. In Vivo 2012;26(3) 411-418.

[20] Iwata N, Takahashi R, Tomioka H, Takei M, Ishida K, Goto K, Murohashi N, Fujimoto K, Kurihara H, Koya S. Anti-oxidant activity of Shojusen. (in Japanese) J New Remedies & Clinics 1999;48 (11) 7-23.

[21] Wang S, Ichimura K, Matsuzaki S, Koya S. Preventive effects of Shojusen on oxidative stress induced by ferric nitrilotriacetate (FNT). (in Japanese) Dokkyo J Med Sci 2000;27 (3) 487-491.

[22] Ye S-F, Koya S, Matsuzaki S. Inhibitory effects of Shojusen on the activity of hepatic and renal ornithine decarboxylase induced by ferric nitrilotriacetate in rat. (in Japanese) Kitakanto Med J 2003;53: 143-148.

[23] Ye S-F, Ichimura K, Matsuzaki S, Koya S. Protective effects of Shojusen on the endocrine disturbances induced by oxidative stress. (in Japanese) Dokkyo J Med Sci 2004;31(1) 91-97.

[24] Sakai A, Watanabe K, Koketsu M, Akuzawa K, Yamada R, Li Z, Sadanari H, Matsubara K, Muroyama T. Anti-human cytomegalovirus activity of constituents from *Sasa albo-marginata* (Kumazasa in Japan). Antiviral Chemistry & Chemotherapy 2008;19, 125-132.

[25] Tsunoda S, YamamotoK, Sakamoto S, Inoue H, Nagasawa H. Effects of Sasa Health, extract of bamboo grass leaves, on spontaneous mammary tumorigenesis in SHN mice. Anticancer Research 1998;18: 153-158.

[26] Ren M, Reilly RT, Schhi N. Sasa health exerts a protective effect on Her/NeuN mammary tumorigenesis. Anticancer Research 2004;24: 2879-2884.

[27] Sakagami H, Hashimoto K, Suzuki S, Ogiwara T, Satoh K, Ito H, Hatano T, Yoshida T, Fujisawa S. Molecular requirement of lignin for expression of unique biological activity. Phytochemistry 2005;66 (17) 2107-2119.

[28] Sakagami H, Kushida T, Oizumi T, Nakashima H, Makino T. Distribution of lignin carbohydrate complex in plant kingdom and its functionality as alternative medicine. Pharmacology & Therapeutics 2010;128(1) 91-105.

[29] Davin L; Wang HB, Crowell AL,Bedgar DL, Martin DM, Sarkanen S, Lewis NG.. Stereoselective biomolecular phenoxy radical coupling by an auxiliary (dirigent) protein without an active center. Science 1997;275, 362-366.

[30] Emiliani G, Fondi M, Fani R, Gribaldo S. (2009). A horizontal gene transfer at the origin of phenylpropanoid metabolism: a key adaptation of plants to land. Biology Direct 2009;4, 4 (https://www.biology-direct.com/content/4/1/7)

[31] Matsuta T, Sakagami H, Sugiura T, Kitajima M, Oizumi H, Oizumi T. Structural characterization of anti-UV components from Sasa senanensis Rehder extract. *In Vivo* 2013; 27 (1) in press.

[32] Matsuta T, Sakagami H, Satoh K, Kanamoto T, Terakubo S, Nakashima H, Kitajima M, Oizumi H, Oizumi T. Biological activity of luteolin glycosides and tricin from *Sasa senanensis* Rehder. In Vivo 2011;25(5) 757-762.

[33] Manabe H, Sakagami H, Ishizone H, Kusano H, Fujimaki M, Wada C, Komatsu N, Nakashima H, Murakami T, Yamamoto N. Effects of Catuaba extracts on microbial and HIV infection. In Vivo 1992;6,,161-166.

[34] Sakagami H. Satoh K, Fukamachi H, Ikarashi T, Simizu A, Yano K, Kanamoto T, Terakubo S, Nakashima H, Hasegawa H, Nomura A, Utsumi K, Yamamoto M, Maeda Y, Osawa K. Anti-HIV and vitamin C-synergized radical scavenging activity of cacao husk lignin fractions. In Vivo 2008;22(3) 327-33.

[35] Sakagami H, Kawano M, May Maw Thet, Hashimoto K, Satoh K, Kanamoto T, Terakubo S, Nakashima H, Haishima Y, Maeda Y, Sakurai K. Anti-HIV and immunomodulation activities of cacao mass lignin carbohydrate complex. In Vivo 2011;25(2) 229-236.

[36] Kawano M, Sakagami H, Satoh K, Shioda S, Kanamoto T, Terakubo S, Nakashima H, Makino T. Lignin-like activity of *Lentinus edodes* mycelia extract (LEM). In Vivo 2010;24(4) 543-552.

[37] Sakagami H, Asano K., Satoh K, Takahashi K, Kobayashi M, Koga N, Takahashi H, Tachikawa R, Tashiro T, Hasegawa A, Kurihara K, Ikarashi T, Kanamoto T, Terakubo S, Nakashima H, Watanabe S, Nakamura, W. Anti-stress, anti-HIV and vitamin C-synergized radical scavenging activity of mulberry juice fractions. In Vivo 2007;21(3) 499-506.

[38] Sakagami H, Watanabe S. Beneficial effects of mulberry on human health. In: Farooqui AA (ed.) Phytotherapeutics and Human Health: Pharmacological and Molecular Aspects, New York, Nova Science Publishers, Inc. 2012 p257-273

[39] Nakashima H, Murakami T, Yamamoto N, Naoe T, Kawazoe Y, Konno K, Sakagami H. Lignified materials as medicinal resources. V. Anti-HIV (human immunodeficiency virus) activity of some synthetic lignins. Chemical & Pharmaceutical Bulletin 1992;40, 2102-2105.

[40] Nakashima H, Murakami T, Yamamoto N, Sakagami H, Tanuma S, Hatano T, Yoshida T, Okuda T. Inhibition of human immunodeficiency viral replication by tannins and related compounds. Antiviral Research 1992; 18, 91-103.

[41] Fukai T, Sakagami H, Toguchi M, Takayama F, Iwakura I, Atsumi T, Ueha T, Nakashima H, Nomura T. Cytotoxic activity of low molecular weight polyphenols against human oral tumor cell lines. Anticancer Research 2000;20, 2525-2536.

[42] Koizumi N, Sakagami H, Utsumi A, Fujinaga S, Takeda M, Asano K, Sugawara I, Ichikawa S, Kondo H, Mori S, Miyatake K, Nakano Y, Nakashima H, Murakami T, Miyano N, Yamamoto, N. Anti-HIV (human immunodeficiency virus) activity of sulfated paramylon. Antiviral Research 1993;21, 1-14.

[43] Kato T, Horie N, Matsuta T, Umemura N, Shimoyama T, Kakeno T, Kanamoto T, Terakubo S, Nakashima H, Kusama K, Sakagami H. In Vivo 2012;submitted.

[44] Nanbu T, Matsuta T, Sakagami H, Shimada J, Maki J, Makino T. Anti-UV activity of *Lentinus edodes* Mycelia Extract (LEM). In Vivo 2011;25(5) 733-740.

[45] Numbu T, Shimada J, Kobayashi M, Hirano K, Koh T, Machino M, Ohno H, Yamamoto M and Sakagami H. Anti-UV activity of lignin-carbohydrate complex and related compounds. 2013;27(1), in press.

[46] Sakagami H, Satoh K, Hakeda Y, Kumegawa M. Apoptosis-inducing activity of vitamin C and vitamin K. Cell and Molecular Biology 2000;46, 129-143.

[47] Sakagami H, Kuribayashi N, Iida M, Hagiwara T, Takahashi H, Yoshida H, Shiota F, Ohata H, Momose K, Takeda M. The requirement for and mobilization of calcium during induction by sodium ascorbate and by hydrogen peroxide of cell death. Life Sciences 1996;58, 1131-1138.

[48] Sakagami H, Satoh K, Ohata H, Takahashi H, Yoshida H, Iida M, Kuribayashi N, Sakagami T, Momose K, Takeda M. Relationship between ascorbyl radical intensity and apoptosis-inducing activity. Anticancer Research 1996;16, 2635-2644.

[49] Satoh K, Ida Y, Ishihara M, Sakagami H. Interaction between sodium ascorbate and polyphenols. Anticancer Research 1999;19(5B), 4177-4186.

[50] Sakagami H, Satoh K, Aiuchi T, Nakaya K, Takeda M. Stimulation of ascorbate-induced hypoxia by lignin. Anticancer Research 1997;17 (2A), 1213-1216.

[51] Cervoni E. Hepatitis C. Lancet 1998;351, 1209-1210.

[52] Nagao Y, Sata M, Tanikawa K, Itoh K, Kameyama T. High prevalence of hepatitis C virus antibody and RNA in patients with oral cancer..Journal of Oral Pathology & Medicine 1995;24, 354-360.

[53] Nagao Y, Sata M. High incidence of multiple primary carcinomas in HCV-infected patients with oral squamous cell carcinoma. Medical Science Monitor 2009;15, 453-459.

[54] Sand LP, Jalouli J, Larsson PA, Hirsch JM. Prevalence of Epstein-Barr virus in oral squamous cell carcinoma, oral lichen planus, and normal oral mucosa. Oral Surgery Oral Medicine Oral Pathology Oral Radiology Endodontology 2002;93, *93:* 586-592.

[55] Matsuta T, Sakagami H, Tanaka S, Machino M, Tomomura M, Tomomura A, Yasui T, Kazuyoshi I, Sugiura T, Kitajima M, Oizumi H, Oizumi T. Pilot clinical study of *Sasa senanensis* Rehder leaf extract treatment on lichenoid dysplasia. *In Vivo* 2012;26, in press.

[56] Sakagami H, Ikeda M, Unten S, Takeda K, Murayama J, Hamada A, Kimura K, Komatsu N, Konno K. Antitumor activity of polysaccharide fractions from pine cone extract of *Pinus parviflora* Sieb. et Zucc. Anticancer Research 1987;7, 1153-1160.

[57] Lai PK, Donovan J, Takayama H, Sakagami H, Tanaka A, Konno K, Nonoyama M. Modification of human immunodeficiency viral replication by pine cone extacts. AIDS Research and Human Retroviruses 1990;6 205-217

[58] Lai PK, Oh-hara T, Tamura Y, Kawazoe Y, Konno K, Sakagami H, Tanaka A, Nonoyama M. Polymeric phenylpropenoids are the active components in the pine cone extract that inhibit the replication of type-1 human immunodeficiency virus *in vitro*. Journal of General and Applied Microbiaology 1992;38, 303-323.

[59] Ichimura T, Otake T, Mori H, Maruyama S. HIV-1 protease inhibition and anti-HIV effect of natural and synthetic water-soluble lignin-like substances. Bioscience Biotechnology, and Biochemistry 1999;63, 2202-2024.

[60] Nagata K, Sakagami H, Harada H, Nonoyama M, Ishihara A, Konno K. Inhibition of influenza virus infection by pine cone antitumor substances. Antiviral Research 1990;13, 11-22.

[61] Harada H, Sakagami H, Nagata K, Oh-hara T, Kawazoe Y, Ishihama A, Hata N, Misawa Y, Terada H, Konno K. Possible involvement of lignin structure in anti-influenza virus activity. Antiviral Research 1991;15, 41-50.

[62] Sakagami H, Nagata K, Ishihama A, Oh-hara T, Kawazoe Y. Anti-influenza virus activity of synthetically polymerized phenylpropenoids. Biochemical and Biophysical Research Communications 1990;172, 1267-1272.

[63] Fukuchi K, Sakagami H, Ikeda M, Kawazoe Y, Oh-hara T, Konno K, Ichikawa S, Hata N, Kondo H, Nonoyama M: Inhibition of herpes simplex virus infection by pine cone antitumor substances. Anticancer Research 1989;9, 313-318.

[64] Thakkar JN, Tiwari V, Dessai UR. Nonsulfated, cinnamic acid-based lignins are potent antagonists of HSV-1 entry into cells. Biomacromolecules 2010;11, 1412-1416.

[65] Zhang Y, But PP, Ooi VE, Xu HX, Delaney GD, Lee SH, Lee SF. Chemical properties, mode of action, and *in vivo* anti-herpes activities of a lignin-carbohydrate complex from Prunella vulgaris. Antiviral Research 2007;75(3), 242-249

[66] López BSG, Yamamoto M, Utsumi K, Aratsu C, Sakagami H. Clinical pilot study of lignin-ascorbic acid combination treatment of herpes simplex virus. In Vivo 2009;23(6) 1011-1016.

[67] López BSG, Yamamoto M, Sakagami H. Treatment of herpes simplex virus with lignin-carbohydrate complex tablet, an alternative therapeutic formula. In: Patrick Arbuthnot, (ed.) Antiviral Drugs – Aspects of Clinical Use and Recent Advances, Rijeka: InTech; 2012. p171-194.

[68] Sakagami H, Asano K, Yoshida T, Kawazoe Y. Organ distribution and toxicity of lignin. In Vivo 1999;13, 41-44.

[69] Lewis NG, Yamamoto E. Lignin. Occurrence, biogenesis and biodegradation. Annual Review of Plant Physiology and Plant Molecular Biology 1990;41, 455-496.

[70] Azuma J-I, Koshijima T. Lignin-carbohydrate complexes from various sources. Methods Enzymol 1988;161, 12-18.

[71] Kushida T, Makino T, Tomomura M, Tomomura A, Sakagami H. Enhancement of dectin-2 gene expression by lignin-carbohydrate complex from *Lentinous edodes* extract (LEM) in mouse macrophage-like cell line. Anticancer Research 2011;31(4) 1241-1248

[72] Brown GD, Gordon S. Immune recognition. A new receptor for beta-glucans. Nature 2001;413(6851)36-37.

[73] Gross O, Gewies A, Finger K, Schäfer M, Sparwasser T, Peschel C, Förster I., Ruland J. Card9 controls a non-TLR signalling pathway for innate anti-fungal immunity. Nature 2006;442(7103) 651-656.

[74] McGreal EP, Rosas M, Brown GD, Zamze S, Wong SY, Gordon S, Martinez-Pomares L, Taylor PR. The carbohydrate-recognition domain of Dectin-2 is a C-type lectin with specificity for high mannose. Glycobiology 2006;16(5) 422-430.

[75] Saijo S, Ikeda S, Yamabe K, Kakuta S, Ishigame H, Akitsu A, Fujikado N, Kusaka T, Kubo S, Chung SH, Komatsu R, Miura N, Adachi Y, Ohno N, Shibuya K, Yamamoto N, Kawakami K, Yamasaki S, Saito T, Akira S, Iwakura Y. Dectin-2 recognition of alpha-mannans and induction of Th17 cell differentiation is essential for host defense against Candida albicans. Immunity 2010;32(5), 681-691.

[76] Vautier S, Sousa Mda G, Brown GD. C-type lectins, fungi and Th17 responses. Cytokine Growth Factor Rev 2010;21(6) 405-412.

Section 4

Action Mechanism and Future Direction

Chapter 9

Promotion of Blood Fluidity Using Electroacupuncture Stimulation

Shintaro Ishikawa, Kazuhito Asano and
Tadashi Hisamitsu

Additional information is available at the end of the chapter

http://dx.doi.org/10.5772/53036

1. Introduction

Acupuncture is an alternative medicine originating in ancient China that treats patients by manipulating thin, solid needles that have been inserted into acupuncture points in the skin. Current several scientific research supports acupuncture's efficacy in the relief of certain types of pain and post-operative nausea [1,2].

Acupuncture's greatest effectiveness appears to be in symptomatic control of pain and nausea. The World Health Organization and the United States' National Institutes of Health (NIH) have stated that acupuncture can be effective in the treatment of neurological conditions and pain [3]. Moreover, it is thought that acupuncture regulates various biological functions. It was presented that acupuncture stimulus influences the cytokine level, hormone level [4] and leukocyte number [5] as effects for blood.

Blood roles in organisms include waste product removal, body temperature adjustment, as well as oxygen and nutritive supply. Physiologically the first priority driving force of blood circulation is cardiac pressure.

Blood flow is determined by co-action of the cardiovascular system and blood fluidity. However, blood flow is also controlled by a blood hydrodynamic characteristic. It is established that changes in the cardiovascular system will cause changes in blood properties as well [6-9]. Changes of blood cell composition and plasma components may influence blood fluidity in the long term [7], and blood cell activity, such as red blood cell agglutination, leukocyte adherence, and platelet aggregation, in the short term [8,9].

It is believed that variations in blood fluidity result in disorders of the circulatory system such as arterial sclerosis or embolism, damage to vascular endothelium cells by hypertension, glucose tolerance degradation and chronic inflammation, degradation of blood vessel flexibility by hyperlipemia and aging, weakness of blood cells, and degradation of plasma plasticity [10,11].

Recently it is assumed that cerebral infarction, myocardial infarction, and pulmonary infarction are caused by an increase of thrombus generation. Common treatments and recurrence prevention for these illnesses include administration of antithrombotic agent such as warfarin and aspirin [12,13].

In the world today Western medicine is sometimes complemented with alternative methods of treatment although this trend is somewhat stalled due to the lack of the scientific evidence for the efficacy of alternative medicine. Western medicine has shown to have a direct effect on cell and metabolic function.

In oriental medicine, the state in which blood is stagnant is called "oketsu (Yu xie)," meaning preceding state or symptomatic of sickness. Acupuncture stimulation is often clinically used for treatment of "oketsu." The degree of "oketsu" is indicated by tongue color and form, swelling, paroxysmal blushing, and dark circles under the eyes [14]. However, these indexes do not reflect the real hemogram.

"oketsu" is now regarded as physiological blood flow and is studied from the point of view of blood fluidity and vascular resistance. We previously reported [15,16] that (1) various types of stress applied to rats cause blood fluidity to decline drastically, as the platelet adhesion increases, (2) acupuncture stimulation increases blood fluidity by the depression of platelet adhesion, and (3) the effects of acupuncture stimulation vary according to the stimulus location (acupoint). Thus, acupuncture stimulus were much effective to improve the decrease of blood fluidity such as "oketsu." The mechanisms that interact between acupuncture stimulus and blood fluidity, however, have not yet been identified.

In this chapter, we first describe our original finding on these topics, and then propose the possible action mechanisms of the improvement of blood fluidity by electroacupuncture.

2. Materials & methods

2.1. Experimental animals

Specific pathogen-free 7-8 weeks old male Wister rats were purchased from Japan Bio-Supply Center (Tokyo, Japan). The animals were maintained at 25 ± 2 ℃, humidity 55 ± 5 %, and a light and dark cycle of 12 hour in our animal facilities. The rats were randomly divided into control group or each experiment group, fed a regular show diet and water during experiments. Each group has 7 animals..

2.2. Acupuncture stimulus

The modality of acupuncture needle used was 0.20 × 40 mm (SEIRIN Co. Japan). Punctures were pricked at acupoints to apply the needle equivalency locus of humans (Figure 1): Zusanli (ST-36) on the outside crus superior, Sanyinjiao (SP-6) on the inside crus lower part, Hegu (LI-4) between the thumb and the forefinger of the arm, Neiguan (P-6) on the distal inside arm, and Shenshu (BL-23) on the outside dorsum spine. Acupuncture was 5 mm deep and stimulated electrically (3-5V, 30-200μA, rectangular and bi-phasic) at a stimulation frequency of 1 or 100 Hz to permit the muscle to shrink slightly. An Ohm Palser LFP-4000A (Zen Iryoki Co. Japan) was used as the device of acupuncture stimulus.

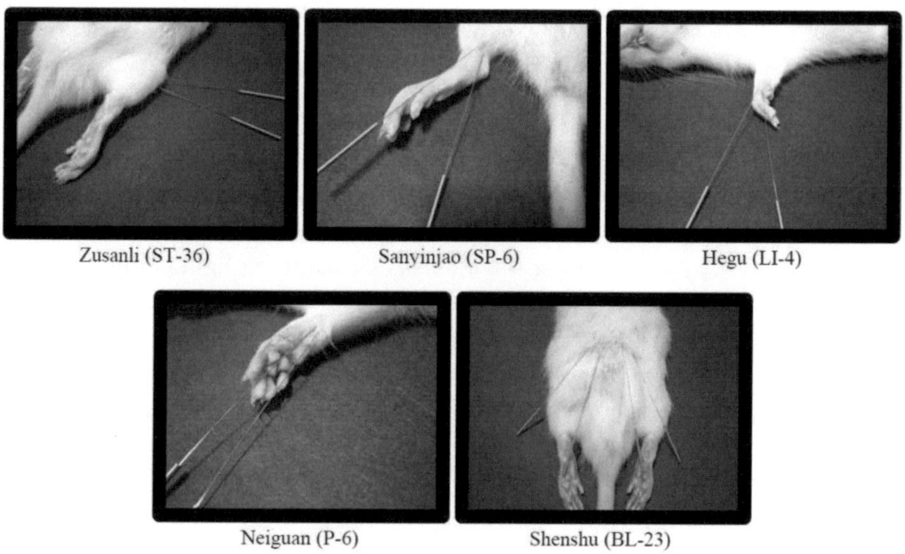

Figure 1. Locations of the acupoints. Cited from [15], with permission

2.3. Measurement of blood fluidity

We determined the blood fluidity using a Micro Channel array Flow Analyzer KH-6 (MC-FAN; MC Laboratory Inc. Japan). Coagulation of blood was blocked by Heparin sodium. We used 100μl of the blood to measure the flow time to the silicon tip of the analyzer (Figure 2)

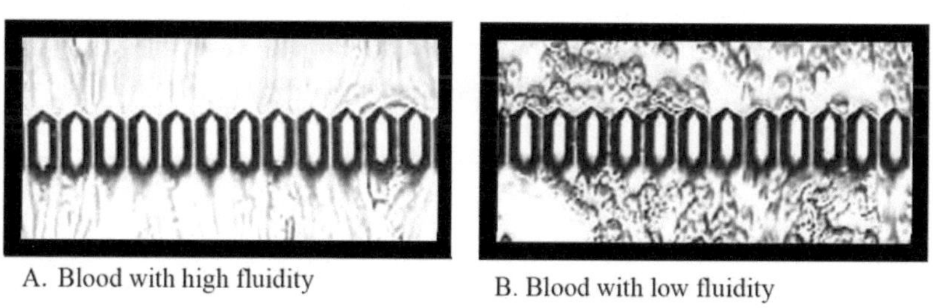

Figure 2. Images of blood flow by MC-FAN MC-FAN measures passing time of blood (100μL).A. Blood flow velocity is rapid. Blood cells are not observed. B. Blood flow velocity is slow. Platelet agglutination is observed.

We assumed that the flow time in the analyzer imitated the capillary blood fluidity index [17]. In an MC-FAN assay, the prolongation of flow time indicates a decrease of blood fluidity and a short flow time, an increase of blood fluidity [18].

2.4. Measurement of platelet aggregation ability

The ability of platelet aggregation was measured with a platelet coagulation measuring system, a platelet aggregometer (PA-20; Kowa Company. Ltd., Tokto, Japan). Blood samples were collected from the inferior vena cava under pentobarbital anesthesia. The blood sample treated with 3.2 % of sodium citrate (2.0 mL) was centrifuged to obtain platelet-rich plasma (PRP) and platelet-poor plasma (PPP).

PRP in a cuvette was pre-warmed to 37 ℃; adenosine 5′-diphosphate (ADP) was added as an agonist and the aggregation level was measured. This PA-20 device can measure platelet aggregation by the light scattering method. This light scattering method can measure the platelet aggregate size by determining the intensity of scattered light emitted from a particle, the light intensity directly corresponding to the particle size. The platelet aggregation curve was separately recorded for each size range as the voltage of light scattering intensity. The aggregates measured were divided into three categories according to size: small (diameter 9-25 μm), medium (diameter 26-50 μm), and large-sized aggregates (diameter 50-70 μm) [19,20].

2.5. Affirmation of blood cell count

In blood fluidity experiments, it is important to consider factors which influence blood properties: the number of erythrocytes, leukocytes, platelets and hematocrit.

Therefore, we confirmed that the above-mentioned blood properties showed no significant differences in both the experiment and control groups.

2.6. The experimental profile

This experiment is divided into three parts. The first is the examination of modality of acupuncture stimulus. The second is the examination of action mechanisms. The third examination focuses on the decreasing state of blood fluidity by the restraint stress method. And finally we reviewed whether acupuncture improves blood fluidity.

3. Results & discussion

3.1. Effects of stimulus approach

At first, blood fluidity was reviewed in several acupuncture stimulus approaches (Figure 3).

http://dx.doi.org/10.5772/53036

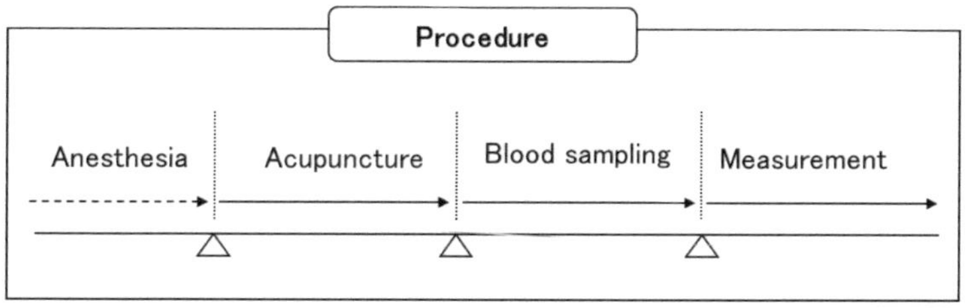

Figure 3. Procedure of study 1-7

3.1.1. Study 1. The influence of prickle acupuncture locus

We applied acupuncture stimulation to determine the influence of acupuncture stimulus on blood fluidity for 60 minutes for only 1 day at 1 Hz, 3-5 V [21]. Acupuncture was performed under anesthesia. Blood samples were collected from the abdominal vein after acupuncture stimulus. The blood samples were pretreated with anticoagulant (heparin sodium). The control group was anesthetized the same as the experimental groups but did not receive stimulation. Because the effects of acupuncture vary according to stimulus locus (acupoint), acupuncture was applied to various loci of the trunk, arm and lower extremities. Results showed that blood flow time shortened significantly in the group with stimulation to the Zusanli, Hegu and Sanyingao; however, there were no significant changes in the group with stimulation to Neiguan and Shenshu acupoints.

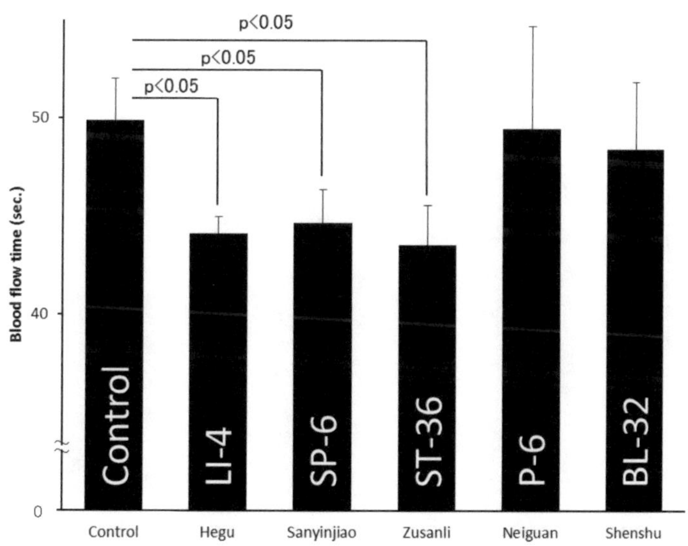

Figure 4. The influence of prickle acupuncture locus

Figure 4 shows that when acupuncture stimulation was applied to the Hegu, Sanyinjao and Zusanli acupoints, blood fluidity was enhanced in comparison with the control. In addition, the results reveal that blood fluidity is not altered by stimulation of any of the acupoints in this study suggesting specificity of acupoints contributing to blood fluidity. Heparin sodium is combined with antithrombin III and inhibits thrombin activity, coagulation factor Xa and XIIa. In other words heparin sodium does not inhibit agglomeration of platelets directly. When heparin was used as an anticoagulant, MC-FAN blood fluidity observation showed the influence of platelet aggregation ability and erythrocyte deformability.

3.1.2. Study 2. The influence of stimulus time

This shows the effect of differences of stimulation period (Figure 5). Acupuncture was stimulated for 15 or 60 minutes at 1 Hz, 3-5 V to the Zusanli acupoint under anesthesia. Acupuncture stimulation by Zusanli enhanced the blood fluidity (reduced the blood flow time (Figure 4). Blood samples were collected from the abdominal vein after acupuncture stimulus. The blood samples were preprocessed with an anticoagulant (heparin sodium).

The control group was anesthetized in the same manner as the experimental groups but did not receive stimulation.

As shown in this result, both stimulation time of 15 minutes and 60 minutes represented similar effect. Even with a short stimulation time, blood fluidity was enhanced suggesting the immediate effect of acupuncture stimulation contributing to blood fluidity.

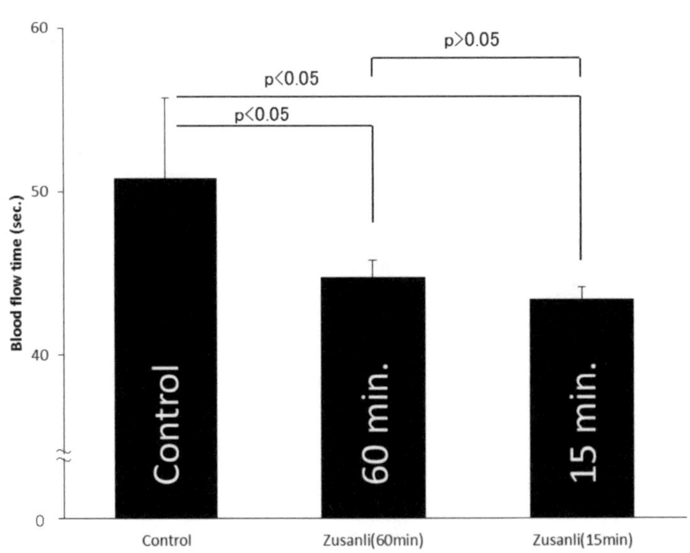

Figure 5. The influence of stimulus tome on blood fluidity. Cited from [16], with permission.

http://dx.doi.org/10.5772/53036

3.1.3. Study 3. The influence of stimulus frequency

The influence of stimulation frequency was investigated (Figure 6). Acupuncture was stimulated for for 60 minutes at 1 Hz or 100 Hz, 3-5 V to Zusanli acupoint under anesthesia. When acupuncture stimulus frequency changed, the blood fluidity was enhanced at both 1 Hz and 100 Hz. This result indicates that blood fluidity is not affected by change of stimulus frequency.

It is known that a low-frequency (1-2 Hz) or a high-frequency (more than 100Hz) stimulus influences mechanisms other than those of acupuncture analgesia [22]. When these two acupuncture analgesic system influences, even an operation is enabled only by acupuncture anesthesia. We think that a decrease of nociception affects blood fluidity. Electric acupuncture of low frequency stimulus (1-5 Hz) secretes arterenol, serotonin and β-endorphin in the central nervous system. In other words, it is thought that the secretion of these transmitters has analgesic and sedative effects on the descending pain modulatory system or the endogenic opioid system [22-24]. In addition, as mechanism through the endogenous opioid system, precedence study shows acupuncture analgesic system of diffuse noxious inhibitory controls (DNIC) participated in acupuncture and moxibustion induced-analgesia [25]. In addition, spinal segment-related analgesia occurs at high-frequency (more than 100Hz) electric acupuncture. This analgesic system produces an analgesic effect in concurrence with the start of the stimulus. It is thought that the gate control theory applies because this system does not compete with naloxone administration [23,24,26,27].

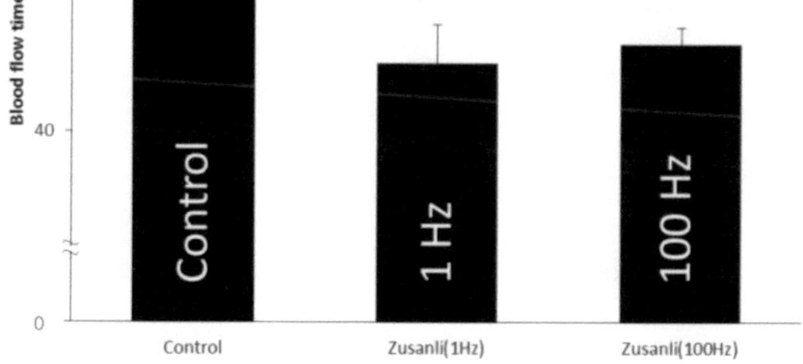

Figure 6. The influence of stimulus frequency on blood fluidity. Cited from [16], with permission.

3.2. Effects of action mechanism

In the second set of experiments, we reviewed the mechanism of acupuncture with medicine.

3.2.1. Study 4. Influence of naloxone

The influence of Naloxone, an antagonist of endogenous opioid was investigated (Figure 7). Acupuncture on the Zusanli was stimulated 60 minutes while injecting naloxone (5 mg/kg, i.p.) into the abdominal cavity every 10 minutes.

Neither acupuncture stimulus nor naloxone was given to the control groups. Physiological saline was injected into the abdominal cavity every 10 minutes of the only acupuncture and the control groups. Results showed that blood flow time decreased significantly in the Zusanli-stimulated and the Zusanli-stimulated plus naloxone groups, although there was no significant difference between these two groups.

The results of figure 5 show that blood fluidity changes with short time electro acupuncture suggesting the intervention of the nervous system. However, when we consider the fact that blood fluidity was not affected by a difference of stimulus frequency nor naloxone administration, it can be surmised that the endogenic opioid system and the spinal segment system do not contribute to blood fluidity. We speculate that acupuncture stimulus changes blood fluidity by the automatic nervous system and axon reflex, and does not influence the opioid system and the spinal segment analgesia system.

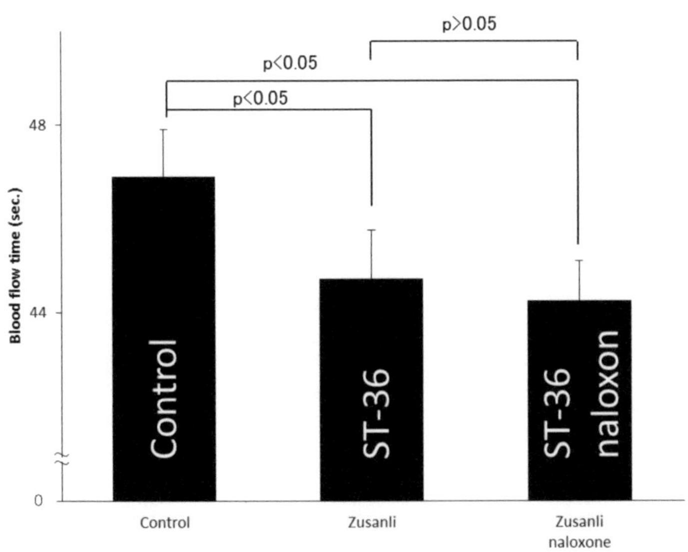

Figure 7. Influence of naloxone on blood fluidity. Cited from [16], with permission.

http://dx.doi.org/10.5772/53036

3.2.2. *Study 5. Influence of β antagonist*

A. The effect of intraperitoneal administered adrenergic drugs on blood fluidity

The influence of sympathetic agonists and antagonists on the blood flow was investigated (Figure 8). We used phenylephrine at 200 μg/kg as an α-agonist, phentolamine at 100 μg/kg as an α-antagonist, isoproterenol at 4 μg/kg as a β-agonist, and propranolol at 40 μg/kg as a β-antagonist. In these experiments, the drugs were dissolved in 1 mL of physiological saline and were administered by intraperitoneal (i.p.) into the rats. Physiological saline (1 mL) was administered by i.p. to the control animals.

The blood flow time was increased with α-agonist and β-antagonist, and the blood flow time was decreased with β-agonist and α-antagonist.

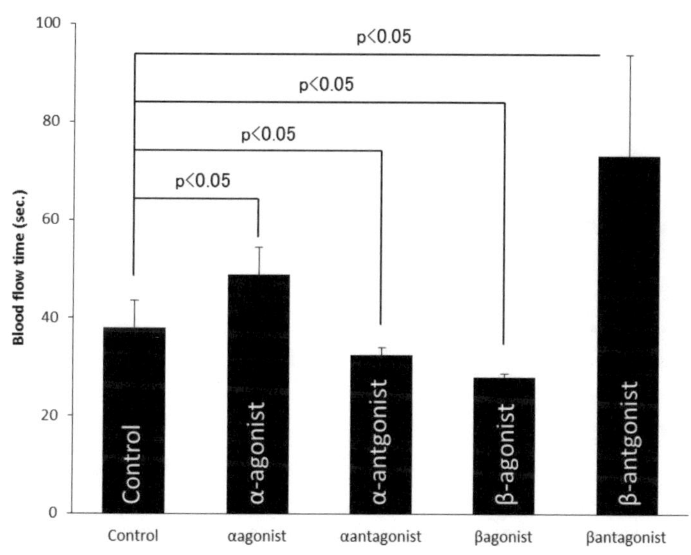

Figure 8. Influence of sympathetic agonists and antagonists on blood fluidity. Cited from [16], with permission.

B. Effect of β-antagonist on the blood fluidity enhanced by acupuncture

Effect of acupuncture together with an adrenergic drug on the blood fluidity was investigated to get the insight into the reaction mechanism (Figure 9). β-antagonist, propranolol at 40 μg/kg, was dissolved in 1 mL of physiological saline and administered before the acupuncture stimulation by i.p into the rats. Acupuncture was stimulated at 1 Hz, 3-5 V for 60 minutes to Zusanli acupoint under anesthesia.

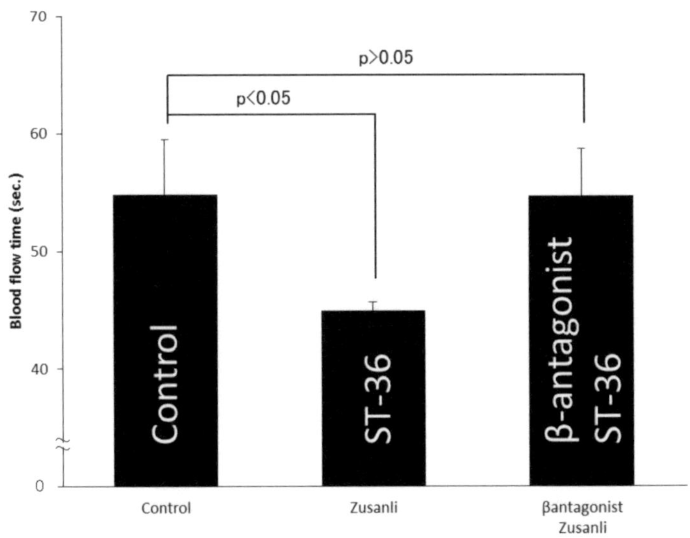

Figure 9. The relevance with βantagonist and blood fluidity. Cited from [16], with permission.

As a result, the β-antagonist canceled the enhancement effect of blood fluidity with acupuncture stimulus. There was no significant difference between the β-antagonist plus acupuncture and the control groups. This result indicates that the sympathetic nervous system influences blood fluidity with an acupuncture stimulus.

3.2.3. Study 6. Inhibition of platelet aggregation

Effect of platelet aggregation was investigated (Figure 10). An ADP an agonist was added in the PRP and the aggregation level was measured by the light scattering method. Acupuncture decreased the formation of large aggregates. In addition, medium and small-sized aggregates in the stimulated experimental group increased significantly. However, in animals previously administered with β-antagonist, the decrease of platelet aggregation by acupuncture was significantly reversed. This result indicates that platelet aggregation may contribute to the blood fluidity enhanced by acupuncture.

3.2.4. Study 7. Influence of acupuncture and β-antagonist on the platelet aggregation

Erythroid deformability was measured by blood fluidity using erythrocyte suspension (Figure 11). Physiological saline (2.0 ml) was added to the blood sample treated with heparin sodium (2.0 ml) and centrifuged (400 g × 5 minutes), resulting in a deposition layer of erythrocyte suspension and removal of the supernatant. Phosphate-buffered saline (PBS) was added to this erythrocyte rich liquid and re-centrifuged twice in the same manner [28]. The layer of erythrocyte was adjusted to 30 % with hematocrit, and this erythrocyte suspension was used for this experiment. The erythrocyte suspension was examined with the MC-FAN.

The fluidity of erythrocyte suspension was not altered by acupuncture. (Figure 11), indicating that erythrocyte deformability does not contribute to blood fluidity strengthened by acupuncture.

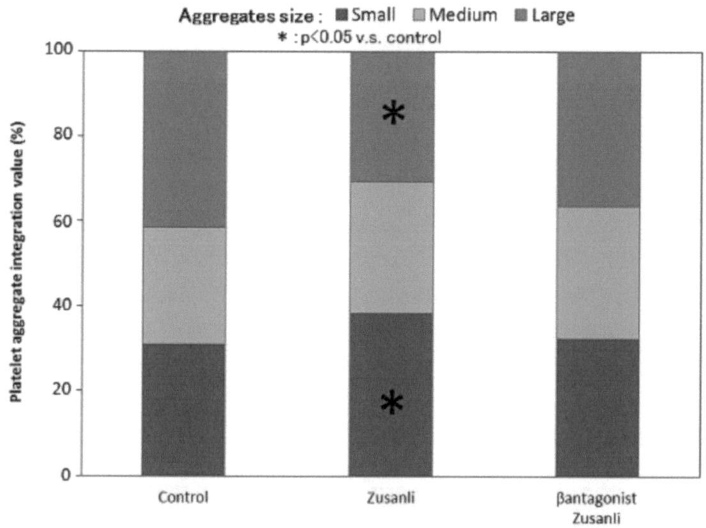

Figure 10. Observation of platelet aggregation Cited from [16], with permission

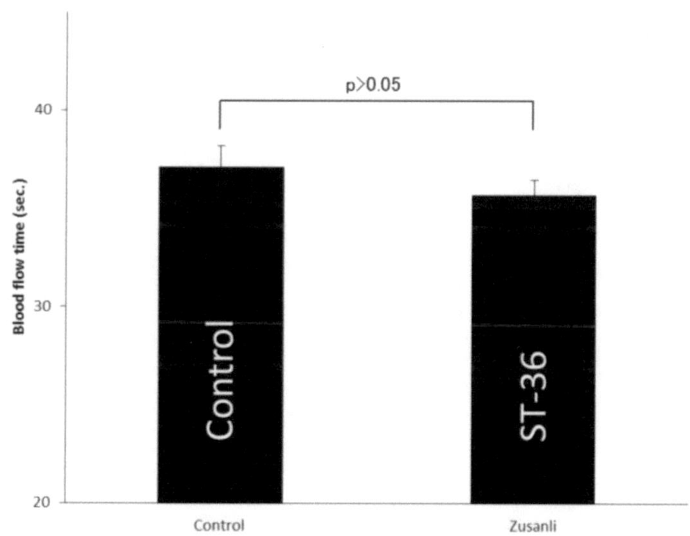

Figure 11. Examination of erythrocyte suspension fluidity. Cited from [15], with permission.

3.3. Influence of restraint stress

Finally, we also focused on the acupuncture stimulus mechanism with the restraint stress method. As preliminary research, we hypothesized that various stressors decrease blood fluidity. Restraint in a rectangular acrylic box for six hours was used as the stressor. Acupuncture stimulation was given for 1 hour (after 5 hours of restriction) at 1 Hz, 3-5V to the Zusanli acupoint with arousal (Figure 12).

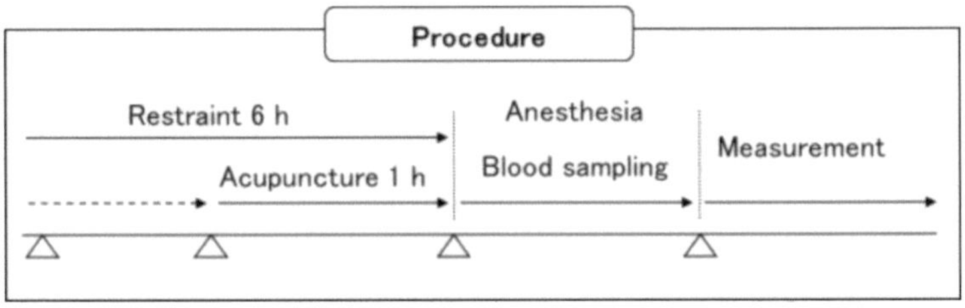

Figure 12. Experimental procedures for the study 8 and 9

3.3.1. Study 8. Observation of blood fluidity and platelet aggregation

Effect on the blood fluidity and platelet aggregation was investigated (Figure 13). In the restraint group, the blood fluidity decreased and the platelet aggregation increased. However, the acupuncture stimulus reversed these changes.

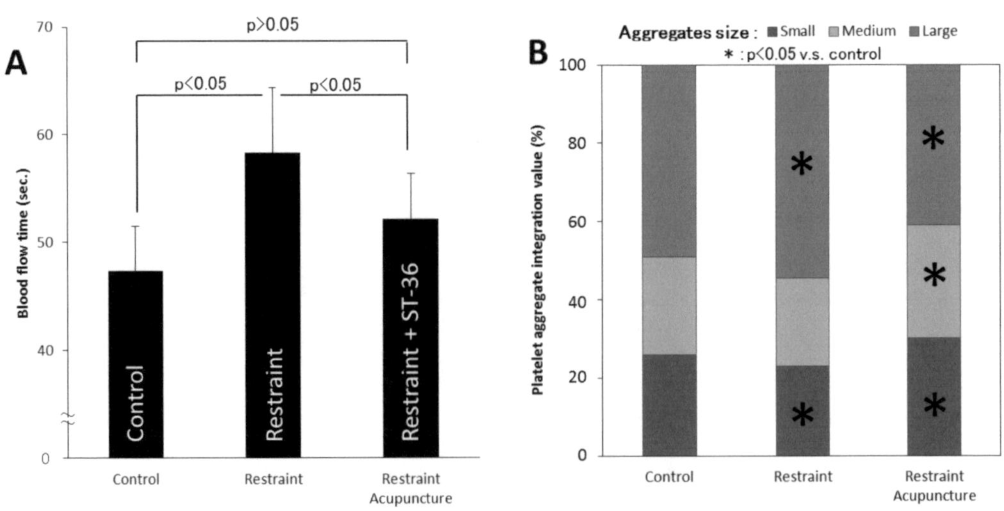

Figure 13. Influence of restraint stress on the bloody fluidity (A) and platelet aggregation (B)

3.3.2. Study 9. Affecters that are involved in platelet aggregation

(a) Blood noradrenalin level

Changes in the blood noradrenaline level after restraing stress and acupuncture was monitored by 2-CAT (A-N) Research ELISA (Labor Diagnostika Nord GmbH & Co. KG) (Figure 14).

In the restraint group, the blood noradrcnalin level increased. In the restraint and acupuncture group, the adrenalin level decreased. These results suggest that acupuncture stimulus inhibits noradrenalin release.

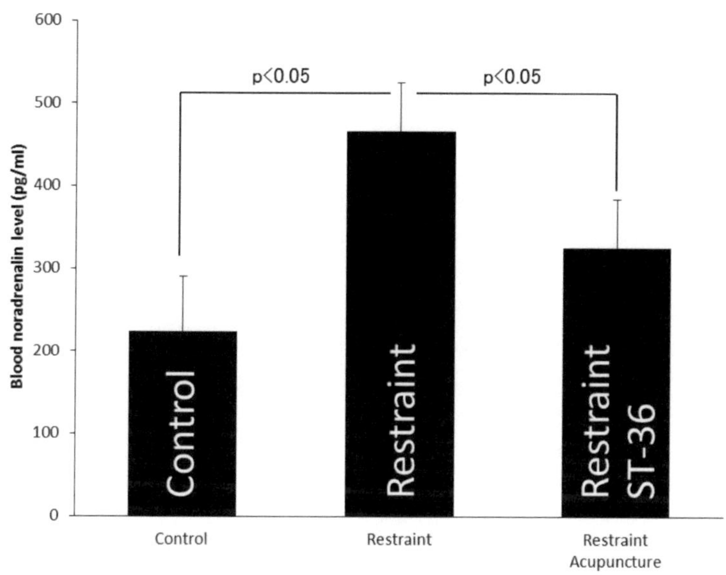

Figure 14. Blood noradrenalin level

(b) Blood ATP level

Changes in the blood ATP level after restraint and acupuncture was monitored by AMERIC ATP kit (Applied Medical Enzyme Research Ins. Co.) (Figure 15).

In the restraint group, the blood ATP level increased. In the restraint and acupuncture group, the ATP level decreased, indicating that acupuncture stimulus most likely inhibits ATP release.

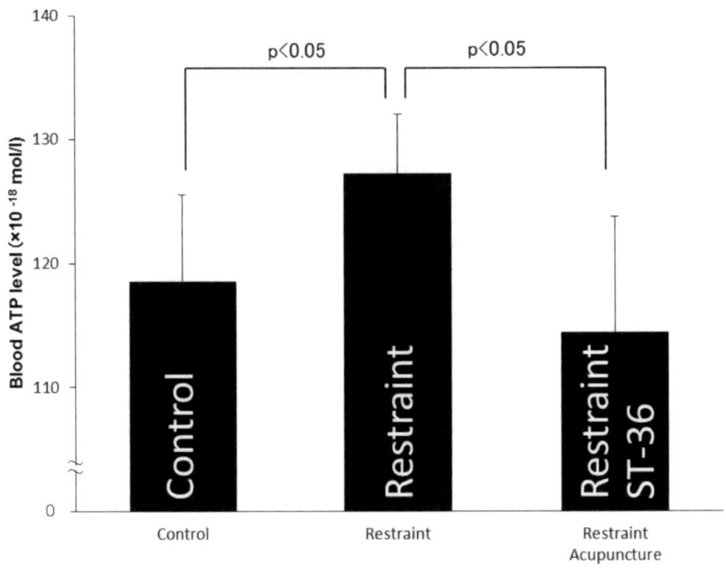

Figure 15. Blood ATP level

(c) Blood NO level

Changes in blood nitric oxide (NO) level after restraint and acupuncture was monitored by Greies test (NO2/NO3 assay kit, Dojindo Molecular Technologies, Inc) (Figure 16). NO is produced by a vascular endothelial cells, and regulates a vascular endothelium function. NO is a molecular mediator of many physiological processes, including vasodilation, inflammation, thrombosis, immunity and neurotransmission [29,30]. Half-life of NO is very short (for 3-6 seconds). It is thought that NO_2^- reflects production of NO. Therefore a level of NO_2^-, which occurred by the oxidation of NO, was examined by the Griess test (NO_2 /NO_3 Assay Kit, Dojindo Molecular Technologies, Inc.).

In the restraint group, the blood NO_2^- level decreased. In the restraint and acupuncture group, the NO_2^- level increased. indicating that acupuncture stimulus most likely improves NO_2^- release.

Stimulation of α1-adrenoceptor with noradrenaline elicits increases in intracellular Ca^{2+} concentration and induces platelet aggregation and vasoconstriction. Furthermore, high-shear-rate conditions activates von Willebrand factor (vWF) in plasma and vascular sub endothelium and produces platelet aggregation [31]. Vascular smooth muscle is controlled between contraction (induced via α_1-adrenoceptor) and relaxation (induced via β_2-aderno-ceptor). It seems that platelet aggregation is enhanced as α_1-adrenoceptor function is more remarkable than β_2-adrenoceptor function. Therefore acupuncture stimulus down-regulates catecholamine secretion from adrenal medulla and may relax with blood vessels.

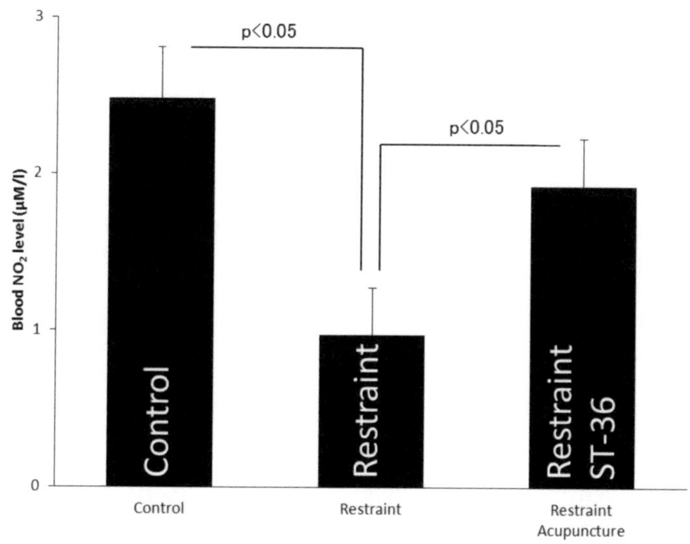

Figure 16. Blood NO_2 level

There is widespread appreciation that ATP also acts as an extracellular mediator. The extracellular ATP is released from nerve endings and various secretory cells in an exocytotic manner, from non-excitable cells by mechanical shear stress and from the cytosol of damaged cells. Extracellular ATP activates multiple cell surface P2 receptors and increases intracellular Ca^{2+}, thereby inducing diverse physiological effects, such as regulation of neurotransmitter release, smooth muscle contraction, prostaglandin formation and platelet aggregation [32].

Nitric oxide (NO) which decreases intracellular Ca^{2+} plays an important role in the regulation of vasoconstriction, inhibition of platelet aggregation, and suppression of smooth muscle cell proliferation. Noradrenalin and ATP increase intracellular Ca^{2+} in vasucular smooth muscle and platelets [33]. However NO inhibits these functions by depression of intracellular Ca^{2+}.

We think that acupuncture stimulus may control intracellular Ca^{2+} level of a blood platelet and vasucular smooth muscle generally.

The cardiovascular system are controlled at least in part by blood fluidity. In addition, it is important that blood circulates smoothly for the removal of reactive oxygen and waste products. When pain results from a bruise, distortion and muscle ache, it is known that acupuncture desensitizes the pain. Many preliminary researches have shown that acupuncture inhibits the nerve action of pain.

The present study suggests that acupuncture stimulus changes blood fluidity separately by the cardiovascular system and a new blood flow improvement system that removes pain in response to a lesion, although the precise mechanisms are still a question for future investigation.

4. Conclusion

We conclude that acupuncture stimulation increases blood fluidity. And several points as follows seem to be important to understand the mechanism.

1. There is specificity of stimulus locus.
2. The acupuncture analgesic system seems to be independent from this mechanism that acupuncture increase blood fluidity.
3. Inhibition of the sympathetic nervous activity by the acupuncture stimulation is suggested to have important role in the mechanism.
4. It seems that acupuncture stimulus has a stronger influence on platelets than erythrocytes, and changes blood fluidity.

It is thought that the acupuncture stimulation changes platelet aggregation by various factors, including the presence of catecholamine, ATP and NO.

Author details

Shintaro Ishikawa[1], Kazuhito Asano[1,2] and Tadashi Hisamitsu[1]

1 Department of Physiology, School of Medicine, Showa University, Tokyo, Japan

2 Division of Physiology, School of Nursing and Rehabilitation Sciences, Showa University, Kanagawa, Japan

References

[1] Lee A, Fan, LTY. Lee, Anna. Stimulation of the wrist acupuncture point P6 for preventing postoperative nausea and vomiting. Cochrane Database of Systematic Reviews (Online) (2): CD003281. doi:10.1002/14651858.CD003281.pub3. 2009

[2] Ernst E, Lee MS, Choi TY. Acupuncture: does it alleviate pain and are there serious risks? A review of reviews. Pain. 152(4):755-64. 2011

[3] McCarthy M. Critics slam draft WHO report on homoeopathy. Lancet, 366: 705-6. 2005.

[4] Sakuma M, Arai M, Matsuba S, Yamaguchi N. Effects of Acupuncture on Intracellular Cytokine and Hormone Levels in Human Peripheral Blood. Cytometry research, 20(1): 41-8, 2010 (in Japanese)

[5] Yamaguchi N, Hashimoto H, Arai M, Takeda S, Kawada N, Taru A, Li AL, Izumi H, Sugiyama K. Effect of Acupuncture on Leukocyte and Lymphocyte Subpopulation in Human Peripheral Blood: Quantitative discussion. BCPM, 65(4): 199-206, 2002

[6] Hirata C, Kobayashi H, Mizuno N, Kutsuna H, Ishina K, Ishii M. Effect of Normal Human Erythrocytes on Blood Rheology in Microcirculation. Osaka City Medical Journal, 53(2): 73-85, 2007

[7] George JN. Platelets. Lancet, 355: 1531–9, 2000

[8] Fusegawa Y, Hashizume H, Okumura T, Deguchi Y, Shina Y, Ikari Y, Tanabe T. Hypertensive patients with carotid artery plaque exhibit increased platelet aggregability. Thrombosis Research, 117: 615-22, 2006

[9] Lee CY, Kim KC, Park HW, Song JH, Lee CH. Rheological properties of erythrocytes from male hypercholesterolemia. Microvascular Research, 67: 133–8, 2004

[10] Ohno H, Kimu CK, Kim JH, Jung YS, Bae SY, Toshinai K, Miyazaki H, Esaki K, Takemasa T, Kinugasa T, Kizaki T, Hitomi Y, Ookawara T, Oh-Ishi S, Haga S. Hematological Response in Juveniles after Training at Moderate Altitude. Advances in Exercise and Sports Physiology, 10(2): 31-5, 2004

[11] Kikuchi Y. Effect of leukocytes and platelets on blood flow through a parallel array of microchannels: micro- and macroflow relation and rheological measures of leukocyte and platelet activities. Microvasc Res., 50(2): 288-300, 1995

[12] Horn NA, Anastase DM, Hecker KE, Baumert JH, Robitzsch T, Rossaint R. Epinephrine enhances platelet-neutrophil adhesion in whole blood in vitro. Anesth Analg., 100(2): 520-6, 2005

[13] Ochi N, Tabara Y, Igase M, Nagai T, Kido T, Miki T, Kohara K. Silent cerebral microbleeds associated with arterial stiffness in an apparently healthy subject. Hypertension Research, 32(4): 255-60, 2009

[14] Horibe Y, Ishino S, Hisamitsu N, Thein Lain, Ishikawa S, Sato T, Hisamitsu T. "Oketsu" and Hemorheological Changes : Examination by Micro Channel Array Flow Analyzer. Japanese Journal of Oriental Medicine, 55(5): 645-8, 2004 (in Japanese)

[15] Ishikawa S, Murai M, Sato T, Sunagawa M, Tokita E, Aung SK, Asano K, Hisamitsu T. Promotion of blood fluidity by inhibition of platelet adhesion using electroacupuncture stimulation., J Acupunct Meridian Stud., 4(1): 44-53, 2011

[16] Ishikawa S, Suga H, Fukushima M, Yoshida A, Yoshida Y, Sunagawa M, Hisamitsu T. Blood fluidity enhancement by electrical acupuncture stimulation is related to an adrenergic mechanism, J Acupunct Meridian Stud., 5(1): 21-28, 2012

[17] Kikuchi Y, Sato K, Ohki H. Optically accessible microchannels fomed in a single - crystal silicon substrate for studics of blood rhcology.Microvasc Res., 44: 226-40, 1992

[18] Seki K, Sumino H, Murakami M. Study on blood rheology measured by MC-FAN. Rinsho Byori, 51(8): 770-5, 2003 (in Japanese)

[19] Matsuno H, Tokuda H, Ishisaki A, Zhou Y, Kitajima Y, Kozawa O. P2Y12 receptors play a significant role in the development of platelet microaggregation in patients with diabetes. J Clin Endocrinol Metab., 90(2): 920-7, 2005:

[20] Yamamoto T, Kamei M, Yokoi N, Yasuhara T, Tei M, Kinoshita S. Platelet aggregates in various stages of diabetic retinopathy: evaluation using the particle-counting light-scattering method. Graefes Arch Clin Exp Ophthalmol, 243(7): 665-70, 2005

[21] Gao YZ, Yin QZ, Hisamitsu T, Jianf XH. An individual variation study of eectroacupuncture anagesia in rats using microarray. Am J Chinese Med., 35(5): 767-78, 2007

[22] Fukazawa Y, Maeda T, Hamabe W, Kumamoto K, Gao Y, Yamamoto C, Ozaki M, Kishioka S. Activation of Spinal Anti-analgesic System Following Electroacupuncture Stimulation in Rats. Journal of Pharmacological Sciences, 99(4): 408-14, 2005

[23] Uchida S. Acupuncture: Is there a physiological basis. Journal of Japan Society of Acupuncture and Moxibustion, 53(4): 555-60, 2003

[24] Okada K. Acupuncture stimulation and Analgesia. Proceedings of the Symposium on Biological and Physiological Engineering, 20: 223-4, 2005

[25] Murase K., Kawakita K. Diffuse noxious inhibitory controls in anti-nociception produced by acupuncture and moxibustion on trigeminal caudalis neurons in rats, Japanese J. Physiol., 50(1): 133-40, 2000

[26] Sumiya E, Kitade K. The theory of transcutaneus electrical nerva stimulation therapy and TENS stimulator. Treatment instruments for pain clinic, 30(2): 148-55, 2009

[27] Toda K. Mechanisms of descending antinociceptive system. Treatment instruments for pain clinic, 28(7): 975-87, 2007

[28] Wan J, Ristenpart WD, Stone HA. Dynamics of shear-induced ATP release from red blood cells. Proc Natl Acad Sci U S A., 105(43): 16432-7, 2008

[29] Hans Oberleithner. Nanophysiology of vascular endothelium. Kitasato Med. J., 40:97-102, 2010

[30] Higashi Y, Noma K, Yoshizumi M, Kihara Y. Endothelial function and oxidative stress in cardiovascular diseases. Circ J., 73(3):411-8, 2009

[31] Sugimoto M, Miyata S. Functional property of von Willebrand factor under flowing blood. Int J Hematol., 75(1):19-24, 2002

[32] Matsuoka I. ATP Receptor-mediated Cellular Responses and Their Regulation by Ecto, Nucleotidases, Fukushima Med. J. 53(2): 125-42, 2003

[33] Tang Y, Wang M, Chen C, Le X, Sun S, Yin Y. Cardiovascular protection with danshensu in spontaneously hypertensive rats. Biol Pharm Bull., 34(10):1596-601, 2011

Chapter 10

Enormous Potential for Development *Liriope platyphylla Wang et Tang* as a Therapeutic Drug on the Human Chronic Disease

Dae Youn Hwang

Additional information is available at the end of the chapter

http://dx.doi.org/10.5772/53520

1. Introduction

Liriope platyphylla Wang et Tang (*L. platyphylla*) is named *Liriope muscari* with Binomial name and called big blue lilyturf, lilyturf, border grass and monkey grass with common name [1]. It is widely used as one of the 50 fundamental herbs in traditional Oriental medicine; the species is one member of low, herbaceous flowing plats, which grows commonly in the shady forests of East Asia including China, Korea and Japan at elevation of 100 to 1400 m. Also, it typically grows 30-45 cm tall and have grass-like evergreen foliage and lilac-purple flowers which produce single seeded berries on spike in the fall [1,2]. Their roots are long fibrous with terminal tubers. Its flower is showy form which an erect spikes with tiered whorls of dense, white to violet-purple flowers rising above the leaves as like grape hyacinth. This flower differents into blackish berries which can maintain their status into winter season (Fig. 1A). Furthermore, *L. platyphylla* bear a strong likeness to *L. spicata* (creeping lilyturf) which is the most common species in this genus. Although the prominent flower spike extending above the leaves is alike, the leaves of *L. platyphylla* were wider and longer than those of *L. spicata* [3,4].

L. platyphylla is easily well grown in most condition of soil including average, medium, well-drained type in full sun shines to partial shade although the ideal condition for it growth are fertile and moist soils with partial shade. Furthermore, it has a wide range of tolerance for light, heat, humidity, drought and soil condition. Because of these advantages, they widely used as one of the most popular border plant and groundcover in southeastern USA [1].

Of several parts in *L. platyphylla*, only roots have generally been used for a variety of purposes, including as a therapeutic drug and in teas (Fig. 1B and C) [1]. However, there are a few studies which purified and elucidated constituents in *L. platyphylla*. Total 13 chemical constituents were isolated from the chloroform fraction and *n*-BuOH fraction from EtOH extract of *L. platyphylla*. These constituents included beta-sitosterol-3-*O*-beta-D-glucopyranosile, palmic acid, ruscogenin, LP-C, LP-D, 25 (S) -ruscogenin 1-*O*-beta-D-xylopyranoside-3-*O*-alpha-L-rhamnopyranoside, lupenone, lupeol, ursolic acid, beta-sitosterol, diosgenin, LP-A and LP-B [5,6].

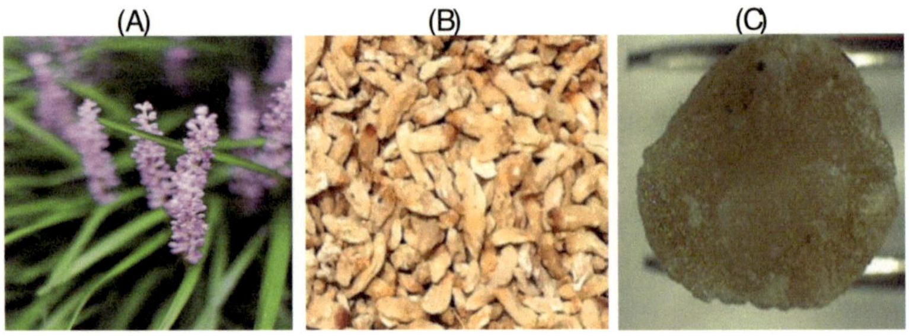

Figure 1. Flowers and roots of *L. platyphylla*. (A) The violet-purple flowers of *L. platyphylla* rise above the leaves as like grape hyacinth. (B) Its dried roots generally used to therapeutic effects. (C) A cross section of *L. platyphylla* root.

A variety of previous pharmacological studies have suggested that *L. platyphylla* may exert beneficial biological effects on inflammation, diabetes, neurodigenerative disorder, obesity and atopic dermatitis (Table 1). However, there are no reviews to publish the report for the therapeutic effects of *L. platyphylla* on the human chronic disease. Therefore, this chapter describes the important results of an experiment using *L. platyphylla* which may prove valuable in the development of a therapeutic drug for the treatment of human chronic disease.

Target Disease	Functional effects	References
Inflammation	-Inhibition of bacteria activity -Inhibition of airway inflammation and hyperresponsiveness	[7,8]
Diabetes	-Worked as insulin sensitizer -Stimulation of insulin secretion -Relief of diabetes symptom	[9-14]
Neurodigenerative disorder	-Stimulation of NGF expression and secretion -Induction of neurite outgrowth -Improvement of learning and memory ability -Induction of neuronal cell survival and neuritic outgrowth	[15-18]
Obesity	-Prevention of obesity and hypertriglyceridemia	[19]
Atopic dermatitis	-Relief of atopic dermatitis	[20]

Table 1. Summary of the pharmacological activities of *L. platyphylla*.

2. Therapeutic effects of *L. platyphylla* on human chronic disease

This main section described experimental results regarding the biological effects of *L. platyphylla* on five chronic disease including inflammation, diabetes, neurodigenerative disorder, obesity and atopic dermatitis.

2.1. Effects of *L. platyphylla* on inflammation

L. platyphylla has been long-used for the treatment against asthma and bronchial and lung inflammation. Firstly, the inhibitory activity of recombinant sortase was evaluated in 80 medicinal plants. In order to test these effects, a total 240 medicinal plant fractions were sequentially purified from 80 plants with *n*-hexane, ethyl acetate and water. As show Table 2, the high inhibition activity was detected in the ethyl acetate fractions of *Cocculus trilobus, Fritillaria vertillata, L. platyphylla* and *Rhus verniciflua.* Especially, the greatest activity was observed in the ethyl acetate fractions of *Cocculus trilobus* [7].

Medicinal plants(part of use)	IC_{50}(μg/ml)
p-Hydroxymercuribenzoic acid	40.55
Achyranthes bidentata (root)	15.48[a]
Benincasa cerifera (seed)	21.57[a]
Cibotium barometz (rhizome)	39.40[a]
Cimicifuga heracleifolia (rhizome)	26.58[a]
Cocculus trilobus (rhizome)	1.52[a]
Coptis chinensis (rhizome)	16.73[a]
Cuscuta austrailia (fruit)	21.12[a]
Ecodia offcinalis (fruit)	13.51[a]
Fritillaria verticillata (tuber)	8.41[a]
Gleditsia japonica (fruit)	27.74[a]
Liriope platyphylla (tuber)	7.96[a]
Rhus verniciflua (bark)	3.22[a]
Zanthoxylum bungeanum (fruit)	27.29[a]

Table 2. Inhibition effects of medicinal plat extracts on recombinant sortase [7] a Ethyl acetate fraction, b Water fraction

Furthermore, anti-asthmatic effects of *L. platyphylla* were investigated in ovalbumin (OVA)-induced airway inflammation and asthma murine model. OVA treatment induced significant accumulation of eosinophils into the airway, but co-administration if *L. platyphylla* induced the decrease of eosinophils and total lung leukocytes (Fig. 2). Also, the level of several important cytokines such as IL-5, IL-13, IL-4 and IgE concentration in Broncho Alveolar

Lavage Fluid (BALF) and serum dramatically decreased in *L. platyphylla* treated group compare to control group (Fig. 3). Therefore, these experiments suggested that *L. platyphylla* has anti-inflammation and anti-asthmatic activity through regulating the correlation between Th1/Th2 cytokine imbalance [8].

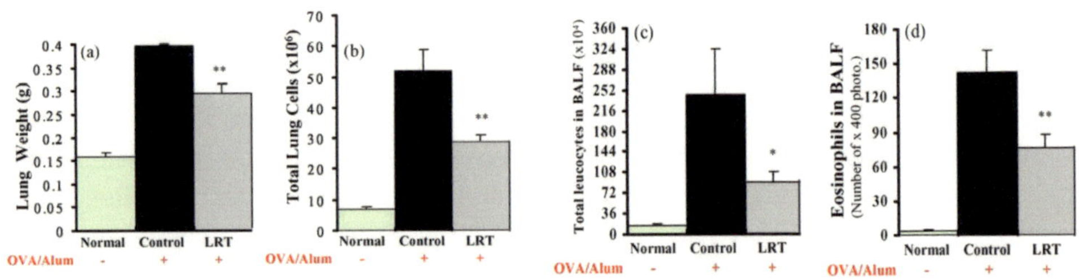

Figure 2. Effect of *L. platyphylla* on total leucocytes number and lung cells in OVA-induced murine model of asthma. *L. platyphylla* was treated into C57BL/6 mice injected with OVA for 8 weeks. Normal: normal C57BL/6 mice; OVA-control: ovalbumin inhalation (control); OVA+ *L. platyphylla* (150 mg/kg) [8].

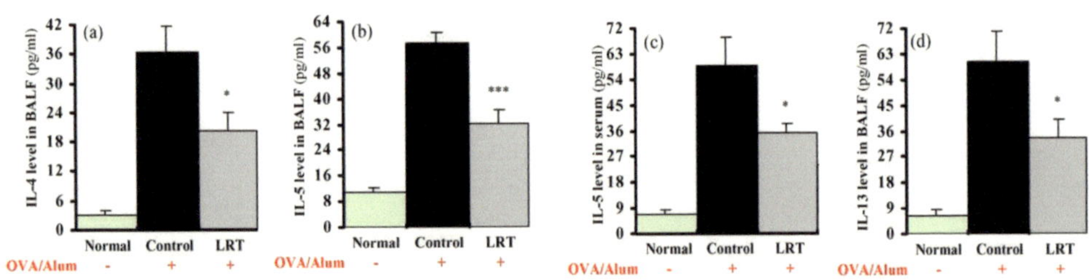

Figure 3. Effect of *L. platyphylla* cytokine level in BALF and serum in OVA-induced murine model of asthma. After final treatment, the BALF and serum were collected from animals of three groups and cytokine concentration were analyzed by ELISA kit. Normal: normal C57BL/6 mice; OVA-control: ovalbumin inhalation (control); OVA+ *L. platyphylla* (150 mg/kg) [8].

2.2. Effects of *L. platyphylla* on diabetes

2.2.1. Role as insulin sensitizer

The therapeutic effects of *L. platyphylla* on diabetes have been well studied for short period. Early study on insulin action was firstly reported by Choi et al. [9]. In this study, the extract of *L. platyphylla* was extracted with 70% methanol for 12 hours. And then, this extracts was further separated by passage through a Diaion HP-20 and silica gel column chromatography a stepwise elution by the gradients of chloroform and methanol (9:1, 6:1, 3:1, 2:1 and 1:1). Of these fractions, the 9:1 fraction induced the increase of glucose uptake 1 ng/mL up to glucose uptake 50 ng/mL insulin in 3T3-L1 adipocytes (Fig. 4). Also, this fraction contained several active compounds including homoisoflavones, methylophiopogonone A, ophiopogonone A, methylophiopogonanone A and ophiopogonanone A. Furthermore, this study showed that the insulin stimulated glucose uptake has been regulated by the increase of glucose transporter (Glut 4) contents in plasma membrane and insulin receptor substrate 1 (IRS1)-PI3 kinase-Akt signalling mechanism (Fig. 5). Particularly, Gluts are a group of membrane protein that facilitate the transport of glucose molecule across a cell membrane. Isoform of Glut was classified by a specific role in glucose metabolism including the expression pattern in tissue, substrate specificity, transport kinetics and expression in different physiological conditions [21]. Until now, 13 members of Gluts have been identified on the basis of sequence similarities [22]. Of these, four Gluts (1-4) were well characterized. Glut-1 highly expressed in erythrocytes and endothelial cells of barrier tissues, and was responsible for the low-level of basal glucose uptake. Glut-2 was widely distributed in renal tubular cells, small intestinal epithelial cells, liver cells and pancreatic beta cells. Especially, in the liver cells, it was required to uptake glucose for glycolysis and release the glucose produced from gluconeogenesis. Most of Glut-3 was expressed in neurons and placenta and Glut-4 was founded in adipose tissue and striated muscle [23]. Therefore, this study suggested possibility that homoisoflavone-enriched fraction of *L. platyphylla* may have the potential role as an insulin sensitizer [9].

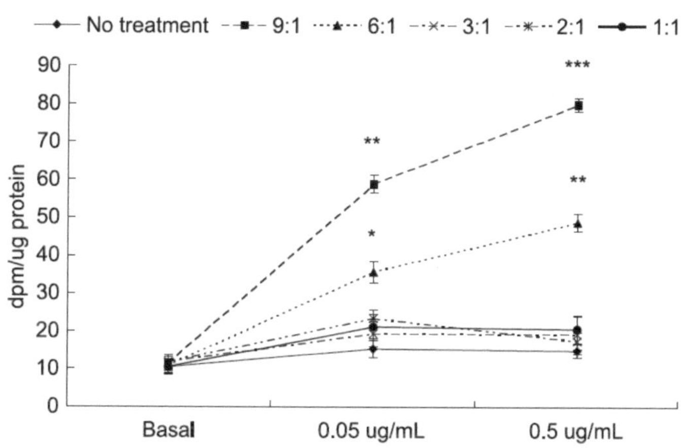

Figure 4. Glucose uptake pattern with 1 ng/mL insulin and fractionated extracts of *L. platyphylla* in 3T3-L1 adipocytes. The basal state was not treated both of insulin and extracts. *Significantly different from no treatment group in 0.05 ug/mL or 0.5 ug/mL treatment group at a=0.01. ** at a=0.001.

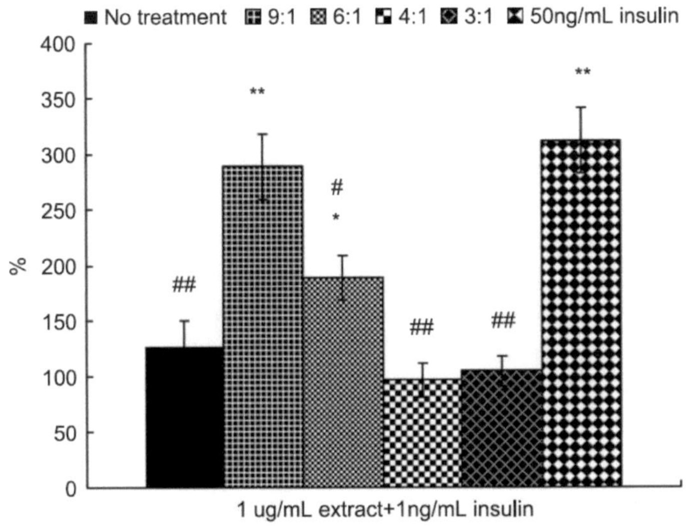

Figure 5. Glut-4 contents in plasma membrane of 3T3-L1 adipocytes. **Significantly different from no treatment group at a=0.001. #Significantly different from 50 ng/mL insulin treated group at a=0.01. ## at a=0.001.

2.2.2. Role as insulin stimulator in vitro

Recently, a role as insulin stimulator of *L. platyphylla* is being extensively researched with our group. Ten novel extracts including LP-H, LP-E, LP-M, LP-M80, LP-M50, LP-H20, LP9M80-H, LP9M80-C, LP9M80-B, LP9M80 were newly extracted from *L. platyphylla* with MeOH, EtOH, BuOH and hexan. The insulin secretion ability of these extracts was measured through the detection of insulin concentration in supernatant of HIT-T15 cells (hamster pancreatic beta cells). Of then extacts, the highest concentration of insulin was detected in LP9M80-H treated group, followed by the LP-H, LP-M, LP-E and LP9M80-C treated group. Furthermore, the optimal concentration of LP9M80-H was determined at approximately 100-125 μg/ml using cell viability test and insulin ELISA in HIT-T15 cells (Fig. 6)[12]. This study suggested that novel extracts, LP9M80-H could be considered as potential candidate for enhancement of insulin secretion.

In addition, the new approach such as steaming had applicated to *L. platyphylla* in order to to increase the level or efficacy of their functional components and to induce chemical transformation of specific components. In our previous study, Red *L. platyphylla* (RLP) has been manufactured with steaming technique under different steaming time and frequencies. Among these, maximum insulin secretion was induced by RLP steamed for 3 hours with two repeated steps (3 hours steaming and 24 hours air-dried) carried out 9 times (Fig. 7). Also, the expression and phosphorylation levels of most components in insulin receptor signalling pathway were significantly enhanced in INS cells (rat pancreatic beta cells) treated with RLP. Furthermore, a significant alteration of glucose transporter expression was detected in same group. Meanwhile, in the study using streptozotocine-induced diabetic model

(Type I), the treatment of RLP for 14 days induced the down-regulation of glucose concentration and upregulation of insulin concentration (Fig. 8)[13]. These data showed that steaming processed *L. platyphylla* may be regared as a potential candidate for a relief and treatment of diabetes.

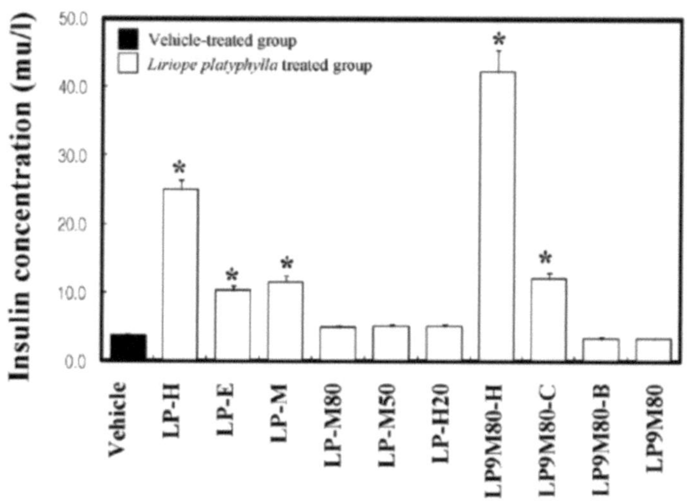

Figure 6. An insulin secretion ability of ten extracts in HIT-T15 cells. Cells were cultured with one of the ten extracts in DMSO at 500 µg/ml concentrations for 24 hr. An insulin concentration in the supernatants was measured using anti-insulin ELISA kit. The values of data represented mean±SD of three experiments. *$p<0.05$ is the significance level compared to the vehicle treated group.

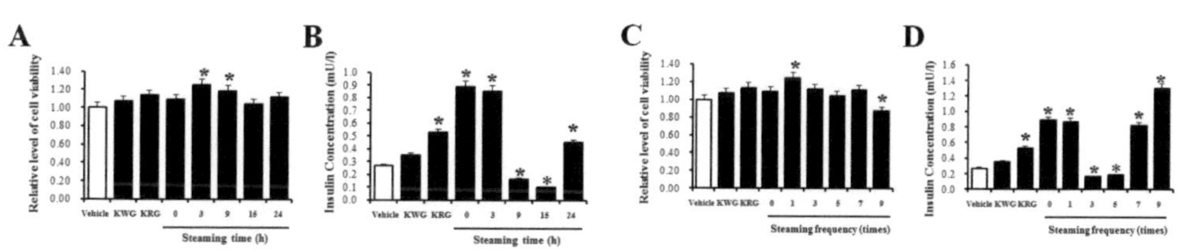

Figure 7. Effects of the different steaming time (A and B) and frequency (C and D) of *L. platyphylla* on toxicity and insulin secretion in INS cells. INS cells were cultured with one of the 5 different extracts manufactured under the different concentrations for 24 hrs. INS cell viability was measured via MTT assays (A and C). Insulin concentration in the supernatant was measured using an anti-insulin ELISA kit (B and D). The values of data represented the means±SD of three experiments. *$P<0.05$ is the significance level relative to the vehicle-treated group.

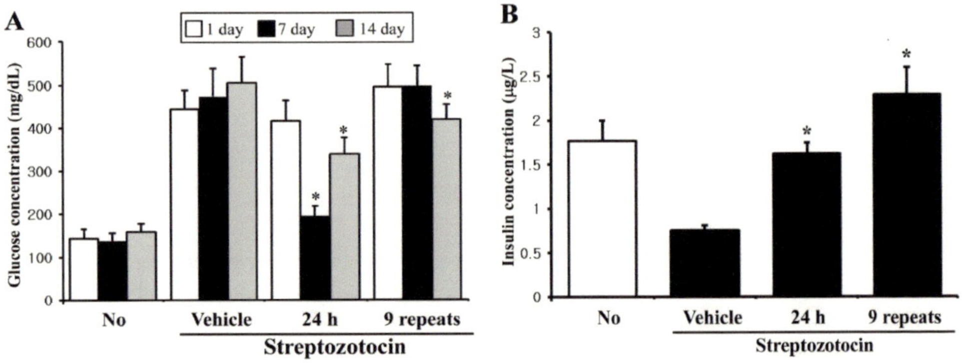

Figure 8. Effects of RLP on glucose and insulin regulation of streptozotocin-induced diabetic mice. During the treatment of RLP for 14 days, the glucose concentration was measured at three different times using the sensitive strip of the Blood Glucose Monitoring System (A). The insulin concentration was detected in the serum of streptozotocin-induced diabetic mice on the final day (B). The values of data were expressed as the means±SD of three experiments. *P<0.05 is the significance level compared to the vehicle-treated group.

2.2.3. Role as insulin stimulator in vivo

Early work was performed with aqueous extract of *L. platyphylla* (AELP). In this study, AELP was administrated into nonobese diabetic (NOD) mice showing type I diabetes with 200 mg/kg body weight for 14 weeks. Glucose concentration was significantly suppressed in NOD mice treated with AELP, while this level was increased in vehicle-treated NOD mice (Fig. 9). Also, AELP treated NOD mice showed higher insulin concentration than control NOD mice, although IL-4 and IFN-γ level was decreased in AELP treated NOD mice (Table 3)[13]. Therefore, these results indicated that AELP have a components down-regulating glucose concentration via enhancement insulin concentration.

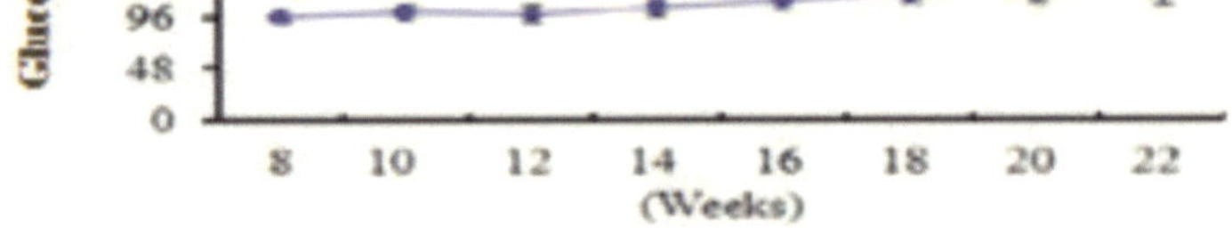

Figure 9. Alteration of glucose concentration in serum of NOD mice after AELP treatment. Glucose concentration was measured in whole blood collected from tail vein of NOD. CT indicated control group, LT indicated AELP treated group.

	C57	NOD(Control)	LT
IL-4(pg/ml)	9.1±0.41	13.4±1.1	11.0±0.7
IFN-γ(pg/ml)	4.2±0.20	45.2±2.5	12.5±3.1
Insulin(pg/ml)	9.8±0.4	3.8±0.8	25.3±0.6

Table 3. Concentration of insulin and cytokines in serum of NOD mice after AELP treatment. C57 indicated 22-week-old C57BL/6 mice, control indicated vehicle-treated group, LT indicated AELP treated group.

In addition, the therapeutic effects of LP9M80-H which had insulin secretion ability in HIT-T15 cells [12] had been investigated in normal animals and diabetic model by our group. Firstly, LP9M80-H was administrated into ICR mice for 4 days to investigate the correlation between Glut biosynthesis and the insulin signalling pathway activated by LP9M80-H. The ICR mice treated with LP9M80-H showed lower glucose concentration and higher insulin concentration than vehicle-treated group, although their body weight was remained constant over 5 days (Fig. 10). Also, the expression of Glut-3 was significantly down-regulated through p38 MAP kinase signalling pathway in liver, while the expression of Glut-1 was up-regulated by Akt and PI3-K pathway in liver and brain of LP9M80-H treated mice (Fig. 11) [10]. Thus, these study showed the first evidences that LP9M80-H could regulate Glut-1 and Glut-3 biosynthesis through the Akt and p38 MAPK signalling pathway in ICR mice.

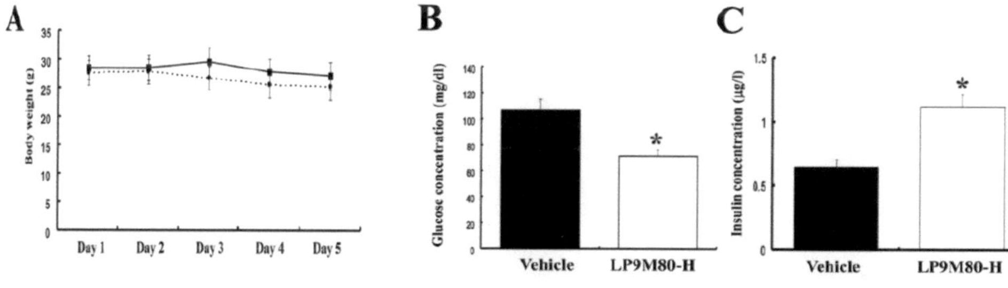

Figure 10. Effects of LP9M80-H on body weight (A), glucose concentration (B) and insulin concentration (C) of ICR mice. After oral gavage with LP9M80-H (10 µg/g body weight/day) for 5 days, blood glucose and insulin concentration were determined with Blood glucose monitoring system and Insulin ELISA kit. Values are means ± SD. *p<0.05 is the significance level compared to the vehicle-treated group.

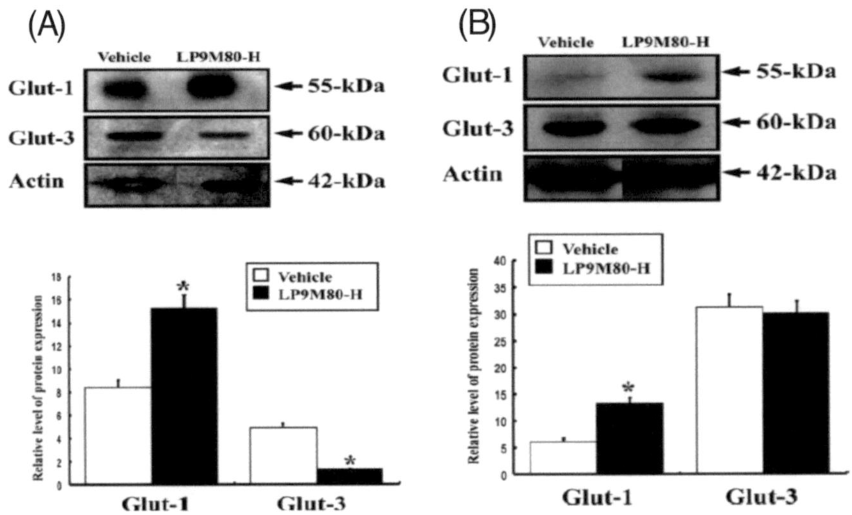

Figure 11. Effects of LP9M80-H on Glut expression in liver (A) and brain of ICR mice. The Glut-1 and Glut-3 protein expression in the liver and brain was detected with anti-Glut-1, anti-Glut-3 primary antibodies, and horseradish peroxidase-conjugated goat anti-rabbit IgG. The intensity of the Glut protein was calculated using an imazing densitometer. The values are the mean ± SD. *p<0.05 is the significance level compared to the vehicle-treated group.

Furthermore, the effects of LP9M80-H were also investigated in OLEFT rats showing type II diabetes to determine whether or not the therapeutic effects on the pathology of diabetes and obesity. After the oral administration for 2 week, the abdominal fat mass were significantly lower in LP9M80-H treated group than vehicle treated group, although there are no difference in body weight between two group. Also, a significant alteration on glucose and insulin concentration was detected in LP9M80-H treated OLETF rats compare with vehicle treated rats (Fig. 12). Furthermore, LP9M80-H treated OLETF rats showed the decrease of lipid and adiponectin concentration as well as the enhanced expression of insulin receptor and insulin receptor substrate. Especially, the Glut-2 and Glut-3 expression was decreased whereas Glut-4 expression increased by LP9M80-H in liver tissue of OLETF rats (Fig. 13) [14]. Therefore, this paper showed that LP9M80-H may also relief the symptoms of diabetes and obesity in Type II model.

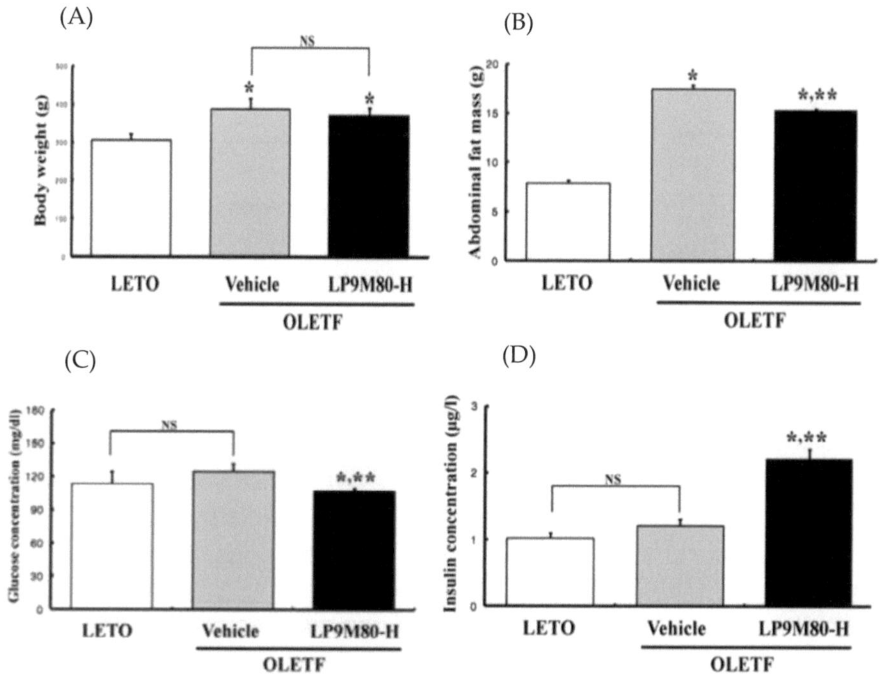

Figure 12. Effects of LP9M80-H on body weight (A), abdominal fat (B), blood glucose (C) and insulin concentration (D) of OLETF rats. At 24 hr after final LP9M80-H treatment, the body weight and abdominal fat mass of OLETF rats were measured with an electronic balance. Glucose level and insulin was measured using blood collected from the abdominal veins of rats. The data represents the mean±SEM from three replicates. *p<0.05 is the significance level compared to LETO group. **p<0.05 is the significance level compared to the vehicle-treated group.

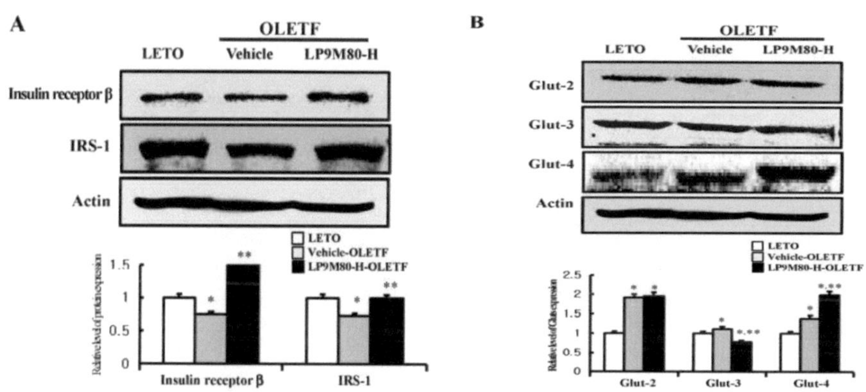

Figure 13. Effects of LP9M80H on insulin receptor-related factors and Gluts expression in liver of rats. Insulin receptor, IRS-1 and Gluts protein expression was detected with each primary antibody and horseradise peroxidase-conjugated goat anti-rabbit IgG. The intensity of each protein was calculated using an imaging densitometer. The data represents the mean±SEM from three replicates. *p<0.05 is the significance level compare to the LETO rats. **p<0.05 is the significance level compare to the vehicle-treated OLETF rats.

2.3. Effects of *L. platyphylla* on neurodegenerative disorder

2.3.1. *Induction effects of Nerve Growth Factor (NGF) secretion in vitro*

NGF was one of neurotrophic factors that regulated the neuronal development and maintenance within central nervous system (CNS) and peripheral nervous system (PNS)[16]. Many perivous studies showed that NGF could reduce the cholinergic neuronal damage induced from surgical injury [16] and prove the cognitive ability of aged rodents [24]. Therefore, NGF was considered as a therapeutic drug for the treatment of neurodegenerative disorder such as Alzheimer's disease and cerebrovascular dementia [25,26].

Firstly, the effects of butanol extract isolated from *L. platyphylla* (BELP) were investigated in undifferentiated PC12 cells (pheochromocytoma of the rat adrenal medulla) using conditional medium of C6 and primary astrocytes [15]. In order to collect conditional medium, C6 and primary astrocytes were incubated with BELP during 24 hr and then media harvested from these cells. In these results, the neuritic outgrowths of PC12 cells were significantly induced with dose-dependent manner. The maximum length of neurite-bearing cells was observed at a concentration of 10 μg/ml of BELP conditional medium (Fig. 14). Furthermore, the expression and secretion of NGF was determined in C6 cells and primary astrocytes. The NGF concentration was higher in the culture media of BELP-treated C6 and primary astrocytes than these of control. The RT-PCR results showed that BELP treatment induced the increase of the expression level of NGF mRNA (Fig. 15). Therefore, these results suggested that BELP may induce the enhancement of the expression and secretion of NGF in astrocytes.

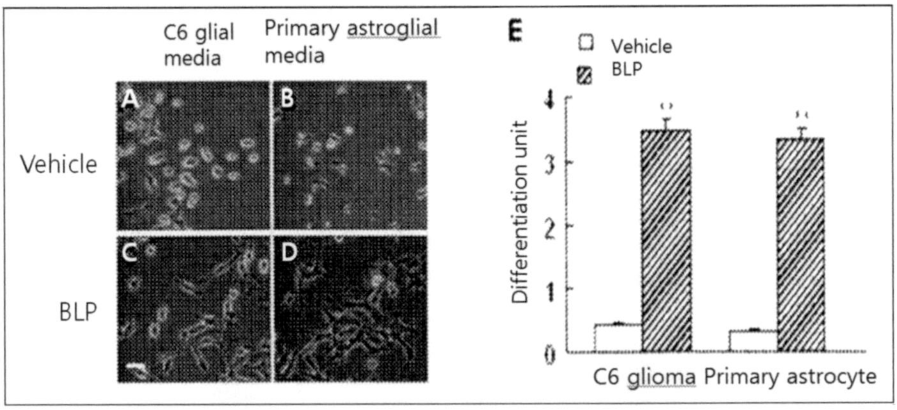

Figure 14. Effect of BELP-conditioned media on the neurite outgrowth of PC12 Cells. After 48 h incubation with four different conditioned media including (A) C6 glial media conditioned by vehicle (DMSO, 0.01%), (B) Primary astroglial media conditioned by vehicle (DMSO, 0.01%), (C) C6 glial media conditioned by BLP (10μ g/ml), (D) Primary astroglial media conditioned by BLP (10μ g/ml), the morphology of PC12 cells were detected using a camera attached to a microscope. (E) The differentiation of PC12 cells was scored as follows: cells without neurite outgrowth; 0, cells bearing neurite as long as one cell diameter; 1, cells bearing neurite two times longer length than their diameter; 2, and cells which had a synapse-like neurite. The results are expressed as the mean± SEM. The asterisks indicate a significant difference from the treatment with media conditioned by vehicle (** $p < 0.01$).

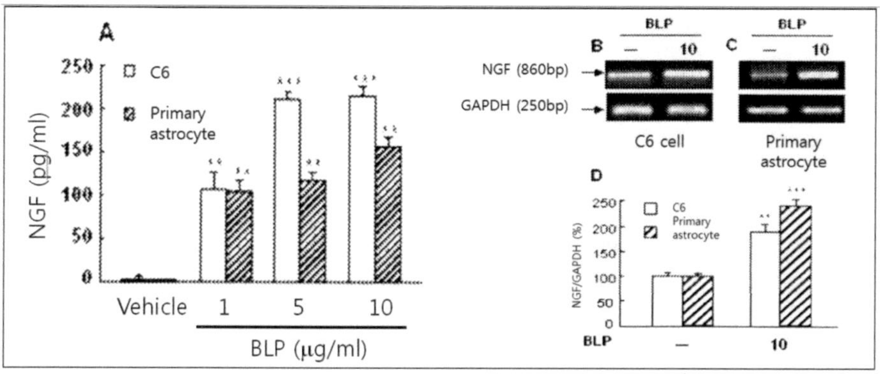

Figure 15. Effect of BELP on NGF synthesis and secretion of astrocytes. After BELP treatment for 6 h, NGF secretion and mRNA expression was measured using an ELISA kit (A) and RT-PCR analysis (B-D). The results are expressed as the mean± SEM. The asterisks indicate a significant difference from the treatment with media conditioned by vehicle (** $p<0.01$).

Meanwhile, Hur et al [16] studied the effects of spicatoside A on NGF secretion and NGF receptor signalling pathway. Spicatoside A used in this study was isolated from dried tubers of *L. platyphylla* using bioactivityguided isolation techniques and their structure was determined with 1H NMR and 13C NMR analysis (Varian U1500, 500 MHz, CD3OD)(Fig. 16). Then, their effects on neurite outgrowth in undifferentiated PC12 cells were investigated. The neuritic outgrowth was significantly increased in PC12 cells treated with spicatoside A and their effects observed at 10 μg/ml were very similar to that of NGF at 50 ng/ml (Fig. 17). In most of animal cells, Trk, a high affinity NGF receptor regulated the cell survival and neuritic outgrowth via ERK1/2 and PI3-kinase signaling pathway [27]. Therefore, the effects of spicatoside A on NGF receptor and their downstream signaling pathway in undifferentiated PC12 cells were examined using western blot analysis to investigate NGF ability. The high level of TrkA phosphorylation was detected in the spicatoside A-treated PC12 cells (Fig. 18). Also, spicatoside A-treated PC12 cells showed the increase level of ERK1/2 and Akt phosphorylation level compare with control group (Fig. 18). In conclusion, spicatoside A may induce the neuritic outgrowth of PC12 cells through TrkA signaling pathway including ERK1/2 and PI3-kinase pathway.

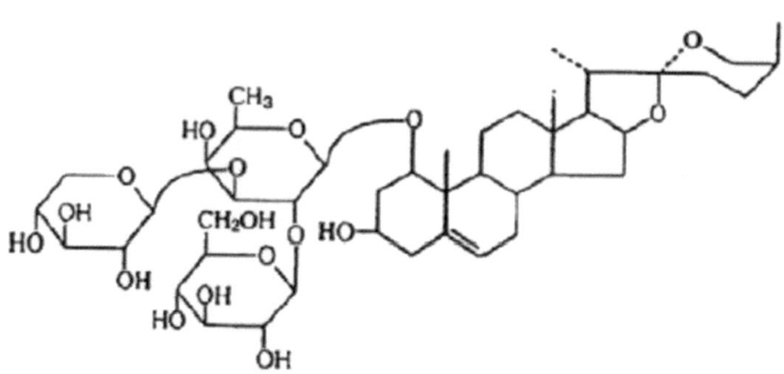

Figure 16. Chemical structure of spicatoside A isolated from *L. platyphylla*.

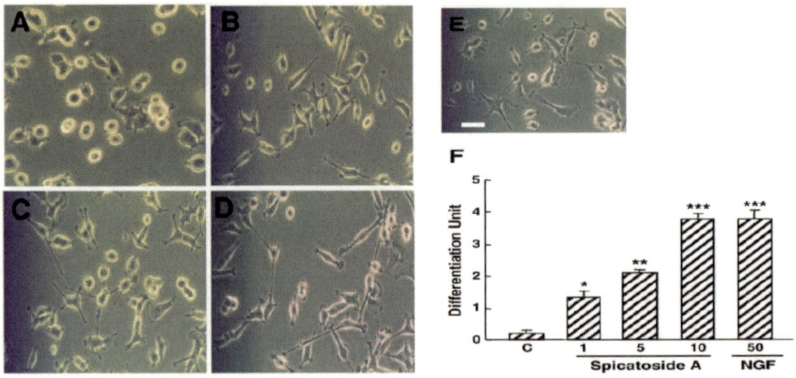

Figure 17. Effects of spicatoside A on the neurite outgrowth of PC12 cells. The morphology of PC12 cells were were observed using a camera attached to a microscope (×100) under the different treatment condition. (A) Vehicle, (B) Spicatoside A (1 μg/mL), (C) Spicatoside A (5 μg/mL), (D) Spicatoside A (10 μg/mL), (E) NGF (50 ng/mL). (F) indicates the length of the PC12 cell neurite outgrowth. The results are expressed as the mean±SEM. The asterisks indicate a significant difference from the control (*P<0.01, **P<0.005, and ***P<0.001).

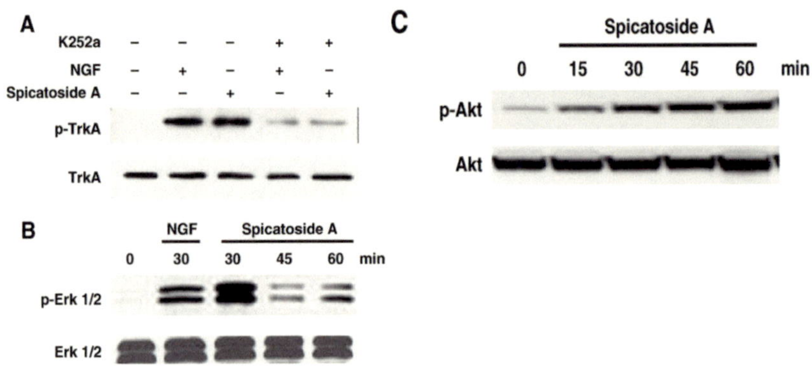

Figure 18. Effects of spicatoside A on NGF receptor signaling pathway. (A) The phosphorylation level of the TrkA receptor was detected in undifferentiated PC12 cells stimulated for 30 min with either spicatoside A (10 μg/mL) or NGF (50 ng/mL) with or without K252a (potent inhibitor of various protein kinases)(100 nM). (B) The intracellular ERK1/2 phosphorylation was measured in the undifferentiated PC12 cells stimulated with spicatoside A (10 μg/mL) for 30, 45, and 60 min or with NGF (50 ng/mL) for 30 min. (C) After the PC12 cells were stimulated with spicatoside A (10 μg/mL) for 30, 45, 60, and 120 min, the proteins containing phosphotyrosine were immunoprecipitated using anti-phosphotyrosine antibody agarose beads. The Akt phosphorylation was detected in the PC12 cells stimulated with spicatoside A (10 μg/mL) for 15, 30, 45, and 60 min.

2.3.2. Induction effects of NGF secretion in vivo

The NGF stimulation effects of *L. platyphylla* observed in several cell lines was further investigated base on behavioural and physiological features in mice. Firstly, the effects of ethanol (70%) extract of roots of *L. platyphylla* (EELP) on learning and memory was measured in ICR mice using the passive avoidance task. The sub-chronic treatment of four different concentrations of EELP induced a significant group effect on the step-through latency in retention trial. Especially, these latencies were significantly loger in EELP-treated group than those in vehicle-treated group (Fig. 19). In addition, EELP effect on the BDNF and NGF expression was detected in brain of ICR mice using immunohistochemistry. BDNF immunoreative cells were dramatically increased in CA1 region of hippocampus and dentate gyrus region in a dose dependent manner. Furthermore, NGF immunostaining cells were increased by treatment of EELP in dentate gyrus region of ICR mice, while those cells did not detected in CA1 region of hippocampus (Fig. 20). Above results showed that EELP administration could improve the learning and memory of mice through the increase of BDNF and NGF expression.

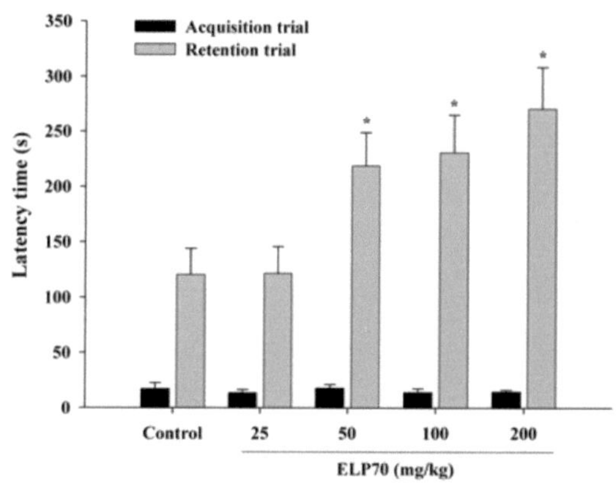

Figure 19. Effects of EELP administration on learning and memory of ICR mice. After final administration of four different concentrations EELP, the retention trials were carried out 24 hr after acquisition trials. The results data are expressed as the mean±SEM. *P<0.005, compare with the vehicle control group.

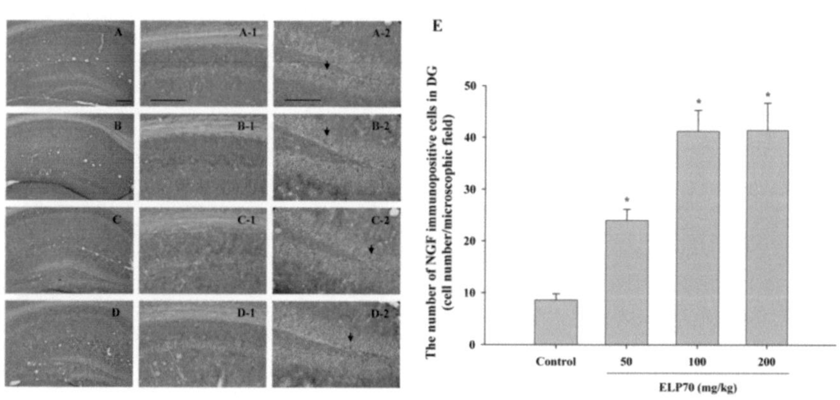

Figure 20. Effects of EELP administration on NGF expression. The NGF positive cells were detected in the hippocampa (A-D), dentate gyrus (A-1, B-1, C-1, D-1), CA1 region (A-2, B-2, C-2, D-2) of brain after administration of vehicle (A, A-1, A-2), EELP 50 mg/kg (B, B-1, B-2), EELP 100 mg/kg (C, C-1, C-2) or EELP 200 mg/kg (D, D-1, D-2). (E) The number of NGF positive cells in the dentate gyrus was calculated in mice treated with three different concentration (50, 100, 200 mg/kg). The results data are expressed as the mean±SEM. *P<0.005, compare with the vehicle control group.

Meanwhile, Nam et al. [18] reported the 100% methanol extracts isolated from *L. platyphylla* (MELP) on NGF metabolism. Firstly, they collected a total 13 novel extract from the roots of *L. platyphylla* using various solvent such as ethylacetate, methanol, hexan, butanol and chloroform. Of these extracts, only four extracts (LP-E, LP-M, LP-M50 and LP2E17P) induced the NGF secretion and mRNA expression in neuroblastoma cells, although the NGF-induced neuritic outgrowth from PC12 cells was only induced by LP-E, LP-M and LP-M50 (Fig. 21). Furthermore, *in vivo* effect of LP-M was investigated in C57BL/6 mice treated with 50 mg/kg of LP-M for 2 weeks. The expression level of NGF mRNA was significantly increased in LP-M treated mice compare with vehicle treated goup. The signaling pathway of TrkA NGF receptor was dramatically activated in hippocampus of mice via LP-M treatment, while the signaling pathway of $p75^{NTR}$ was inhibited in the cortex by LP-M treatment (Fig. 22). Then, these results suggested the possibility that four novel extracts of *L. platyphylla* was considered to be a good candidate for a neurodegenerative disease-therapeutic drug.

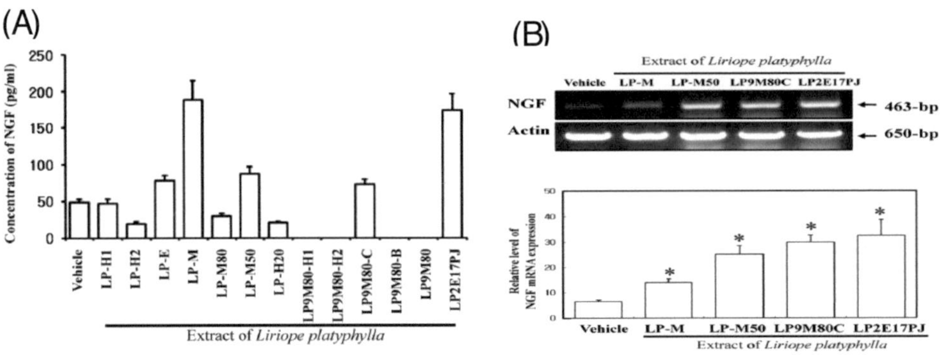

Figure 21. Novel extracts of *Liriope platyphylla* on the NGF secretion and mRNA expression. (A) After the 13 extracts treatment into B35 cells for 24 hr, An NGF concentration in the supernatant was measured using anti-NGF ELISA kit. (B) The density of NGF mRNA was quantified using a Kodak Electrophoresis Documentation and Analysis System 120. The β-actin signal was used as the endogenous control, and the transcript (650-bp) indicates the RNA loading. The values of data represented mean±SD of three experiments. *p<0.05 is the significance level compared to the vehicle treated group.

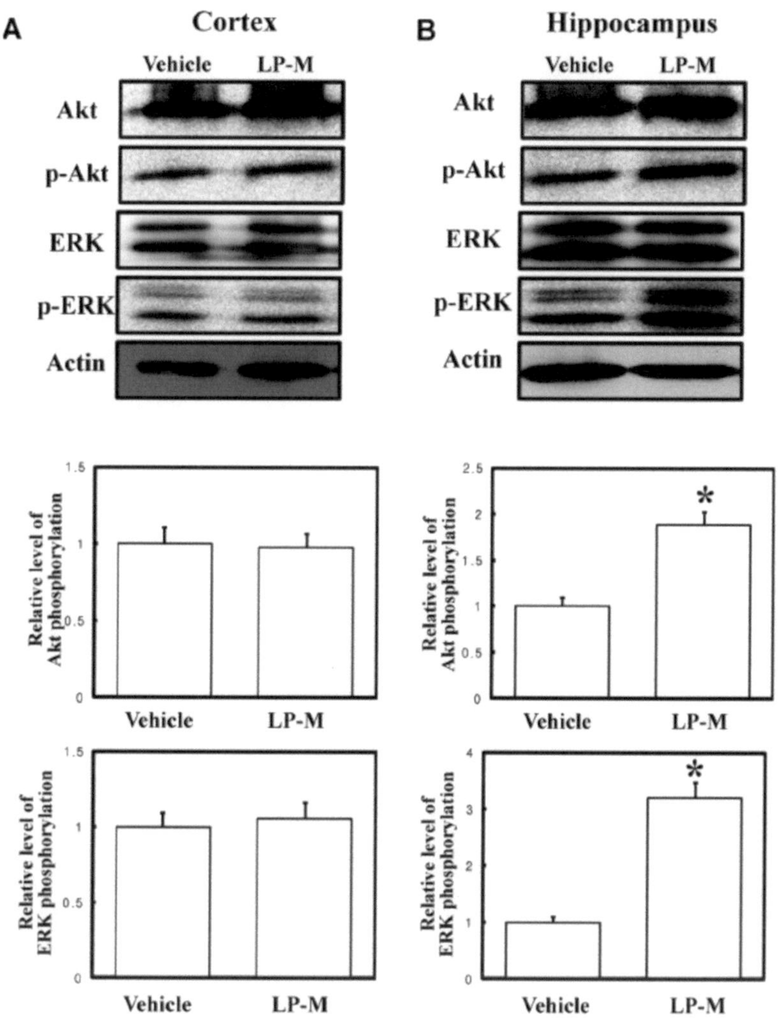

Figure 22. Effect of LP-M on down-stream signaling pathway of NGF high affinity receptor in cortex (A) and hippocampus (B) of C57Bl/6 mice. The values are the mean±SD. *$p<0.05$ is the significance level compared to the vehicle treated group.

2.4. Therapeutic effects on other diseases

2.4.1. Prevent effects on obesity

Obesity was caused by an energy imbalance induced by an increase ration of caloric intake to energy expenditure. Recently, a development of novel drug for obesity has received attention as important topics. In an effort of develop drug for the treatment of obesity, Hur et al. [16] investigated the therapeutic effects of Gyeongshingangjeehwan which composed of four medicinal plants, *L. platyphylla, P. grandiflorum, S chinensis,* and *E. sinica* using OLEFT rats. Firstly, abdominal fat area was significantly decreased by 12.1% in GGEx (X5) treated OLETF rats and 42.8% in GGEx (X10) group (Fig. 23A and B). Compare with the LETO group, the leptin level that reflects changes in body weight and adipose tissue mass [28] were 172% higher in the vehicle treated OLETF rats. But, GGEx treatment decreased leptin levels by 23.5% in vehicle treated OLETF rats with similar level to those in sibutramine (oral anorexiant)-treated obese rats (Fig. 23C). Also, the beneficial effects of GGEx on circulating lipid profile including triglyceride and total cholesterol were examined. GGEx treated OLETF rats showed a reduction of plasma triglycerides by 28.7% although total cholesterol level were unaffected by GGEx treatment (Fig. 24). Furthermore, the hepatic lipid accumulation were markedly lower in GGEx treated OLETF rats than those in vehicle treated OLETF rats (Fig. 25), while the mRNA level of PPARα target enzymes were upregulated by GGEx administration [19]. These results suggest that GGEx including *L. platyphylla* may effectively prevent obesity and hypertriglyceridemia through the inhibition of feeding and the activation of hepatic PPAR.

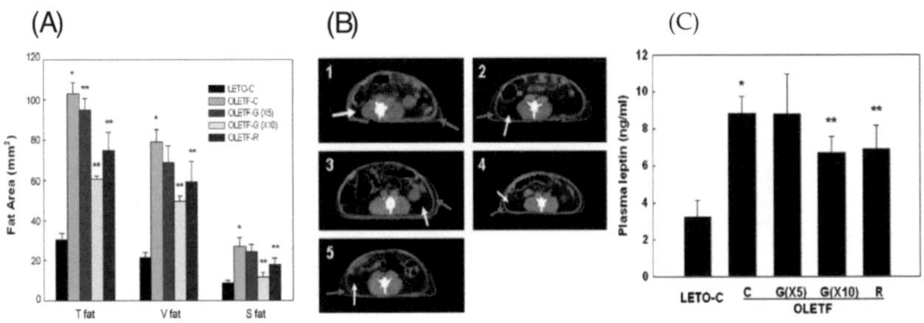

Figure 23. Effects of GGEx on abdominal fat mass and leptin concentration in genetically obese OLETF rats. Adult male LETO and OLETF rats were treated with water, GGEx, or sibutramine for 8 weeks. (A) Rats underwent CT to measure cross-sectional abdominal subcutaneous and visceral fat areas. (B) Representative CT images are shown. Gray and white arrows indicate subcutaneous and visceral fat. (C) The leptin plasma levels were measured by ELISA kit. All values are expressed as the mean±S.D. for *n*=4 rats. **p* < 0.05 is the significance level compared to the LETO control rats. ***p* < 0.05 is the significance level compared to the vehicle treated OLETF rats.

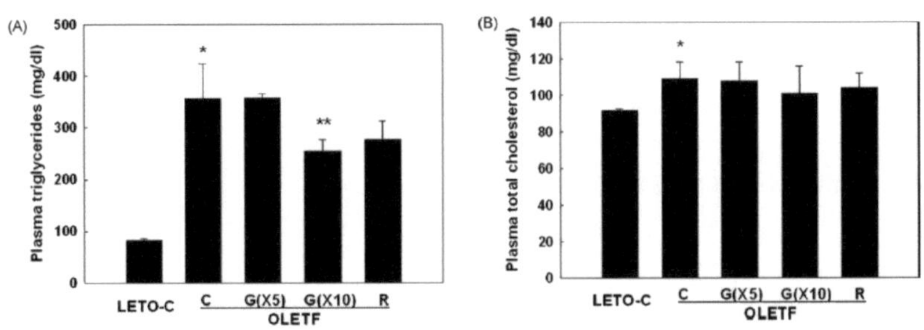

Figure 24. Effects of GGEx on circulating triglycerides and total cholesterol in genetically obese OLETF rats. After water, GGEx, or sibutramine for 8 weeks, Plasma concentrations of triglycerides (A) and total cholesterol (B) were measured and all values are expressed as the mean±S.D. for *n*=4 rats. **p* < 0.05 is the significance level compared to the LETO control rats. ***p* < 0.05 is the significance level compared to the vehicle treated OLETF rats.

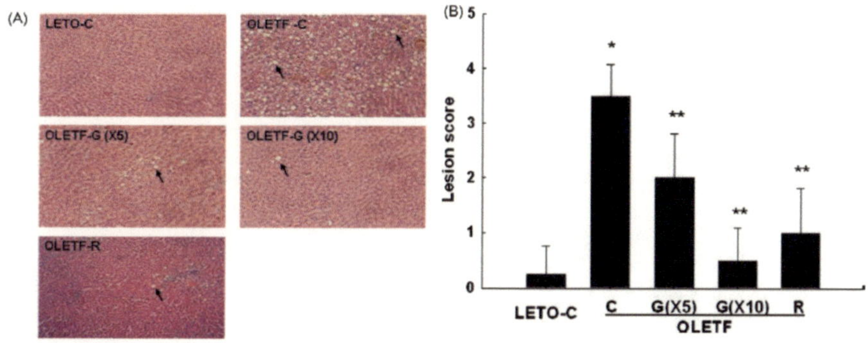

Figure 25. Effects of GGEx on inhibition of hepatic lipid accumulation in genetically obese OLETF rats. (A) Representative hematoxylin- and eosin-stained sections of livers are shown (original magnification 200×). (B) Histological analyses of hepatic lipid accumulation. Pathological scores of hepatic lipid accumulation are as follows: 0, no lesion; 1, mild; 2, moderate; 3, severe; 4, very severe. All values are expressed as the mean±S.D. for n=4 rats. *$p < 0.05$ is the significance level compared to the LETO control rats. **$p < 0.05$ is the significance level compared to the vehicle treated OLETF rats.

2.4.2. Therapeutic effects on atopic dermatitis

Atopic dermatitis was a typical skin disorder showing inflammatory, chronically relapsing, noncontagious and pruritic symptoms. Also, they were induced by several factors such as epidermal barrier dysfunction, allergy, microwave radiation, food allergy, histamine intolerance and other biological factors. Recently, Kim et al. [20] has investigated the effects of aqueous extracts of *L. platyphylla* (AELP) on atopic dermatitis of NC/Nga mice after phthalic anhydride (PA) treatment. In this animal model, 10% AELP treated mice showed the significant decline of the pathological phenotypes of atopic dermatitis such as erythema, ear thickness, edema, scab and discharge compare to control group (Fig. 26). Also, the weight of immune related organs including lymph node and thymus were gradually decreased in AELP treated groups, while the weight of spleen was slightly increased in same group (Fig. 27). The significant histological changes including inflammation, edema, epidermal hyperplasia were observed in 5% and 10% AELP treated group. Furthermore, toluidine blue staining analysis, a method used to specifically identify the mast cell, showed that the decrease of master cell infiltration into the dermis were statistically observed in 5% AELP and 10% AELP treated groups (Fig. 28). The IgE concentration was lower in only 10% AELP treated group than that in control group although this level was not affected in 5% AELP treated group. Therefore, these results indicated that the aqueous extracts of *L. platyphylla* may contribute the relieve of atopic dermatitis symptoms.

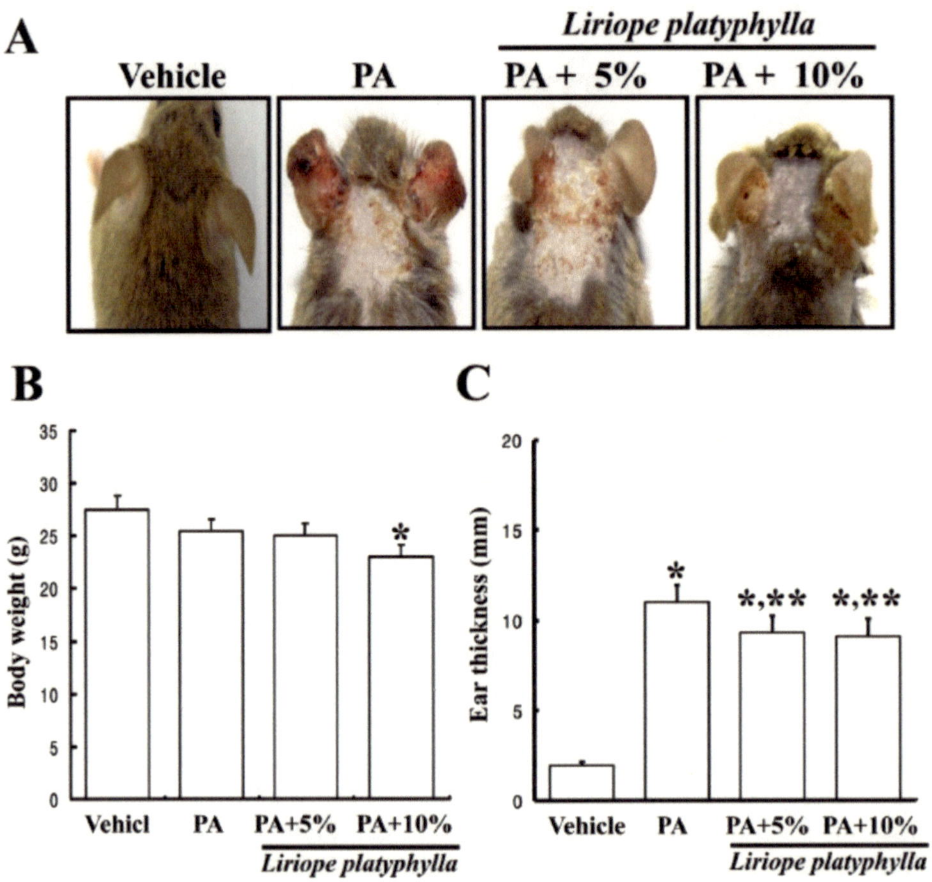

Figure 26. Effects of AELP on the ear pathological phenotypes, the body weight and the ear thickness. PA solution was repeatedly applied to the dorsum of the ear and back skin of NC/Nga mice. After 2 weeks, the change of ear pathological phenotype (A), the body weight (B) and the ear thickness (C) were detected in the mice. Data shown are the means±SD (n=5). *P<0.05 is the significance level compared to the vehicle treated group. **P<0.05 is the significance level compared to the PA treated group.

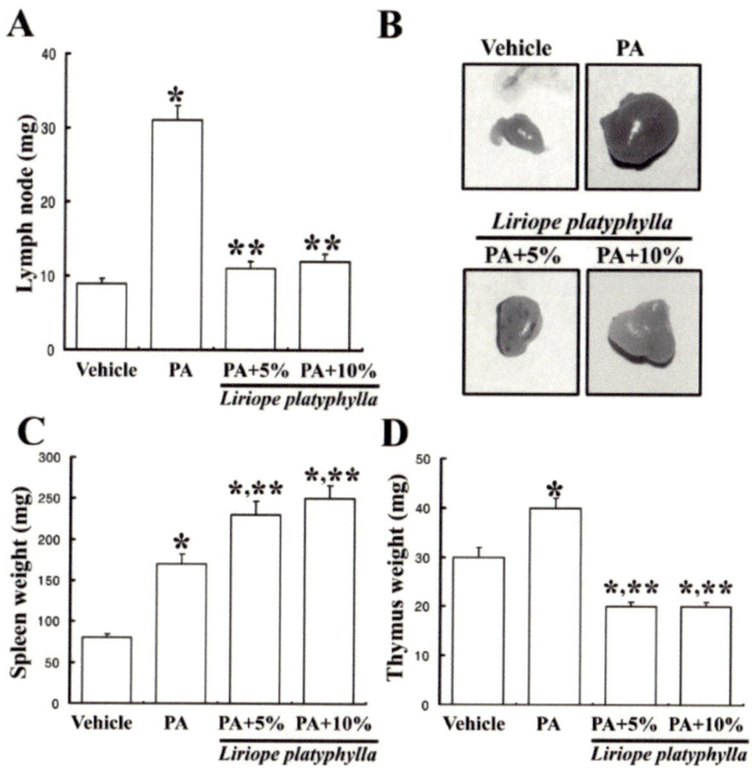

Figure 27. Effects of AELP on weight of three immune organs. After final AELP treatment, all of the animals were immediately sacrificed using CO2 gas in order to prepare the immune organs. The weight of lymph nodes, spleens and thymus were measured using the chemical balances. Data shown are the means±SD (n=5). *P<0.05 is the significance level compared to the vehicle treated group. **P<0.05 is the significance level compared to PA treated group.0

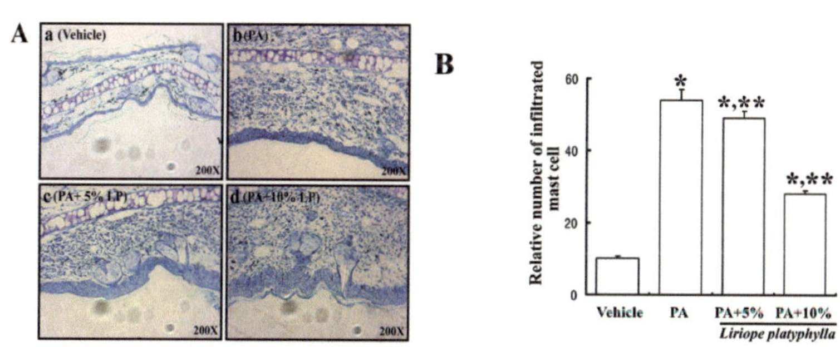

Figure 28. Effects of AELP on the mast cell infiltration. (A) The slide sections of ear tissue were stained with toluidine blue and observed at 400x magnification. Mast cells were stained with purple color in the dermis of ear tissue. (B) In each slide, five fields were randomly chosen and the number of mast cells was counted under a light microscope. Data shown are the means±SD (n=5). *P<0.05 is the significance level compared to the vehicle treated group. **P<0.05 is the significance level compared to the PA treated group.

3. Conclusion

The development and identification of novel therapeutic drugs for human chronic disease was considered as a very important project in the field of pharmacological and clinical research. Among the variety of approaches thus far pursued to develop novel drugs, identification and screening of natural compounds from medicinal herbs has proven a very effective one—not least, because this method saves a great deal of time and cost. Recently, some scientists including our group in Asia countries have reported the therapeutic effects of *L. platyphylla* on the human chronic disease. This chapter introduces some extracts and compound which may prove valuable in efforts to combat chronic diseases such as inflammation, neurodegenerative disorders, diabetes, obesity and atopic dermatitis.

Three extracts prepared with *n*-hexane, ethyl acetate and water was found to significantly induce anti-inflammation and anti-asthmatic effects in model animals. Some extracts of *L. platyphylla* play a role as insulin sensitizer in adipocytes and stimulator in insulinoma cells and the pancreas of mice. Additionally, butanol extracts and spicatoside A markedly induced NGF secretion and expression in some cell lines, while ethanol and methanol extracts induced in mice. Furthermore, recent studies showed that GGEx and water extracts prevented or improved the obesity and atopic dermatitis.

In conclusion, the results of above studies indicated that some extracts and compounds from *L. platyphylla* could contribute the relief and prevent of several chronic diseases including dementia, diabetes, obesity and atopic dermatitis. However, more research was needed to verify the action mechanism and toxicity side effects.

Acknowledgements

I would like to express my gratitude to my students, including JE Kim, SL Choi, IS Hwang, HR Lee, YJ Lee and MH Kwak for helping to compile this paper and with the graphics and charts herein.

Author details

Dae Youn Hwang

Pusan National University, Republic of Korea

References

[1] Wikipedia Foundation Inc. http://en.wikipedia.org/wiki/Liriope_muscari (accessed 20 July, 2012).

[2] Plantforafuture.http://server9.webmania.com/users/pfafardea/database/plants.php?Liriope+muscari (accessed 20 July, 2012).

[3] University of Florida IFAS Extension. http://edis.ifas.ufl.edu/pdffiles/FP/FP34800 (accessed 20 July, 2012).

[4] Broussard MC. A Horticultural Study of Liriope and Ophiopogon: Nomenclature, Morphology and Culture. PhD thesis. Louisiana State University; 2007.

[5] Jiang T, Tang XY, Wu JS, Wang LQ, Huang M, Han T, Qin LP. Study on Chemical Constituents of the Root of *Liriope platyphylla*. Zhong Yao Cai 2011;34(10) 1537-1539.

[6] Jiang T, Huang BK, Zhang QY, Han T, Zheng HC, Qin LP. Studies on Chemical Constituents of *Liriope platyphylla*. Zhong Yao Cai 2007;30(9) 1079-1081.

[7] Kim SW, Chang IM, Oh KB. Inhibition of the Bacterial Surface Protein Anchoring Transpeptidase Sortase by Medicinal Plants. Bioscience, Biotechnology, and Biochemistry 2002;66(12) 2751-2754.

[8] Lee YC, Lee JC, Seo YB, Kook YB. *Liriopis tuber* inhibit OVA-induced Airway Inflammation and Bronchial Hyperresponsiveness in Murine Model of Asthma. Journal of Ethnopharmacology 2005;101(1-3) 144-152.

[9] Choi SB, Wha JD, Park S. The Insulin Sensitizing Effect of Homoisoflavone-enriched Fraction in *Liriope platyphylla Wang et Tang* via PI3-kinase Pathway. Journal of Life Science 2004;75(22) 2653-2664.

[10] Rho SS, Choi HJ, Kim DH, Seo YB Studies of Anti-inflammation of *Liriopis Tuber* to Autoimmune Diabetes in NOD mice. Korean Journal of Oriental Physiology & Pathology 2008;22(4) 766-770.

[11] Kim JH, Kim JE, Lee YK, Nam SH, Her YK, Jee SW, Kim SG, Park DJ, Choi YW, Hwang DY. The Extracts from *Liriope platyphylla* Significantly Stimulated Insulin Secretion in the HIT-T15 Pancreatic β-cell Line. Journal of Life Science 2010;20(7) 1027-1033.

[12] Lee YK, Kim JE, Nam SH, Goo JS, Choi SI, Choi YH, Bae CJ, Woo JM, Cho JS, Hwang DY. Differential Regulation of the Biosynthesis of Glucose Transporters by the PI3-K and MAPK Pathways of Insulin Signaling by Treatment with Novel Compounds from *Liriope platyphylla*. International Journal of Molecular Medicine 2010;27(3) 319-327.

[13] Choi SI, Lee YK, Goo JS, Kim KE, Nam SH, Hwang IS, Lee YJ, Park SH, Lee HS, Lee JS, Jang IS, Son HJ, Hwang DY. Effects of Steaming Time and Frequency for Manufactured Red *Liriope platyphylla* on the Insulin Secretion Ability and Insulin Receptor Signaling Pathway. Laboratory Animal Research 2011;27(2) 117-126.

[14] Kim JE, Hwang IS, Goo JS, Nam SH, Choi SI, Lee HR, Lee YJ, Kim YH, Park SJ, Kim NS, Choi YH, Hwang DY. LP9M80-H Isolated from *Liriope platyphylla* Could Help Al-

leviate Diabetic Symptoms via the Regulation of Glucose and Lipid Concentration. Journal of Life Science 2010;22(5) 634-641.

[15] Hur J, Lee P, Kim J, Kim AJ, Kim H, Kim SY. Induction of Nerve Growth Factor by Butanol Fraction of *Liriope platyphylla* in C6 and Primary Astrocyte Cells. Biological and Pharmaceutical Bulletin 2004;27(8) 1257-1260.

[16] Hur J, Lee P, Moon E, Kang I, Kim SH, Oh MS, Kim SY. Neurite Outgrowth Induced by Spicatoside A, a Steroidal Saponin, via the Tyrosine Kinase A Receptor Pathway. European Journal of Pharmacology 2009;620(1-3) 9-15.

[17] Mun JH, Lee SG, Kim DH, Jung JW, Lee SJ, Yoon BH, Shin BY, Kim SH, Rye JH Neurotrophic Factors Mediate Memory Enhancing Property of Ethanolic Extract of *Liriope platyphylla* in mice. The Journal of Applied Pharmacology 2007;15 83-88.

[18] Nam SH, Choi SI, Goo JS, Kim JE, Lee YK, Hwang IS, Lee HR, Lee YJ, Lee HG, Choi YW, Hwang DY. LP-M, a Novel Butanol-extracts Isolated from *Liriope platyphylla*, Could Induce the Neuronal Cell Survival and Neuritic Outgrowth in Hippocampus of Mice through Akt/ERK Activation on NGF Signal Pathway. Journal of Life Science 2011;9 1234-1243.

[19] Jeong SH, Chae KS, Jung YS, Rho YH, Lee JM, Ha JR, Yoon KH, Kim GC, Shin SS,Yoon MC. The Korean Traditional Medicine Gyeongshingangjeehwan Inhibits Obesity through the Regulation of Leptin and PPARα Action in OLETF Rats. Journal of Ethnopharmacology 2008;119 245-251.

[20] Kim JE, Lee YK, Nam SH, Choi SI, Goo JS, Jang MJ, Lee HS, Son HJ, Lee CY, Hwang DY. The Symptoms of Atopic Dermatitis in NC/Nga Mice Were Significantly Relieved by the Water Extract of *Liriope platyphylla*. Laboratory Animal Research 2010;26(4) 377-384.

[21] Joost H, Thorens B. "The Extended GLUT-family of Sugar/polyol Transport Facilitators: Nomenclature, Sequence Characteristics, and Potential Function of its Novel Members (review)". Molecular Membrane Biology 2001;18(4) 247–256.

[22] Bell G, Kayano T, Buse J, Burant C, Takeda J, Lin D, Fukumoto H, Seino S. "Molecular Biology of Mammalian Glucose Transporters". Diabetes Care 1990;13(3) 198–208.

[23] Thorens B. Glucose Transporters in the Regulation of Intestinal, Renal, and Liver Glucose Fluxes. The American Journal of Physiology 1996;270(4 Pt 1) G541–553.

[24] Mandel RJ, Gage FH, Clevenger DG, Spratt SK, Snyder RO, Leff SE. Nerve Growth Factor Expressed in the Medial Septum Following *in vivo* Gene Delivery Using a Recombinant Adeno-Associated Viral Vector Protects Cholinergic Neurons from Fimbria–formix Lesion-induced Degeneration. Experimental Neurology 1999;155 59–64.

[25] Gustilo MC, Markowska AL, Breckler SJ, Fleischman CA, Price DL, Koliatsos VE. Evidence that Nerve Growth Factor Influences Recent Memory through Structural Changes in Septohippocampal Cholinergic neurons. The Journal of Comparative Neurology 1999;405(4) 491–507.

[26] Pesavento E, Capsoni S, Domenici L, Cattaneo A. Acute Cholinergic Rescue of Synaptic Plasticity in the Neurodegenerating Cortex of Anti-nerve-growth-factor Mice. European Journal of Neuroscience 2002;15(6) 1030-1036.

[27] Jozsef S, Peter E. Cellular Components of Nerve Growth Factor Signaling. Biochimica et Biophysica Acta. Molecular cell research 1994;1222 187-202.

[28] Considine RV, Alexiu A, Lemonnier D. Dietary-induced Obesity: Effect of Dietary Fats on Adipose Tissue Cellularity in Mice. The British Journal of Nurition 1983;49(1)17-26.

Chapter 11

Investigation on the Mechanism of Qi-Invigoration from a Perspective of Effects of Sijunzi Decoction on Mitochondrial Energy Metabolism

Xing-Tai Li

Additional information is available at the end of the chapter

http://dx.doi.org/10.5772/54760

1. Introduction

Traditional Chinese medicine (TCM) is an ancient Chinese medical system that takes a deep understanding of the laws and patterns of nature and applies them to the human body. TCM, which is also considered as an alternative medicine, is gradually being accepted and is practiced even in the Western world, is the quintessence of the Chinese cultural heritage, has made an everlasting contribution to the survival, propagation and prosperity of all ethnic groups in China, thereby enhancing the fertility and prosperity of the nation. TCM has been practiced by the Chinese for five thousands of years and is rooted in meticulous observation of how nature, the cosmos, and the human body are interacting. Major theories include: Qi, Yin and Yang, the Five Phases (Wu Xing), the human body Meridian system (Jingluo) and viscera and bowels (Zang Fu organs) theory.

Western medicine places strong emphasis on the physical structures of the body, which are made up of different organic and inorganic substances, proteins, cells and tissues. These substances form the physiological basis of humans. Western medicine treats disease at microscopic point of view. TCM, on the other hand, views life differently. Instead of emphasizing discrete body components, the body is seen as a whole entity with connecting parts that work together to sustain life. TCM studies the world from the macroscopic point of view, and its target is to maintain the original harmony of human being [1]. Qi, Blood and Body Fluids are the most important fundamental substances necessary for life. Western Medicine is different from TCM because the TCM has a concept of Qi as a form of energy. It is suggested that Qi was "born" at the same instant as the rest of the universe, and that we are all born from the Qi of the universe. The ancient concepts of Qi are the foundation of TCM and accordingly, disease or sickness is caused by a disruptive flow of energy or the imbalance of the Yin and Yang energies around our human bodies. Hence, TCM provides a holistic treatment [2]. Qi is said to be the unseen vital force that nourishes one's body and sustains one's life. An individual would become ill or dies if one's Qi in the body is imbalanced or exhausted [1].

The total loss of Qi is what Chinese medicine refers to as death. And here are Chinese people from all walks of life as they seek relief, through a rebalancing of their Qi, their vital energy, for ailments from colds to cancer. The ultimate goal of Tai Chi is to control and direct the Qi within the body. But does Qi really exist? It has no place in Western medical practice, but is essential to the practice of traditional medicine in China. Have ever you had a dramatic spiritual or emotional experience and felt energy literally rushing through your body? I believe this is Qi energy at work, moving through the body. The two types of medical practice existed side by side in China, and had little intercourse with one another. And from the Chinese perspective, Qi is the origin of true strength and power as well as genuine health—body, mind, and spirit.

All kinds of diseases and ailments are born from Qi in TCM, Qi deficiency is the common cause of a variety of diseases and can lead to energy metabolism dysfunction, and Qi-invigoration is the basic principle for treatment of Qi deficiency. Due to the popularity and therapeutic values of "Qi-invigorating" herbal formulae, the investigation of biological activities and the underlying mechanisms in relation to "Qi-invigoration" is of great pharmacological interest. However, the mechanisms for Qi-invigoration in TCM remain elusive. In this regard, our previous studies show that all the four widely used Qi-invigorating herbal medcines (including ginseng, astragalus root, pilose asiabell root, white atractylodes rhizome) can increase bioenergy level of liver cells *in vivo*. We propose a hypothesis that Qi is closely related to bioenergy according to the ancient concept of Qi and modern bioenergetics [3]. The Qi-invigorating representative prescription Sijunzi Decoction (SD) is widely used for treatment of Qi deficiency. However, the pharmacological basis of "Qi-invigorating" action has yet to be established. This chapter aims to provide a comprehensive overview of Qi and Qi-invigoration in TCM, analyze mitochondrial protection and energy metabolic improvement of SD, find its underlying mechanism, thus further reveal the nature of Qi-invigoration in TCM from mitochondrial energy metabolism perspective, help to interpret the concept of Qi scientifically, and provide a new way of thinking and scientific evidence in guiding Qi-invigorating prescriptions for the treatment of energy metabolism- and mitochondria-related diseases. The mechanism of SD on energy metabolism improvement will be explored from mitochondrial oxidative phosphorylation and intracellular adenylates levels.

2. The ancient Chinese philosophy background in formation of Qi concept in TCM

Perhaps the greatest genius of the ancient Chinese sages, and the insight that has given TCM its uninterrupted longevity and effectiveness as a complete medical system, was their discovery of Qi that gives life to everything in the universe and is everything in the universe at the very root of reality. It's impossible to really understand TCM and its incredible healing power throughout the millennia without realizing the importance of Qi. The unseen power and intelligence that animates and orchestrates all physical and metaphysical processes is Qi. It is Qi that delivers the necessary information and messages between all body structures and systems, and it is Qi that enables us to connect with the natural world and the Universal. Qi is the life force that permeates everything in the universe. Without it there can be no growth and change. Your physical body cannot exist without Qi. When you die your Qi leaves–it's transformed.

The theory of Qi in ancient philosophy was introduced into the medical field, the basic theory of Qi in TCM was formed, i.e., the concept of Qi in TCM was established during the mutual penetration between the materialist philosophy and medicine in ancient China. Qi has been used as a healing technique in China for 4000 years. The origin of the character of Qi was traced back to 3500 years ago. Confucius (who lived approximately 2500 years ago), taught moral and ethical behavior. In his Analects, the character of Qi appeared in four locations. It expressed the concept related to breathe, food and vitality.

Taoism, which was founded by Lao-Tze (who was believed to have lived around the time of Confucius or 100 later), have had more influence on Qi and Qigong. In the book "Zhuangzi", which compiled the thoughts of Lao-Tze in the third century BC, the character of Qi appeared 39 times. What it explained was: "Qi exists throughout the universe, when Qi assembles, it appears as a human life; when Qi disassembles, the human will die. Therefore, do not worry about life and death. Live naturally and freely as you are". When one studies the principle of the Life Force, the Qi and the Tao (Yin and Yang); one would understand how this Life Force manifests in nature. Through self-cultivation, one basically enriches one's Qi for optimum health and longevity. This happens when one subscribes to this Life Force from nature that flows freely into one's mind and body. However, this requires one to live freely from desires, worries and emotions. To live freely, one has to detach from the worldly possessions. For the instance, money is to be spent, there is to-ing and fro-ing, thus a going and a coming of it; and there is a non-attachment to the money or the material things for better flow. Furthermore, one is required to discipline oneself by having a proper diet, sleep and exercise so that one would not disturb and interrupt with the movement of Life Force which may cause the Qi to dissipate in one's body. This dissipation of Qi would result one to fall into sickness, disease, physical and mental sufferings. It is the Taoist's belief that the practice of Qigong, Tai Chi movements and meditation helps one to harmonize one's Life force with one's environment and nature [2].

"Two classic medical texts, the Nei Jing (compiled from 100 B.C. to 100 A.D.) and the Nan Jing (written circa 100 to 200 A.D.) were important early documents that presented the core concepts of TCM, and they have informed generations of scholars and practitioners ever since. These core concepts suggest that disease is the result of imbalances in the flow of the body's Qi, and that the human body is a microcosm of the basic natural forces at work in the universe. Generally speaking, Qi is an essential substance that is full of vigor and flows fast. The Yellow Emperor's Inner Canon (Nei Jing) teaches us: "It is from calm, indifference, emptiness, and nondesiring that true Qi arises. If the spirit is harboured inside, whence can illness arise? When the will is at rest and wishes little, when the heart is at peace and fears nothing, when the body labours but does not tire, then Qi flows smoothly from these states, each part follows its desires, and the whole gets everything it seeks'. The Chinese philosopher, Mencius (372–289 BC) described Qi in terms of moral energy, related to human excellence. This reinforces the argument that Qi is contextual, fluid in nature and not a fixed entity.

3. The concept of Qi

Qi is the hub from basic theory to clinical practice and health longevity in TCM. The true foundation of TCM is Qi. Qi, is an important category in the ancient Chinese philosophy, is a simple understanding of natural phenomena. In TCM, Qi is constantly in motion, is the subtle substance with a strong vitality which constitute the human body and maintain the activities of human life, is one of the most basic material, it is also known as the "essence Qi". When the concept Qi in TCM was used to discuss the human body, it often has the meaning of both life material and physiological functions. Therefore, Qi in TCM is one of the most important basic concepts. Qi is the basis for unifying theories of TCM, and Qi theory is the core of the basic theories of TCM. According to TCM, " Qi is fundamental to human, both life and death of human all depend on Qi, if Qi gets together, it will result to the birth; if Qi is harmonious, then the human body is healthy; if Qi decline, the body is weak; if Qi is disordered, the human will be sick; if Qi is depleted, the human will die; therefore, unharmonious Qi is fundamental to the disease." The concept of Qi is complex and messy, connotation of Qi is colorful, extension of Qi is all-pervasive and unlimited, Qi becomes the enigma of Chinese medicine. Because modern medicine has not the concept of "Qi", Qi is the biggest difference between Chinese and Western medicine, which caused communication barriers between the two systems of medicine.

3.1. The meanings of Qi

What is Qi? The concept of Qi is based on the ancient Chinese initial understanding of natural phenomena. That is, Qi is the most basic substance of which the world is comprised. Everything in the universe results from the movements and changes of Qi. This concept was introduced into TCM and became one of its characteristics. The meaning of Qi in TCM has two aspects. One refers to the vital substances comprising the human body and maintaining its life activities, such as the Qi of water and food (food essence), the Qi of breathing (breathing nutrients) and so on. The other refers to the physiological functions of viscera and bowels, Meridian system, such as the Qi of the heart, the lung, the spleen and the stomach and so on.

The ancient Chinese people believed Qi was the most fundamental entity making up the world. The Chinese character for "Qi" is the same word used for air or gas, and it is thought to have the same properties as these substances. While Qi is often described in the West as energy, or vital energy, the term Qi carries a deeper meaning. Qi has two aspects: one is energy, power, or force; the other is conscious intelligence or information. Qi can be interpreted as the "life energy" or "life force," which flows within us. Sometimes, it is known as the "vital energy" of the body. In fact, it may be difficult to find one equivalent English word or phrase that completely describes the nature of Qi. Most often, Qi is best defined according to its functions and properties. In the human body, Qi flows through meridians, or energy pathways. Twelve major meridians run through the body, and it is over this network that Qi travels through the body and that the body's various organs send messages to one another.

3.2. The sources of Qi

Man depends on nature for his production and growth and must observe the common laws of the world. As everything in the world comes from the interaction of Heaven Qi and Earth Qi, man must breathe to absorb Heaven Qi and eat to absorb Earth Qi. The food Essence transformed and transported by the Spleen[1] must be sent up to the Lung to combine with fresh air to produce the nutrients necessary for man's life activities. Qi of the human body comes from the combination of three kinds of Qi, Primordial Qi inherited from parents, the fresh air inhaled by the Lung and the refined food Essence transformed by the Spleen. Both the inherited and the acquired vital energies are further processed and transformed by the organs. The kidney first sends the innate vital substance upwards where it combines with food essence derived from the spleen. It further mixes with the fresh air from the lungs where it finally forms into Qi of the body.

By understanding how Qi is formed, TCM has identified two important factors necessary for maintaining health. By eating a healthy diet and breathing fresh air, the body extracts their most valuable essences and uses them to help form the vital energy. Following these simple principles are the first steps towards creating a healthy balance in the body. By keeping your daily source of energy—Acquired Qi—strong and balanced, energy is saved because a healthy Spleen and Stomach can extract more Qi from food and drink. Choosing food wisely and eating at regular intervals helps accomplish this.

3.3. The functions of Qi

Generally speaking, Qi of the human body has five functions: promoting, warming, defending, controlling and transforming. Qi provides the active, vital energy necessary for the growth and development of the human body and to perform the physiological functions of the organs, meridians and tissues. In addition, Qi promotes the formation and circulation of blood and

1 Both TCM and western medicine have the name of"spleen" organ, but connections and differences between them were perceived. TCM practitioners pay more attention to the function than the organ entity in the viscera concept. The Spleen is one of the viscera (zàng) organs stipulated by TCM, it is a functionally defined entity and not equivalent to the anatomical organ of the same name in Western medicine. The Spleen transforms and transports food Essence from the food after it has been preprocessed by the Stomach and the Small Intestine, and then distributes it to the whole body, especially upwards to the Lung and Heart, where food Essence is transformed into Qi and Blood. In this spirit, the Spleen is also called "root of the postnatal". Thus, TCM also describes the Spleen as the source of "production and mutual transformation" of Qi and Blood. The function "the Spleen governs transportation and absorption" and that of the pancreas have many things in common, therefore, the Spleen in TCM should include spleen and pancreas in Western medicine. The Spleen also assists the body's water metabolism, exercises control over the blood inside the vessels and governs muscles and limbs. Whereas spleen is the largest lymphoid organ in the human body in Western medicine, and its main function is to participate in the function of the immune response of the lymphoid tissue and it is closely related to cellular and humoral immunity.The author considers that the core connotation of the Spleen in TCM is energy metabolism, i.e.,the process of cellular energy metabolism is the function of the Spleen, where organelles that in charge of the energy metabolism in the cell (i.e., mitochondria) may attribute to the Spleen in TCM.

supports the metabolism of body fluid. If there is a deficiency of Qi, its promoting functions are weakened. As a result, growth and development can be affected or delayed, the organs and meridians cannot function properly and blood formation is hampered, leading to a series of health problems. Qi also contains heat energy for the body. Being a heat source, Qi warms the body and keeps it at a constant temperature so normal physiological functions can take place. Deficiency of Qi can lead to a lowered body temperature, intolerance of cold and cold hands and feet. In TCM, "Evils" are environmental factors that lead to illness. They are classified as wind, summer heat, dampness, dryness, cold and fire. One of the main causes of disease is the invasion of "Evils". By resisting the entry of "illness evils" into the body, Qi defends against their attack and maintains healthy physiological functions.

Qi consolidates and retains the body's substances and organs by holding everything in its proper place. Qi keeps the blood flowing within the vessels and prevents it leaking out, controls and adjusts the secretion and excretion of sweat, urine and saliva, and keeps body fluids from escaping the body, consolidates and stores sperm to prevent premature ejaculation, and consolidates the organs and stops them from descending into a position where they cannot function properly. If Qi is deficient, the consolidating function is weakened, leading to various kinds of health problems such as haemorrhage, frequent urination, premature ejaculation and stomach or kidney prolapses. The promoting and consolidating functions work in a complementary manner. For example, Qi promotes blood circulation and the distribution of body fluids, but it also controls and adjusts the secretion of fluid substances. The balance between these two functions is essential for maintaining a healthy blood circulation and water metabolism. Qi also possesses vaporization or "transformation" functions, which are important for the metabolism of fundamental substances. As suggested by these words, Qi may "vaporize" substances in the body and transform them into essence or vital energy. For example, certain actions of Qi allow food to be changed into food essence, which is in turn transformed into different types of Qi and blood. Indigestible food and waste are also transformed by Qi into urine and stools for excretion.

3.4. The movement of Qi

Qi flows throughout the whole body because of its strength and vigor. The movement of Qi is called Mechanism of Qi, which can be generalized as four aspects: ascending, descending, entering and exiting movements, which are based on directions. Qi was originally a philosophic concept. Through out the ages, the Chinese have developed working constructs which serve to explain the observable phenomenon of the natural world. The idea of Qi is one of the most basic building blocks upon which the Chinese, of both ancient and modern times, conceive the universe. The concept of Qi is a fundamental stratagem in the practice of any Chinese art and is at the root of Chinese medical theory. According to Chinese thought, Qi is an invisible energy-like phenomenon which is present in every animate or inanimate object in the universe. It is a difficult concept to explain but Qi can almost be thought of as an adhesive which holds the cosmos together; the inertia through which all is create and destroyed. The ancient Chinese philosophy holds that Qi is this most basic substance constituting the world. Accordingly, TCM also believes that Qi is the most fundamental substance in the construction of the human body and in the maintenance of its life activities. Therefore, any substantial matter can be regarded as a special process of the movement of Qi, and life, in essence, is the course of Qi's ascending, descending, exiting and entering movements in given conditions.

3.5. The relations between Qi and blood, Yin and Yang

In TCM theory, blood and Qi are inseparable. Blood is the "mother" of Qi; it carries Qi and also provides nutrients for its movement. In turn, Qi is the "commander" of the blood. This means that Qi is the force that makes blood flow throughout the body and provides the intelligence that guides it to the places where it needs to be. Losing too much blood causes an overall Qi deficiency. When there is a Qi deficiency, the body cannot function properly and therefore presents with a fever. In the treatment of such Blood Deficiency, supplementing Qi plays an even more important role than nourishing Blood. Bleeding, for another example, may be the result of Qi deficiency because Qi controls Blood flow, so such bleeding should be treated by strengthening Qi. TCM understands that everything is composed of two complementary energies; one energy is Yin and the other is Yang. They are never separate; one cannot exist without the other. Yin and Yang come from Qi. Qi is required to harmonize Yin and Yang.

4. Mitochondrial energy metabolism – Its related diseases and ageing

After the symbiotic engulfment of aerobic α-proteobacteria by pre-eukaryotic cells more than 1.5 billion years ago, mitochondria evolved as specialized organelles with a plethora of cellular functions. Over recent years, mitochondria have taken center stage as remarkably autonomous and dynamic cellular organelles that are intimately involved in orchestrating a diverse range of cellular activities. Mitochondria regulate the life and death of cells by manipulating several factors, including bioenergetics, mitochondrial permeability transition, and mitochondrial redox-status, they are usually regarded as specialized organelles for cellular respiration and oxidative phosphorylation (OXPHOS). Mitochondria are the driving force behind life, over 80% of the energy which is required by an adult is produced by OXPHOS under normal physiological condition. Energy metabolism would be regulated by the relative amount of adenosine triphosphate (ATP) available, as described by adenylate energy charge (AEC). ATP has been called the energy "currency" of the cell. The electron transport chain (ETC) in the mitochondrial inner membrane is actively involved in ATP synthesis in combination with respiration. The impaired ETC works less efficiently in ATP synthesis and generates more reactive oxygen species (ROS), which will cause further oxidative damage to various biomolecules. In the aging process, oxidative damage ultimately leads to a progressive decline in bioenergetic function and enhanced mitochondrial oxidative stress. Lower ATP levels can decrease the efficiency of energy-dependent processes and ATP-mediated signal transductions. Inadequate ATP availability would initiate and accentuate the adverse consequences of energy-dependent pathways. The energy depletion and enhanced oxidative stress can lead to the aging process. As the "hubs" for cellular metabolism, mitochondria are crucial for both life and death of eukaryotic cells, and are the main switch of cell apoptosis.

Dysfunction of mitochondria has severe cellular consequences and is linked to ageing and neurodegeneration in human. Since discovery of the first case of mitochondrial disease in 1959, with the depth of mitochondrial research and the rapid development of mitochondrial medicine, the number of mitochondria-related diseases is rapidly amplified, mitochondrial dysfunction would undermine the function of cells, tissues and organs, thereby causing cancer, myasthenia gravis, obesity, stroke, cardiovascular disease (ischemic reperfusion injury, hypertension, coronary heart disease, heart failure, diabetes and atherosclerosis, etc.), age-related diseases, neurodegenerative diseases (Parkinson's disease, Alzheimer's disease, depression etc.), and aging etc. These diseases is today's major diseases that threaten human health, mitochondria has become a new target for the treatment of diseases, because mitochondrial oxidative damage is the main reason for cell damage and death, the general treatment program to treat a variety of mitochondrial diseases is the reduction in mitochondrial oxidative damage. Therefore, mitochondrial protection is an important mechanism for the treatment of mitochondrial-related diseases.

Bioenergetics research in life sciences have played an important role, Mitchell's chemiosmotic theory earned the 1978 Nobel Prize in Chemistry, as the coupling between electron transport in the respiratory chain and adenosine diphosphate (ADP) phosphorylation which is caused by electrochemical gradient of protons between inner and outer mitochondrial membrane was expounded; Nobel Prize in Chemistry in 1997 was awarded academician PD Boyer in the U.S. Academy of Sciences for elucidating generation mechanism of ATP—the most important energy molecules. The work was closely related to the energy production and consumption which is required for life activities. According to the modern life science, energy metabolism is the center for life activity, if the energy metabolism is normal, the body can carry out normal vital activities, if no bio-energy is supplied for the body, the life activities cease immediately. Therefore, Qi and bioenergy have identical functions.

4.1. Energy metabolism in mammalian cells

Mitochondria have been described by cytologists since the mid 19th century. According to Scheffler [4], the term mitochondrion was coined by Benda in 1898. However, only in the mid 20th century the role of the mitochondria in oxidative energy metabolism was established in detail [5]. All cells in the body depend on a continuous supply of ATP in order to perform their different physiological and biochemical activities. Mitochondria have a central role in the energy metabolism. Part of the free energy derived from the oxidation of food inside mitochondria is transformed to ATP, energy currency of the cell. This process depends on oxygen. When oxygen is limited, glycolytic products are metabolized directly in the cytosol by the less efficient anaerobic respiration that is independent of mitochondria. The following describes the basic processes occurring in a typical normal cell, using glucose as a major source of energy (Figure 1). The breakdown of glucose into water and CO_2 includes two steps, namely, glycolysis (the anaerobic phase) taking place in the cytoplasm, and OXPHOS (the aerobic phase) occurring in the mitochondria. Of the total yield of 38 ATP per mole of glucose, two are produced in the glycolysis process and 36 during the OXPHOS. It is important to note that oxygen availability in the mitochondrion is a critical factor for the normal ATP production in the cell. The end product of glycolysis, pyruvate, is transported into the mitochondria by a specific carrier protein. The pyruvate is transformed, in the matrix of the mitochondria, into acetyl coenzyme A that activates the tricarboxylic acid (TCA) (Krebs) cycle. In the absence of oxygen, the end product of pyruvate is lactate that may leave the cell and pass into the microcirculatory blood stream via the monocarboxylase transporter located in the plasma membrane [6].

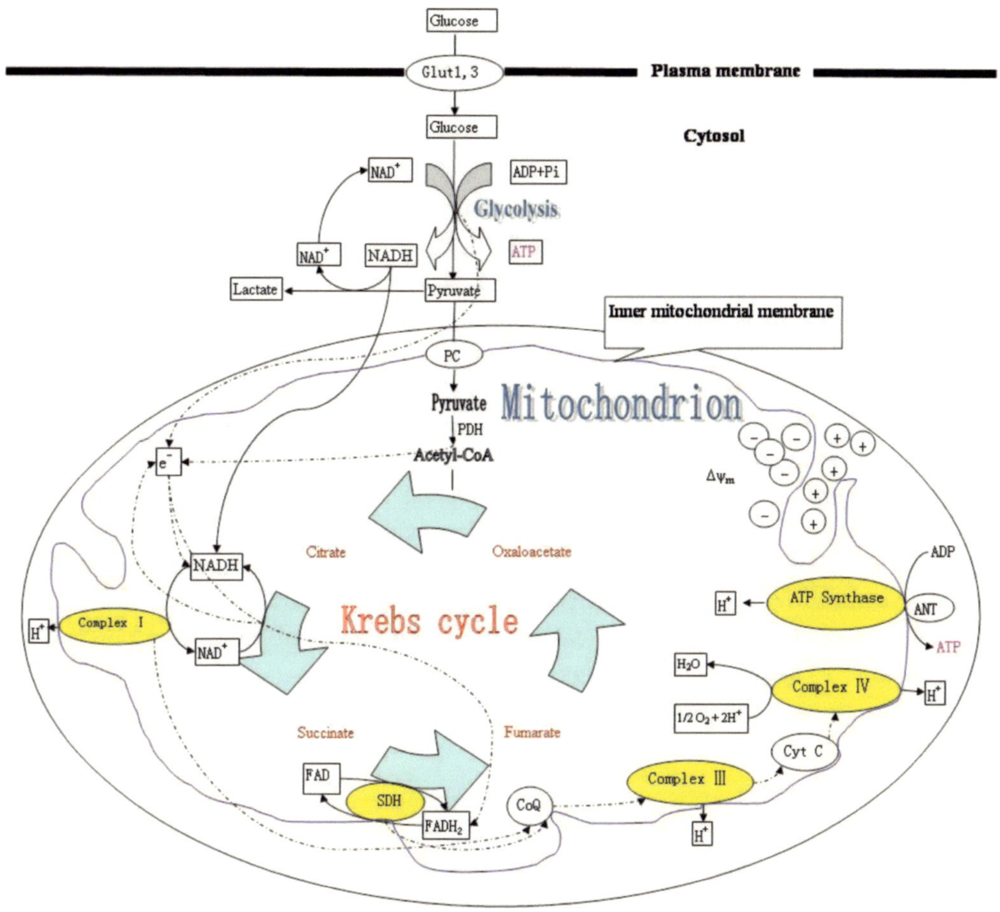

Figure 1. Overview of the cellular energy metabolic pathways. Mitochondria can metabolize fuels, such as fatty acids, amino acids and pyruvate, derived from glucose. When glucose enters the cell via glucose transporters, it is metabolized by glycolysis to pyruvate. Pyruvate prevalently enters mitochondria through its specific carrier (PC), with only a small amount being metabolized to lactate due to the excess of NADH. In mitochondria, pyruvate dehydrogenase complex (PDH) converts pyruvate into acetyl-CoA, which feeds into the Krebs cycle, of which the net reactive result is to generate NADH and $FADH_2$. The respiratory chain consists of four enzyme complexes (complexes I–IV) (yellow), and two mobile carriers (coenzyme Q and cytochrome c) along which the electrons liberated by the oxidation of NADH and $FADH_2$ are passed, and ultimately transferred to oxygen. This respiratory process which electrons pass through generates membrane potential ($\Delta\psi_m$)– the main driving force for ATP synthesis used by the ATP synthase to phosphorylate ADP and produce ATP, that in turn is carried to the cytosol by adenine nucleotide translocase (ANT) in exchange for ADP.

The mitochondrial ATP production relies on the ETC, composed of respiratory chain complexes I–IV, which transfer electrons in a stepwise fashion until they finally reduce oxygen to form water. The NADH and $FADH_2$ formed in glycolysis, fatty-acid oxidation and the citric acid cycle are energy-rich molecules that donate electrons to the ETC. Electrons move toward compounds with more positive oxidative potentials and the incremental release of energy during the electron transfer is used to pump protons (H^+) into the intermembrane space. Complexes I, III and IV function as H^+ pumps that are driven by the free energy of coupled oxidation reactions. During the electron transfer, protons are always pumped from the mitochondrial matrix to the intermembrane space, resulting in a potential of ~150–180 mV. Proton gradient generates a chemiosmotic potential, also known as the proton motive force, which drives the ADP phosphorylation via the ATP synthase (F_oF_1 ATPase i.e., complex V). F_o domain of ATPase couples a proton translocation across the inner mitochondrial membrane (IMM) with the phosphorylation of ADP to ATP [7]. The energy-transducing function is maintained by the mitochondrial inner membrane and over 95% of total cellular ATP is supplied by mitochondrial phosphorylation [8]. Cellular activities can, therefore, be adversely affected by damage to the mitochondrial energy-transducing functions [9]. The rate of mitochondrial respiration depends on the phosphorylation potential expressed as a [ATP]/[ADP] [Pi] ratio across the IMM that is regulated by the adenine nucleotide translocase (ANT). In the case of increased cellular energy demand when the phosphorylation potential is decreased and more ADP is available, a respiration rate is increased leading to an increased ATP synthesis. There is usually a tight coupling between the electron transport and the ATP synthesis and an inhibition of ATP synthase will therefore also inhibit the electron transport and cellular respiration. Under certain conditions, protons can reenter into mitochondrial matrix without contributing to the ATP synthesis and the energy of proton electrochemical gradient will be released as heat. This process, known as proton leak or mitochondrial uncoupling, could be mediated by protonophores (such as FCCP) and uncoupling proteins (UCPs) [10]. As a consequence, uncoupling leads to a low ATP production concomitant with high levels of electron transfer and high cellular respiration [11].

From its role as the cellular powerhouse, the mitochondrion is emerging as a key participant in cell death. Apoptosis and necrosis are two alternative forms of cell death, with well-defined morphological and biochemical differences [12]. One crucial physiological difference between cells that undergo apoptosis or necrosis is intracellular ATP level. Complex I plays a major role in mitochondrial OXPHOS, include oxidizing NADH in the mitochondrial matrix, reducing ubiquinone to ubiquinol and pumping protons across the inner membrane to drive ATP synthesis [13]. Since its inhibition results in incomplete mitochondrial electron transport and disturbance of mitochondrial energy metabolism, dysfunction of Complex I in the hippocampus during the initial prolonged epileptic seizure may conceivably lead to necrosis because of a decrease in ATP production [14]. Mitochondrial creatine kinase is an important component of the cellular energy buffering and transport system, connecting oxidative phosphorylation to ATP consumption. The reduced activity of creatine kinase may lead to a decreased cellular ATP/ADP ratio [15].

4.2. The dysfunction of mitochondrial energy metabolism and human diseases

The role of mitochondria in mammalian cells is generally presented as a "central pathway" for energy metabolism, but mitochondria house many additional metabolic pathways and play a key role in apoptosis, free radical production, thermogenesis and calcium signaling. As a consequence, impairment of mitochondrial function is associated with a clinically heterogeneous group of human disorders, often referred to as mitochondrial cytopathies [16]. In recent years, much attention has been attributed to the dysfunction of mitochondrial energy metabolism, which has not only been associated with cardiac failure but also to numerous other disorders, such as cancer, diabetes, obesity and general senescence. The mitochondrion hosts the enzymes of the Krebs cycle and the complexes of the ETC which generate ATP by oxidation of carbohydrates, fatty acids and amino acids. It therefore functions as the foremost supplier of energy substrate to maintain systemic energy balance and homeostasis [17]. Mitochondrial OXPHOS serves a central role for energy homeostasis in mammals. Impaired mitochondrial OXPHOS contributes to the pathogenesis of a wide range of disease conditions, including metabolic disorders, neurodegeneration, and heart failure. Genetic control of mitochondrial biogenesis and function has been an active area of research in recent years [18].

In addition to the mitochondrial role in cellular bioenergetics, the pivotal role of mitochondrial dysfunction in various human diseases has become increasingly clear. For example, the involvement of the mitochondria in tumor cell pathogenesis was initially described by Warburg 80 years ago, and later followed by many studies. The pioneering work of Warburg on the metabolism of tumors led to the hypothesis that the development of cancer may originate when cellular glycolysis increases, while mitochondrial respiration becomes impaired [19-21]. Warburg's hypothesis, termed the "Warburg effect", explains the significance of cellular energy metabolism in the pathophysiology of cancer cells. Since then, a large body of investigations has shown the involvement of the mitochondria in many human diseases.

Mitochondrial oxidative damage is a major factor in many human disorders, including mitochondrial hepatopathies, chronic hepatitis C, steatosis, early graft dysfunction after liver transplantation, ischemia–reperfusion injury, ageing and inflammatory damage [22]. Oxidative damage accumulates more in mitochondria than in the rest of the cells because electrons continually leak from the respiratory chain to form damaging ROS. This oxidative damage may modify mitochondrial proteins, DNA and lipids which may lead to mitochondrial bioenergetics failure leading to necrotic or apoptotic cell death [23]. Despite the collection of vast knowledge on the mitochondrial function and human health, the accumulated information did not translate into practical clinical tools, such as new drugs or medical devices.

Decreased levels of ATP and phosphocreatine were observed in brains of portacaval-shunted rats infused with ammonia [24] as well as in rats with chronic hepatic encephalopathy (HE) [25]. Reduced brain ATP levels were likewise reported in rats with acute hyperammonemia [26]. Further, decreased levels of ATP were observed in cultured astrocytes treated with ammonium chloride [27]. Recent studies have also indicated reduced levels of AMP and ADP in rats with acute hyperammonemia, and such decrease was found to be due to increased activity of AMP deaminase and adenosine deaminase [28,29]. Another possible mechanism for impaired energy metabolism in HE and hyperammonemia is the mitochondrial permeability transition (MPT). The MPT is characterized by a sudden increase in the permeability of the IMM to small solutes (ions and other molecules <1500 Da). The MPT is due to the opening of the permeability transition pore (PTP) in the IMM, usually in response to an increase in mitochondrial Ca^{2+} levels. This leads to a collapse of the mitochondrial inner membrane potential that is created by the pumping out of protons by the electron transport chain. Loss of the membrane potential leads to colloid osmotic swelling of the mitochondrial matrix, movement of metabolites across the inner membrane (e.g., Ca^{2+}, Mg^{2+}, glutathione, and NADPH), defective OXPHOS, cessation of ATP synthesis, and the generation of ROS. The latter acts to further aggravate the MPT [30,31]. Ca^{2+} is a well known inducer of the MPT [32]. Mitochondrial ATP-sensitive K^+ channel (mitoK_{ATP}) opening results in decreased mitochondrial ROS production. In addition, under energy deprivation conditions, mitoK_{ATP} opening inhibits mitochondrial ATP hydrolysis by ATP synthase, which helps to keep the cytosolic ATP/ADP ratio and also to limit mitochondrial Ca^{2+} uptake, indirectly preventing MPT [15].

As noted in the above sections dealing with glycolysis, TCA cycle and OXPHOS, various animal models of acute liver failure (ALF) have been used to examine bioenergetic events in ALF. These studies described several abnormalities in cerebral energy metabolism, including glucose utilization [33], reduction in TCA cycle enzyme activity [34], decreased rate of respiratory chain activity [35], inhibition of creatine kinase activity [36], and reduced levels of ATP [37]. Studies showing the induction of the MPT in ammonia-treated cultured astrocytes, as well as in brains of rats with ALF suggest that the MPT plays a crucial role in the bioenergetic failure associated with HE and hyperammonemia. Hypertrigliceridemic liver mitochondria have a higher resting respiration rate but normal OXPHOS efficiency. The mild uncoupling mediated by mitoK_{ATP} accelerates respiration rates and reduces ROS generation [38]. Since the mitochondria are involved in a wide range of diseases, a new therapeutic approach was developed 30 years ago, aimed to develop drugs targeting the mitochondria.

4.3. Mitochondrial energy metabolism and ageing

Ageing is a process characterized by a general decline in physiological functions, and it is also considered as a major risk factor for many age-related diseases, including, but not limited to, neurodegenerative diseases, cardiovascular disorders, and metabolic diseases [39-41]. Ageing can be defined as "a progressive, generalized impairment of function, resulting in an increased vulnerability to environmental challenge and a growing risk of disease and death". Ageing is likely a multifactorial process caused by accumulated damage to a variety of cellular components. During the last 20 years, gerontological studies have revealed different molecular pathways involved in the ageing process and pointed out mitochondria as one of the key regulators of longevity. Increasing age in mammals correlates with increased levels of mitochondrial DNA (mtDNA) mutations and a deteriorating respiratory chain function. Experimental evidence in the mouse has linked increased levels of somatic mtDNA mutations to a variety of ageing phenotypes, such as osteoporosis, hair loss, graying of the hair, weight reduction and decreased fertility. A mosaic respiratory chain deficiency in a subset of cells in various tissues, such as heart, skeletal muscle, colonic crypts and neurons, is typically found in aged humans. It has been known for a long time that respiratory chain-deficient cells are more prone to undergo apoptosis and an increased cell loss is therefore likely of importance in the age-associated mitochondrial dysfunction [42]. In this part, I'd like to point out the link between the mitochondrial energy balance and ageing, as well as a possible connection between the mitochondrial metabolism and molecular pathways important for the lifespan extension.

Mitochondrial theory of ageing: Even though the process of oxidative phosphorylation is efficient, a small percentage of electrons may "leak" from the ETC, particularly from complexes I and III, during normal respiration and prematurely reduce oxygen, forming ROS [43]. Mitochondria is a well known source of cellular ROS; when an electron escapes from the mitochondrial electron transport chain, especially at complex I or III, it may react with molecular oxygen to form superoxide ion. Superoxide ion constantly generated during cellular metabolism gets converted to hydrogen peroxide (H_2O_2) and other ROS. Under physiological conditions, the maintenance of an appropriate level of intracellular ROS is important in keeping redox balance and signaling cellular proliferation [44]. ROS produced within mitochondria presents almost 90% of the total ROS produced in the cell. The fact that the mitochondrial ETC is the major ROS production site leads to the suggestion that mitochondria are a prime target for oxidative damage and hence the mitochondrial theory of ageing, a correlate to the free radical theory [45]. Over the years, substantial evidence has emerged from morphological, bioenergetic, biochemical and genetic studies to lend support to this theory [42].

Despite conflicting views concerning the primary role of mitochondrial ROS as a cause of aging [46], the generation of ROS within mitochondria remains the most viable theory to explain the process of aging. Increased levels of ROS within mitochondria are the principal trigger not only for mitochondrial dysfunction, but also for diseases associated with aging in general [47]. The latest results strongly argue that the observed phenotypes in mtDNA mutator mice are a direct consequence of the accumulation of mtDNA point mutations in protein-coding genes, leading to a decreased assembly of mitochondrial ETC complexes, respiratory chain dysfunction and thus to premature ageing [48].

On the other hand, the "uncoupling to survive" theory proposes that energy metabolism is in a positive relation with longevity. This theory is also based on the notion that inefficiency in the mitochondrial ATP generation may be necessary to reduce ROS generation in the cell [49]. High proton motive force that drives an efficient ATP synthesis comes with an additional cost, the production of ROS. Because ROS production is highly dependent on the proton motive force, proton leak might help to limit the oxidative damage. There are a number of articles suggesting that UCPs could play an important role in this process. It has been proposed that UCPs have a role in the protection from oxidative damage by lowering a proton motive force thus causing a "mild" uncoupling and the attenuation of superoxide production from electron chain [49]. During "mild" uncoupling, caused by UCPs activation with superoxide and other ROS products derived upon oxidation of membrane phospholipids, ATP is still synthesized, a respiration rate is increased and in parallel a ROS production is decreased [49,50].

A significant decrease in the mitochondrial bioenergetic capacity with advancing age has been shown in numerous animal models and recently in a study of human volunteers [51]. A study on aged rats showed an increased intra-mitochondrial ROS production and oxidative damage, increased proton leak rates resulting in a depletion of membrane potential and a reduction of ATPase and complex IV activities. Treatment of aged rats with the insulin-like growth factor 1 (IGF1) corrected these parameters indicating that a cytoprotective effect of IGF1 is closely related to the mitochondrial protection [52]. Caloric restriction is the only dietary intervention that consistently increases median and maximal lifespan in organisms ranging from yeast to mammals. This dietary regime implies 20–50% restriction of the overall caloric intake of animals on *ad libitum* regime [53]. The precise molecular mechanisms of the life-extending actions of caloric restriction still remains unclear, but most likely mitochondrial energy metabolism plays a very important role in this process.

The age-related increase in mitochondrial oxidative stress can disrupt mitochondrial structural and functional integrity, thereby triggering a vicious cycle of ROS generation. Experimental findings indicate that the age-related decrease in mitochondrial respiratory efficiency was associated with the significant decline in respiratory complex (I-V) activities, presumably mediated by self-inflicted oxidative damage [54]. In addition, the extent of oxidative damage on key metabolic enzymes increases with age, with consequent decreases in substrate binding affinity and mitochondrial ATP generation capacity [55]. The oxidation of DNA, RNA, protein and lipid molecules in mitochondria and other cellular components can culminate in functional impairment in cells, tissues, and ultimately in vital organs such as brain, heart and liver [56]. Taken together, the capacity to produce ATP and respond to cellular stress decrease as a function of age during the age-associated deterioration of mitochondrial structure and function. The mitochondrial dysfunction results in increased ROS generation, which tilts the cellular environment towards an oxidative state (i.e., impairment of cellular redox balance) and increases the susceptibility to diseases associated with aging [57].

Studies that link mitochondrial respiration/ATP production and longevity are needed to clarify the role of mitochondrial biogenesis, mitochondrial respiration rate and ROS production in different aspects of ageing. However, mitochondria are today in the scientific spotlight and sure hold promises for the future ageing research. That is certainly enough to make mitochondria a center of our attention.

5. Qi-invigoration and Yang-invigoration

According to TCM theory, in order to have good health you must have sufficient Qi and your internal organs must work in harmony with each other, as long as sufficient Qi flows freely through the meridians and your organs work in harmony your body can remain healthy. If there isn't enough Qi, one or more organs can become imbalanced and develop energy function disorders. TCM frequently references several major Qi states of imbalance. One is an overall "Qi deficiency", which is often described in Western medical terms as chronic fatigue syndrome (CFS), may effect the Lungs with symptoms of shortness of breath, the Stomach/Spleen with symptoms such as poor appetite and the body in general with symptoms of fatigue and weakness. Most treated CFS by invigorating Qi and Yang. For an explanation of TCM, the ultimate reasons for the symptoms described earlier are induced by deficiencies in five organs (including Qi, Blood, Yin and Yang deficiencies) caused by the invasion of an exogenous pathogen, excessive physical strain (manual labor, mental labor and sexual intercourse), abnormal emotional states (elation, anger, worry, anxiety, sorrow, fear and terror) or an improper diet.

Chinese tonic herbs that can produce heath-promoting action are used for the treatment of various patterns of deficiency in body function with respect to Qi, Blood, Yin, or Yang, and their combinations. These types of functional imbalance are viewed as sub-healthy conditions in modern medicine. Chinese tonic herbs are generally classified into four categories on the basis of their health-promoting actions, namely, "Qi-invigorating", "Blood-enriching", "Yin-nourishing" and "Yang-invigorating". Of these four types of tonic herbs, the "Qi-invigorating" and "Blood-enriching" herbs are grouped under the "Yang" family and "Yin" family, respectively. Maintaining Yang and Yin in harmony is akin to attaining the homeostatic state in modern medicine [58]. Yang Qi refers to the body's vital force or functional aspects in general. Unlike the Blood or Body Fluids, Qi is an abstract concept in TCM; it can't be seen and belongs to Yang. Yang Qi sometimes refers to some body qualities and functions like superficial, upward direction, hyper-functioning, stimulating and light. It is the opposite of Yin Qi. Yang deficiency indicates insufficiency of Yang Qi inside the body that fails to provide the functions of warmth, motivation and promotion. Symptoms or signs include aversion to cold, cold limbs, bland taste in the mouth, preference for hot drinks, pale complexion, spontaneous sweating, general swelling, profuse and clear urine or loose stool. The tongue is pale, bulky with a white slimy coating, and the pulse is deep and slow or thready on examination.

According to TCM theory, Yang is viewed as a manifestation of body function supported by various organs. A "Yang-invigorating" action therefore involves the general up-regulation of cellular activities. As ATP, an energy-rich biomolecule, is universally used for energizing cellular activities, the "Yang-invigorating" action may be mediated by the enhancement of mitochondrial ATP generation [59]. "Yang-invigorating" Chinese tonic herbs have shown to enhance the myocardial mitochondrial ATP generation capacity in mice *ex vivo* and in H9c2 cardiomyocytes [58,60]. All "Yang-invigorating" Chinese tonic herbs dose-dependently enhanced the mitochondrial ATP generation capacity. The stimulation of ATP generation was associated with an increased extent of mitochondrial electron transport [60]. It is believed that the up-regulation of cellular activities by "Yang-invigoration" in Chinese medicine requires an increased supply of ATP, which is in turn largely supported by mitochondrial OXPHOS [58].

Holistically, it is believed that the Yang-invigorating herbs enhance physiological cellular activities, which is in turn critically dependent on mitochondrial ATP generation through the OXPHOS process at the cellular level. A previous study has shown that short-term oral treatment with the methanol extract of Yang-invigorating herbs, including Cortex Eucommiae, Herba Cistanches, Herba Cynomorii, Rhizoma Curculiginis, Herba Epimedii, Radix Dipsaci, Rhizoma Drynariae, Fructus Psoraleae, Semen Cuscutae, Radix Morindae, and Semen Alliion, enhanced myocardial ATP generation and produced significant stimulatory action on pyruvate-supported mitochondrial electron transport in mice [60]. This finding is corroborated by a recent study involving Yang and Yin tonic herbs using a cell-based assay of ATP-generating capacity, which showed that Yang but not Yin tonic herbs enhanced mitochondrial

ATP generation capacity in H9c2 cardiomyocytes [58]. Moreover, long-term treatment with a Yang-invigorating Chinese herbal formula (VI-28; composed of Radix Ginseng, Cornu Cervi, Cordyceps, Radix Salviae, Semen Allii, Fructus Cnidii, Fructus Evodiae and Rhizoma Kaempferiae) was found to enhance mitochondrial ATP generation in brain, heart, liver and skeletal muscle tissues of male and female rats [61].

Emerging evidence has suggested that in addition to up-regulating mitochondrial functional status, Yang tonic herbs also enhance cellular/mitochondrial antioxidant capacity, and may thus prevent age-related diseases and prolong the healthspan. The proposed biochemical mechanism underlying the antioxidant action of Yang tonic herbs involves a sustained and low level of mitochondrial ROS production, which is secondary to the increased activity of the ETC, with the possible involvement of mitochondrial uncoupling. "Yang invigoration" improves antioxidant defense in the body in the long term and thereby offers a promising prospect for preventing or possibly delaying age-related diseases and the detrimental effects of aging [62]. Studies from various laboratories showed that Yang tonic herbs produced antioxidant actions by free radical-scavenging, inhibition of oxidant production, inhibition of NADPH-dependent lipid peroxidation and increase of antioxidant enzyme activities, with a resultant protection against oxidative tissue damage. These findings were consistent with the earlier study which showed that Yang tonic herbs possessed stronger free radical scavenging activity than that of tonic herbs of other functional categories [63].

A growing body of evidence has revealed the crucial involvement of mitochondrial dysfunction and impaired antioxidant status in the pathogenesis of various age-related diseases and the aging process in general [64,65]. Yang tonic herbs/ formulae, which can induce endogenous mitochondrial antioxidant status and functional capacity enhancement [66], may therefore offer a promising prospect for preventing or possibly delaying age-related diseases and the detrimental effects of aging. With respect to Chinese medicine, more than 50% of the elderly people in China were found to show a deficiency of Yang (or Qi) in body function [67], and Yang (or Qi) tonic herbs/formulae are therefore commonly used for retarding the adverse consequences of aging in the practice of Chinese medicine. According to TCM theory, a deficiency of Yang is believed to be one of the causative factors for the development of Parkinson's disease (PD), a common neurodegenerative disease that severely compromises the quality of life in many elderly individuals [68]. Based on the finding that ViNeuro can enhance the mitochondrial ATP generation capacity (a "Yang-invigoration" property), it is plausible that the relief of Parkinsonian symptoms involves an improvement of cellular energy status that eventually leads to an enhancement of neuronal function [62].

TCM frequently references several major Qi, or energy function, problems. One is an overall "Qi deficiency". Qi deficiency is the common cause of a variety of diseases and Qi-invigoration is the basic principle for treatment of Qi deficiency. Doctors of TCM usually compose prescriptions made up of Qi-invigorating herbal medicines (QIHM) for Qi deficiency, and have accumulated abundant clinical experience for a long time. QIHM is a kind of herbal medicines which can invigorate Qi and treat syndromes of Qi deficiency, they have the effects of invigorating Qi, promoting the production of body fluid and tonifying the Spleen and Lung etc. Within the body, Qi is present in all active aspects of the body, so is considered to be a

Yang substance. Due to the popularity and therapeutic values of "Qi-invigorating" herbs, the investigation of biological activities and the underlying mechanisms in relation to "Qi-invigoration" is of great pharmacological interest. In this regard, our earlier study has demonstrated the relationship between "Qi-invigorating" action and bioenergetic level in skeletal muscle of "Qi-invigorating" herb-treated rats [69]. However, the pharmacological basis of "Qi-invigorating" action has yet to be established. To investigate the mechanism of Qi-invigoration in TCM, the following experiment was performed.

6. Research ideas on Qi-invigoration – Mitochondrial energy metabolism perspective

Sijunzi Decoction (SD), a Chinese recipe issued firstly in the ancient pharmacopeia of the Song Dynasty,"*Taiping Huimin Heji Jufang*", having effects of reinforcing the asthenia Qi, is one of the classic recipes. The recipe consists of ginseng root, white atractylodes rhizome, Poria cocos and honey-fried licorice root. As the traditional Qi-invigorating and spleen-tonifying prescription, SD experienced repeated clinical validation by the many TCM practitioners for hundreds of years, its prescription is concise, compatibility is decent, the effect is exact, and it is highly regarded. A number of Qi-invigorating prescriptions are derived based on it, and it is a basic prescription for Spleen Qi deficiency syndrome, the series of Qi-invigorating prescriptions derived from SD are widely used for clinical treatment of many diseases, not only for digestive diseases, but also for the treatment of chronic hepatitis, chronic nephritis, and coronary heart disease etc. Pharmacological studies show that SD has anti-aging, anti-fatigue, anti-hypoxia, antioxidant and immune-improving function. SD can enhance mitochondrial succinate dehydrogenase, cytochrome oxidase activity and relieve the mitochondrial injury of the Spleen Qi deficiency rats. In such case, SD was selected for investigating Qi-invigorating role to make it more representative.

Our previous studies show that all the four Qi-invigorating herbal medicines (QIHM) (including ginseng, astragalus root, pilose asiabell root, white atractylodes rhizome) can increase levels of ATP, adenylate energy charge (AEC), total adenylate pool (TAP); on the contrary, all the four Qi-flow regulating herbal medicines (QRHM, including immature bitter orange, magnolia bark, green tangerine and lindera root) can decrease levels of ATP, AEC and TAP in liver cells. In a word, QIHM and QRHM increase and decrease bioenergy level of liver cells respectively *in vivo*. Therefore, Qi is closely related to bioenergy [3]. Previous experimental findings have demonstrated that all "Yang-invigorating" herbs are capable of enhancing mitochondrial ATP generation capacity (ATP-GC) in both cell and animal studies [58,70]. As a subcategory of "Yang-invigorating" herbs, "Qi-invigorating" herbs may also stimulate mitochondrial ATP-GC in various tissues. In a study, using Renshen (*Panax ginseng*), Xiyangshen (*Panax quinquefolius*) and Dangshen (*Codonopsis pilosulae*), the effect of "Qi-invigorating" Chinese tonic herbs on mitochondrial ATP-GC using *in situ* and *ex vivo* assay systems were investigated. The results showed that the three tested "Qi-invigorating" Shens in Chinese medicine stimulated the ATP-GC *in situ* in the cell-based assay system [71]. Further investigations should examine whether representative "Qi-invigorating" herbal formula SD can stimulate mitochondrial ATP-GC *in vivo*.

Although Qi of TCM is similar to the concept of modern medical bioenergy in some aspects, the mechanism of Qi-invigoration still lacks convincing evidence. Therefore, I take it as my basic point to approach the characteristics of SD on energy metabolism from the production (oxidative phosphorylation) and regulation (adenylate energy charge) of bioenergy (ATP). Since there is no direct detection method on Qi, the Qi-invigorating representative prescriptions SD were selected to study the effect on dysfunction of energy metabolism caused by Qi deficiency to investigate the mechanism of Qi-invigoration in TCM.

6.1. Materials and methods

6.1.1. Animals and materials

Male Kunming mice were purchased from Experimental Animal Center, Dalian University. Spherisorb C_{18} reversed-phase chromatographic column (4.6 mm×250 mm, 5 μm particle size) was purchased from Dalian Institute of Chemistry and Physics, Chinese Academy of Sciences. Adenosine triphosphate (ATP), adenosine diphosphate (ADP), adenosine monophosphate (AMP), L-glutamic acid, and DL-malate were from Sigma Chemical (St Louis, MO, USA). Ginseng root, white atractylodes rhizome, Poria cocos, honey-fried licorice root, immature bitter orange, magnolia bark and Rhizoma et Radix Rhei Palmat were purchased from Beijing Tongrentang Drugstore, and identified by professor Li Jiashi at Beijing University of Chinese Medicine. They are *Panax ginseng* C.A. Mey (Tongrentang red ginseng), *Atractylodes macrocephala* Koidz, *Poria cocos* (Schw.) Wolf, *Glycyrrhiza uralensis* Fisch., *Citrus aurantium* L., *Magnolia officinalis* Rehd et Wils, and *Rheum palmatum* L. respectively.

6.1.2. Preparation of Sijunzi Decoction (SD) and Xiaochengqi Decoction (XD)

SD and XD were prepared by hot-water extraction. Powdered dry Ginseng root, white atractylodes rhizome, Poria cocos and honey-fried licorice root (1:1:1:1) were immersed in distilled water (the ratio of the drug and distilled water was 1:10) for 2 hours and extracted thrice for 0.5 hour each in a boiling water bath. The filtrate was collected after filtration with gauze, mixed and condensed to 0.5 g crude drug/mL under a reduced pressure and then centrifuged at 3000 rpm for 10 min. The supernatant (SD) was collected and stored at 4°C. XD [Rhizoma et Radix Rhei Palmat, magnolia bark and immature bitter orange (4:5:3)] was prepared by the same way as SD and condensed to 2.5 g crude drug/mL.

6.1.3. Spleen Qi deficiency model

Spleen Qi deficiency model was established by exhaustion, dissipating stagnant Qi and irregular diet which was induced by XD and semi-starvation. Forty mice were randomly divided into four groups: Normal group, model group, SD low dose group (SDL) and SD high dose group (SDH). Normal group mouse was administered normal saline (10 mL/kg/day) for 43 days by oral gavage. All the other group mouse was administered an oral dose of XD (60 g/kg/day) for 15 days and was fed with half-full diet once every other day, then the model group mouse was killed for analysis. SDL and SDH mice were given an oral dose of SD (8 and 16 g/kg/day respectively) for 28 days and were killed on forty-fourth day for detection. All the mice were maintained with free access to drinking water.

6.1.4. Isolation of liver mitochondria

Mitochondria were isolated by differential centrifugation using a modified protocol of Fink et al. [72]. Protein determinations were carried out by Bradford method using BSA as a standard [73].

6.1.5. Measurement of ATP, ADP, and AMP in skeletal muscle cells by HPLC

Briefly, determination of ATP, ADP, and AMP in cells of skeletal muscle from the thigh of mice, which was carried out with our previous method [74], by gradient RP-HPLC (reversed-phase high performance liquid chromatography) with ultraviolet detector at room temperature. ATP, ADP and AMP contents in liver cells was calculated by computing the peak area of standard solutions of nucleotides with known concentrations. Total adenylate pool (TAP) and adenylate energy charge (AEC) were calculated by the following formulas respectively: TAP = [ATP] + [ADP] + [AMP], AEC = ([ATP] + 0.5[ADP])/TAP.

6.1.6. Measurement of liver mitochondrial respiratory function

Respiratory function of liver mitochondria was measured using the Clark-type oxygen electrode method described by Estabrook [75] with slight modifications [3]. Respiratory state 3 and 4 can be calculated according to the OXPHOS curve. Respiration rates were expressed in nanomoles atom O per minute per milligram of protein. Respiratory control ratio (RCR) was the ratio of state 3 to state 4 respiration. P/O ratio is the number of ADP molecules phosphorylated per oxygen atom reduced.

6.1.7. Statistical analysis

Data were expressed as means ± SD and statistical differences between groups were analyzed by one-way analysis of variance (ANOVA) followed by least significant difference (LSD) *post hoc* multiple comparisons test using the statistical software package SPSS 16.0 for Windows (SPSS Inc., Chicago, Illinois, USA). Results were considered statistically significant at the probability (P) values < 0.05 level.

6.2. Results and discussion

6.2.1. Effects of SD on energy state in skeletal muscle cells of mice under Qi deficiency in vivo

The Spleen and the Stomach—especially the Spleen—are in charge of producing Qi and blood to nourish the body, particularly the muscles. In Chinese medicine, the Spleen is related to the muscles. Qi is closely related to bioenergy according to the ancient concept of Qi and modern bioenergetics [3]. Therefore, skeletal muscle was used for investigating energy level change of Qi deficiency mice. Impaired mitochondrial ATP formation may be the key characteristic of Qi deficiency. I found that Qi deficiency led to a marked fall in cellular ATP, and a rise in cellular AMP associated with decreases in ATP/ADP and ATP/AMP ratios. The changes in ATP/ADP ratio might significantly influence mitochondrial membrane potential ($\Delta\psi_m$) [76]. The cellular AMP/ATP ratio was monitored as an index of metabolic stress [77]. Through the action of adenylate kinase (AK), any decrease in the cellular ATP/ADP ratio is converted into a decrease in the ATP/AMP ratio [78]. Qi deficiency elicits a marked decrease in the ATP/AMP ratio. The ATP/AMP ratio reduced from 27.4 of normal group to 6.25 under Qi deficiency conditions, whereas the ATP/ADP ratio reduced from 4.95 to 3.38. Qi deficiency has altered cellular energy state.

Adenylate energy charge (AEC) represents a linear measure of the metabolic energy stored in the adenine nucleotide system. Energy metabolism would be regulated by the relative amount of ATP available, as described by AEC. ATP has been called the "energy currency" of the cell, TAP is a measure of the cell energy status. TAP levels and AEC in muscle cells of model group were decreased compared with normal group. The AMP level in model group remained twofold higher than in normal group. SD treatment could increase ATP, TAP levels and ATP/ADP, ATP/AMP ratio, AEC in muscle cells in a dose-dependent manner. ATP/AMP ratio in SDH (16 g/ kg/day) group increased over fivefold than in model group (Table 1).

Group	Dose (g/kg/day)	ATP (mM)	ADP (mM)	AMP (mM)	TAP (mM)	AEC	ATP/ADP	ATP/AMP
Model	-	1.01±0.21	0.29±0.13	0.16±0.08	1.46±0.29	0.78±0.07	3.38±0.84	6.25±4.3
Normal	-	1.66±0.31^c	0.34±0.11	0.06±0.04^b	2.06±0.38^b	0.89±0.08^b	4.95±0.69^c	27.4±7.8^c
SDL	8	1.35±0.23^b	0.32±0.12	0.09±0.06^a	1.76±0.34^a	0.85±0.05^a	4.26±0.74^a	14.8±5.7^b
SDH	16	1.68±0.28^c	0.35±0.15	0.05±0.05^b	2.08±0.40^b	0.90±0.07^b	4.82±0.85^b	33.8±8.3^c

All values are mean±SD (n=10). $^aP<0.05$, $^bP<0.01$, $^cP < 0.001$ compared to model group.

Each value expressed in mM (ATP, ADP, AMP, TAP) or as a ratio (AEC, ATP/ADP, ATP/AMP).

SDL: SD low dose group; SDH: SD high dose group; ATP: adenosine triphosphate; ADP: adenosine diphosphate; AMP: adenosine monophosphate; TAP: total adenylate pool; AEC: adenylate energy charge.

Table 1. Effects of Sijunzi Decoction on adenylates level in skeletal muscle cells of mice *in vivo*.

Recently, a second mechanism of respiratory control has been found in eukaryotes. This control is based on the intramitochondrial ATP/ADP ratio, with a high ratio inhibiting oxidative phosphorylation through allosteric binding of ATP to a subunit of Complex IV. This inhibition is reversed when the concentration of ADP increases [79]. Energy metabolism would be regulated by AEC. In this study, we found that Qi deficiency significantly decreased AEC, which was reversed by SD accompanied by an increase in ATP. Thus, stimulation of ATP production by SD may be achieved through the regulation of the mitochondria by affecting the AEC response. This is consistent with the ability of *P. ginseng* in increasing ATP [75]. SD was able to enhance ATP production, cellular ATP levels are closely linked to mitochondrial function, which is regulated perhaps by AEC. SD was able to regulate AEC, possibly linked to mitochondrial ATP production. Data showed SD to be an enhancer of ATP production under

Qi deficiency induced anti-ATP circumstance. ATP levels were drastically lowered by Qi deficiency but SD stimulated an increased output of ATP.

The Spleen Qi-deficiency mice are characterized by lassitude of the limbs and poor appetite etc. In short, the TCM therapeutic approach of invigorating Qi and tonifying the spleen by SD can improve the mitochondrial energy metabolism of muscle cells as well as symptoms for the Spleen Qi-deficiency of experimental animals.

6.2.2. *The effects of SD on liver mitochondrial respiratory function in vivo*

Liver plays important role in metabolism to maintain energy level and structural stability of body. It is also site of biotransformation by which toxic compounds get transformed into less harmful products to reduce toxicity [80]. The state 3 respiration (oxygen consumption), the respiratory control ratio (RCR) values and P/O ratio of liver mitochondria of model mice driven by complex I substrates were all significantly decreased compared with the normal. Liver mitochondria isolated from SD treated rats showed significant decrease in state 3 respiration, RCR and P/O ratio, compared to the rates in mitochondria from models (Table 2). State 4 respiration was not significantly altered in SD treated rats. It showed that the efficiency of ATP production via ADP phosphorylation was decreased. Qi deficiency allows tissues to minimize their energy needs. In perfectly coupled mitochondria, there would be no proton leak across the IMM, and the entire gradient generated by the respiratory chain would be used to generate ATP [81]. Control of OXPHOS allows a cell to produce only the precise amount of ATP required to sustain its activities. Recall that under normal circumstances, electron transport and ATP synthesis are tightly coupled. The value of P/O ratio (the number of moles of Pi consumed for each oxygen atom reduced to H_2O) reflects the degree of coupling observed between electron transport and ATP synthesis [82]. Oxygen consumption increase dramatically when ADP is supplied. The control of aerobic respiration by ADP is referred to as respiratory control. Substrate oxidation accelerates only when an increase in the concentration of ADP signals that the ATP pool needs to be replenished. This regulation matches the rates of phosphorylation of ADP and of cellular oxidations via glycolysis, the citric acid cycle, and the electron transport chain to the requirement for ATP [79].

Group	Dose (g/kg/day)	State 3 (nmol/min/mg) [d]	State 4 (nmol/min/mg) [d]	RCR	P/O ratio
Model	-	66±10	18.8±2.5	3.5±0.5	2.08±0.33
Normal	-	82±12[b]	19.4±1.8	4.2±0.6[a]	2.59±0.28[b]
SDL	8	60±14	18.7±2.3	3.2±0.7	1.90±0.24
SDH	16	56±11[a]	18.3±2.2	2.9±0.6[a]	1.78±0.22[a]

[d] nanomole O_2 per minute per milligram protein (nmol O_2 min^{-1} mg $protein^{-1}$).

All values are mean±SD (n=10). [a]$P < 0.05$, [b]$P < 0.01$ compared to model group.

RCR: respiratory control ratio; SDL: SD low dose group; SDH: SD high dose group.

Table 2. Effects of SD on liver mitochondrial respiratory function *in vivo*.

Mitochondria produce significant amounts of cellular ROS via aberrant O_2 reaction during electron transport. This process in physiological conditions is tightly controlled with majority of ROS produced remaining inside intact mitochondria. The rate of mitochondrial respiration and ROS formation is largely influenced by the coupling state of the mitochondria [83]. SD decrease oxygen consuming rate and RCR of liver mitochondria maybe by improving of mitochondrial energy status (Figure 2), therefore, reduce mitochondrial ROS production. We consider this is appearance of lowering standard metabolic rate and is a kind of protective adaptation. Qi deficiency patients need nutritional supplements, adequate rest, and should reduce energy consumption, SD can just achieve this goal. It is conceivable that impairment of mitochondrial ATP production and the resulting energy depletion can lead to apoptosis. Aging-associated declines in mitochondrial respiratory function can lead to lower ATP production and higher oxidative stress. Lower ATP levels can decrease the efficiency of energy-dependent processes and ATP-mediated signal transductions [84]. An explanation of the protective effects of SD on mitochondria is based on the improvement of cellular energy status.

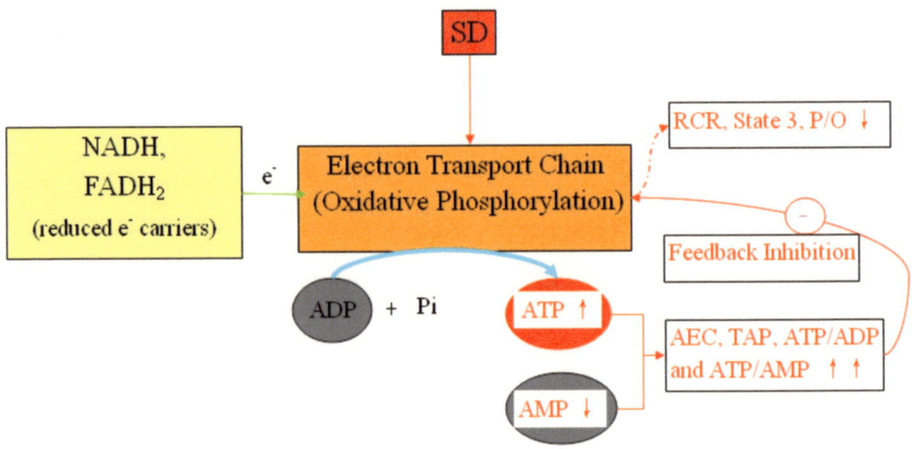

Figure 2. The action site of mitochondria as potential targets for SD therapy. SD treatment could increase ATP and TAP, decrease AMP levels and increase ATP/ADP, ATP/AMP ratio, AEC in muscle cells which feedback inhibit OXPHOS by decreasing RCR, state 3 respiration and P/O ratio of liver mitochondria. This is the result of improved mitochondrial energy metabolism and bioenergetic level and the potential Qi-invigoration mechanism of SD.

7. Conclusion

Qi is the hub from basic theory to clinical practice and health longevity in TCM. The true foundation of TCM is Qi. All kinds of diseases and ailments are born from Qi, Qi deficiency is the common cause of a variety of diseases and can lead to mitochondrial energy metabolism dysfunction, and Qi-invigoration is the basic principle for treatment of Qi de-

http://dx.doi.org/10.5772/54760

ficiency. However, the mechanisms for Qi-invigoration in TCM remain elusive. We propose a hypothesis that Qi is closely related to bioenergy according to the ancient concept of Qi and modern bioenergetics [3], which is the entry point; all the QIHM have the regularity of same pharmacological effects, such as exercise capacity improvement, anti-fatigue, anti-oxidation and anti-apoptosis, etc. which are all closely related to mitochondrial function, which is the basis of study; Qi-invigorating prescriptions and QIHM have a good effect in improving the energy metabolism and for treatment of mitochondria-related diseases, and the Qi-invigorating representative prescriptions Sijunzi Decoction (SD) was used for treatment of Qi deficiency, which is the object of study. The mechanism of energy metabolism improvement has been explored from mitochondrial oxidative phosphorylation, intracellular adenylates levels, and the mechanism of mitochondrial protection of SD were investigated. In summary, SD was able to improve mitochondrial function by enhancing cellular bioenergetics and had the pharmaceutical activities of mitochondrial protection. The study provides scientific evidence for the mechanism of Qi-invigoration in TCM which is achieved by improving mitochondrial energy metabolism.

Acknowledgements

This work was supported by the Fundamental Research Funds for the Central Universities in China (grant number: DC12010210); the Post-doctoral Research Station of Daxing'anling Beiqishen Green Industry Group, Doctoral Research Center of Heilongjiang University of Chinese Medicine (No.LRB10-316); and the Talents Project of Dalian Nationalities University (No.20116126).

Author details

Xing-Tai Li

College of Life Science, Dalian Nationalities University, Dalian, China

References

[1] Zhang YS. Mathematical Reasoning of Treatment Principle Based on "Yin Yang Wu Xing" Theory in Traditional Chinese Medicine (II). Chinese Medicine 2011; 2: 158-170.

[2] Low PKC, Ang S-L. The Foundation of Traditional Chinese Medicine. Chinese Medicine 2010; 1: 84-90.

[3] Li XT, Zhao J. An Approach to the Nature of Qi in TCM—Qi and Bioenergy. In: Kuang H. (ed.) Recent Advances in Theories and Practice of Chinese Medicine. Rijeka: InTech; 2012. p79-108.

[4] Scheffler IE. Mitochondria. New York: Wiley–Liss Inc; 1999.

[5] Kennedy EP, Lehninger AL. Oxidation of Fatty Acids and Tricarboxylic Acid Cycle Intermediates by Isolated Rat Liver Mitochondria. Journal of Biological Chemistry 1949; 179: 957–972.

[6] Mayevsky A. Mitochondrial Function and Energy Metabolism in Cancer Cells: Past Overview and Future Perspectives. Mitochondrion 2009; 9: 165–179.

[7] Reid RA, Moyle J, Mitchell P. Synthesis of Adenosine Triphosphate by a Protonmotive Force in Rat Liver Mitochondria, Nature 1966; 212: 257–258.

[8] Weiss L. The cell. In: Weiss L. (ed.) Cell and Tissue Biology: A Textbook of Histology (6th ed.). Baltimore: Urban & Schwarzenberg; 1988. p1-65.

[9] Nishihara Y, Utsumi K. 2,2',5,5'-Tetrachlorobiphenyl Impairs the Bioenergetic Functions of Isolated Rat Liver Mitochondria. Biochemical Pharmacology 1986; 35: 3335–3339.

[10] Mozo J, Emre Y, Bouillaud F, Ricquier D, Criscuolo F. Thermoregulation: What Role for UCPs in Mammals and Birds? Bioscience Reports 2005; 25: 227–249.

[11] Cannon B, Shabalina IG, Kramarova TV, Petrovic N, Nedergaard J. Uncoupling Proteins: a Role in Protection against Reactive Oxygen Species—or Not? Biochimica et Biophysica Acta 2006; 1757: 449–458.

[12] Majno G, Joris I. Apoptosis, Oncosis, and Necrosis. An Overview of Cell Death. American Journal of Pathology 1995; 146: 3–15.

[13] Hatefi Y. The mitochondrial Electron Transport and Oxidative Phosphorylation System. Annual Review of Biochemistry 1985; 54: 1015–1069.

[14] Chuang Y-C, Lin J-W, Chen S-D, Lin T-K, Liou C-W, Lu C-H, Chang W-N. Preservation of Mitochondrial Integrity and Energy Metabolism during Experimental Status Epilepticus Leads to Neuronal Apoptotic Cell Death in the Hippocampus of the Rat. Seizure 2009; 18: 420–428.

[15] Melo DR, Kowaltowski AJ, Wajner M, Castilho RF. Mitochondrial Energy Metabolism in Neurodegeneration Associated with Methylmalonic Academia. Journal of Bioenergetics and Biomembranes 2011; 43: 39–46.

[16] Rocher C, Taanman J-W, Pierron D, Faustin B, Benard G, Rossignol R, Malgat M, Pedespan L, Letellier T. Influence of Mitochondrial DNA Level on Cellular Energy Metabolism: Implications for Mitochondrial Diseases. Journal of Bioenergetics and Biomembranes 2008; 40: 59–67.

[17] Schulz TJ, Westermann D, Isken F, Voigt A, Laube B, Thierbach R, Kuhlow D, Zarse K, Schomburg L, Pfeiffer AFH, Tschöpe C, Ristow M. Activation of Mitochondrial Energy Metabolism Protects against Cardiac Failure. Aging 2010; 2 (11): 843-853.

[18] Lin JD. The PGC-1 Coactivator Networks: Chromatin-Remodeling and Mitochondrial Energy Metabolism. Molecular Endocrinology 2009; 23(1): 2–10.

[19] Warburg O. The Metabolism of Tumours. London: Constable & CO LTD; 1930.

[20] Warburg O. On Respiratory Impairment in Cancer Cells. Science 1956; 124: 269–270.

[21] Warburg O. On the Origin of Cancer Cells. Science 1956; 123: 309–314.

[22] Fiskum G, Starkov A. Mitochondrial Mechanisms of Neural Cell Death and Neuroprotective Interventions in Parkinson's Disease. Annals of the New York Academy of Sciences 2003; 991: 111–119.

[23] Smith R, Porteous CM, Murphy CM. Selective Targeting of an Antioxidant to Mitochondria. European Journal of Biochemistry 1999; 263: 709–716.

[24] Hindfelt B, Plum F, Duffy TE. Effect of Acute Ammonia Intoxication on Cerebral Metabolism in Rats with Portacaval Shunts. Journal of Clinical Investigation 1977; 59: 386–396.

[25] Astore D, Boicelli CA. Hyperammonemia and Chronic Hepatic Encephalopathy: an *in vivo* PMRS Study of the Rat Brain. Magnetic Resonance Materials in Physics, Biology and Medicine 2000; 10: 160–166.

[26] McCandless DW, Schenker S. Effect of Acute Ammonia Intoxication on Energy Stores in the Cerebral Reticular Activating System. Experimental Brain Research 1981; 44: 325–330.

[27] Haghighat N, McCandless DW, Geraminegad P. The Effect of Ammonium Chloride on Metabolism of Primary Neurons and Neuroblastoma Cells *in vitro*. Metabolic Brain Disease 2000; 15: 151–162.

[28] Kaminsky Y, Kosenko E. AMP Deaminase and Adenosine Deaminase Activities in Liver and Brain Regions in Acute Ammonia Intoxication and Subacute Toxic Hepatitis. Brain Research 2010; 1311: 175–181.

[29] Kosenko EA, Kaminsky YG. Activation of AMP Deaminase and Adenosine Deaminase in the Liver during Ammonia Poisoning and Hepatitis. Bulletin of Experimental Biology and Medicine 2011; 150: 36–38.

[30] Bernardi P, Colonna R, Costantini P, Eriksson O, Fontaine E, Ichas F, Massari S, Nicolli A, Petronilli V, Scorrano L. The Mitochondrial Permeability Transition. Biofactors 1998; 8: 273–281.

[31] Norenberg MD, Rao KV. The Mitochondrial Permeability Transition in Neurologic Disease. Neurochemistry International 2007; 50: 983–997.

[32] Kristal BS, Dubinsky JM. Mitochondrial Permeability Transition in the Central Nervous System: Induction by Calcium Cycling-dependent and-independent Pathways. Journal of Neurochemistry 1997; 69: 524–538.

[33] Mans AM, DeJoseph MR, Hawkins RA. Metabolic Abnormalities and Grade of Encephalopathy in Acute Hepatic Failure. Journal of Neurochemistry 1994; 63: 1829–1838.

[34] Zwingmann C, Chatauret N, Leibfritz D, Butterworth RF. Selective Increase of Brain Lactate Synthesis in Experimental Acute Liver Failure: Results of a [H–C] Nuclear Magnetic Resonance Study. Hepatology 2003; 37: 420–428.

[35] Boer LA, Panatto JP, Fagundes DA, Bassani C, Jeremias IC, Daufenbach JF, Rezin GT, Constantino L, Dal-Pizzol F, Streck EL. Inhibition of Mitochondrial Respiratory Chain in the Brain of Rats after Hepatic Failure Induced by Carbon Tetrachloride is Reversed by Antioxidants. Brain Research Bulletin 2009; 80: 75–78.

[36] Pacheco GS, Panatto JP, Fagundes DA, Scaini G, Bassani C, Jeremias IC, Rezin GT, Constantino L, Dal-Pizzol F, Streck EL. Brain Creatine Kinase Activity Is Inhibited after Hepatic Failure Induced by Carbon Tetrachloride or Acetaminophen. Metabolic Brain Disease 2009; 24: 383–394.

[37] Bates TE, Williams SR, Kauppinen RA, Gadian DG. Observation of Cerebral Metabolites in an Animal Model of Acute Liver Failure *in vivo*: a ^{1}H and ^{31}P Nuclear Magnetic Resonance Study. Journal of Neurochemistry 1989; 53: 102–110.

[38] Alberici LC, Vercesi AE, Oliveira HCF. Mitochondrial Energy Metabolism and Redox Responses to Hypertriglyceridemia. Journal of Bioenergetics and Biomembranes 2011; 43: 19–23.

[39] Shigenaga MK, Hagen TM, Ames BN. Oxidative Damage and Mitochondrial Decay in Aging. Proceedings of the National Academy of Sciences of the United States of America 1994; 91(23): 10771-10778.

[40] Ames BN, Shigenaga MK, Hagen TM. Oxidants, Antioxidants, and the Degenerative Diseases of Aging. Proceedings of the National Academy of Sciences of the United States of America 1993; 90(17): 7915-7922.

[41] Harman D. Aging: A Theory Based on Free Radical and Radiation Chemistry. Journal of Gerontology 1956; 11(3): 298-300.

[42] Bratic I, Trifunovic A. Mitochondrial Energy Metabolism and Ageing. Biochimica et Biophysica Acta 2010; 1797: 961–967.

[43] Liu Y, Fiskum G, Schubert D. Generation of Reactive Oxygen Species by the Mitochondrial Electron Transport Chain. Journal of Neurochemistry 2002; 80: 780–787.

[44] Dwivedi N, Mehta A, Yadav A, Binukumar BK, Gill KD, Flora SJS. MiADMSA Reverses Impaired Mitochondrial Energy Metabolism and Neuronal Apoptotic Cell Death after Arsenic Exposure in Rats. Toxicology and Applied Pharmacology 2011; 256: 241–248.

[45] Harman D. The Biologic Clock: the Mitochondria? Journal of the American Geriatrics Society 1972; 20(4): 145–147.

[46] Lapointe J, Hekimi S. When a Theory of Aging Ages Badly. Cellular and Molecular Life Sciences 2010; 67(1): 1-8.

[47] Wanagat J, Dai DF, Rabinovitch P. Mitochondrial Oxidative Stress and Mammalian Healthspan. Mechanisms of Ageing and Development 2010; 131(7-8): 527-535.

[48] Edgar D, Shabalina I, Camara Y, Wredenberg A, Calvaruso MA, Nijtmans L, Nedergaard J, Cannon B, Larsson NG, Trifunovic A. Random Point Mutations with Major Effects on Protein-coding Genes are the Driving Force behind Premature Ageing in mtDNA Mutator Mice. Cell Metabolism 2009; 10: 131–138.

[49] Brand MD. Uncoupling to Survive? The Role of Mitochondrial Inefficiency in Ageing. Experimental Gerontology 2000; 35: 811–820.

[50] Echtay KS, Roussel D, St-Pierre J, Jekabsons MB, Cadenas S, Stuart JA, Harper JA, Roebuck SJ, Morrison A, Pickering S, Clapham JC, Brand MD. Superoxide Activates Mitochondrial Uncoupling Proteins. Nature 2002; 415: 96–99.

[51] Short KR, Bigelow ML, Kahl J, Singh R, Coenen-Schimke J, Raghavakaimal S, Nair KS. Decline in Skeletal Muscle Mitochondrial Function with Ageing in Humans. Proceedings of the National Academy of Sciences of the United States of America 2005; 102: 5618–5623.

[52] Puche JE, Garcia-Fernandez M, Muntane J, Rioja J, Gonzalez-Baron S, Castilla Cortazar I. Low Doses of Insulin-like Growth Factor-I Induce Mitochondrial Protection in Ageing Rats. Endocrinology 2008; 149: 2620–2627.

[53] Lambert AJ, Wang B, Yardley J, Edwards J, Merry BJ. The Effect of Ageing and Caloric Restriction on Mitochondrial Protein Density and Oxygen Consumption. Experimental Gerontology 2004; 39: 289–295.

[54] Navarro A, Boveris A, Brain R. Liver Mitochondria Develop Oxidative Stress and Lose Enzymatic Activities on Aging. American Journal of Physiology-Regulatory, Integrative and Comparative Physiology 2004; 287(5): R1244-R1249.

[55] Moghaddas S, Hoppel CL, Lesnefsky EJ. Aging Defect at the Q_o Site of Complex III Augments Oxyradical Production in Rat Heart Interfibrillar Mitochondria. Archives of Biochemistry and Biophysics 2003; 414(1): 59-66.

[56] Liu J, Atamna H, Kuratsune H, Ames BN. Delaying Brain Mitochondrial Decay and Aging with Mitochondrial Antioxidants and Metabolites. Annals of the New York Academy of Sciences 2002; 959: 133-166.

[57] Ugidos A, Nystrom T, Caballero A. Perspectives on the Mitochondrial Etiology of Replicative Aging in Yeast. Experimental Gerontology 2010; 45(7-8): 512-515.

[58] Wong HS, Leung HY, Ko KM. 'Yang-Invigorating' Chinese Tonic Herbs Enhance Mitochondrial ATP Generation in H9c2 Cardiomyocytes. Chinese Medicine 2011; 2: 1-5.

[59] Ko KM, Mak DHF, Chiu PY, Poon MKT. Pharmacological Basis of 'Yang-Invigoration' in Chinese Medicine. Trends in Pharmacological Sciences 2004; 25(1): 3-6.

[60] Ko KM, Leon TYY, Mak DHF, Chiu PY, Du Y, Poon MKT. A Characteristic Pharmacological Action of 'Yang-Invigorating' Chinese Tonifying Herbs: Enahcnement of Myocardial ATP-Generation Capacity. Phytomedicine 2006; 13(9-10): 636-642.

[61] Leung HY, Chiu PY, Poon MK, Ko KM. A Yang-Invigorating Chinese Herbal Formula Enhances Mitochondrial Functional Ability and Antioxidant Capacity in Various Tissues of Male and Female Rats. Rejuvenation Research 2005; 8(4): 238-247.

[62] Lam PY, Wong HS, Chen J, Ko KM. A Hypothetical Anti-Aging Mechanism of "Yang-Invigorating" Chinese Tonic Herbs. Chinese Medicine, 2012; 3: 72-78.

[63] Yim TK, Ko KM. Antioxidant and Immunodulatory Activities of Chinese Tonifying Herbs. Pharmaceutical Biology 2002; 40(5): 329-335.

[64] Beal MF. Mitochondria Take Center Stage in Aging and Neurodegeneration. Annals of Neurology 2005; 58(4): 495-505.

[65] Chan DC. Mitochondria: Dynamic Organelles in Disease, Aging, and Development. Cell 2006; 125(7): 1241-1252.

[66] Chiu PY, Leung HY,Siu AH, Chen N, Poon MK, Ko KM. Long-Term Treatment with a Yang-Invigorating Chinese Herbal Formula Produces Generalized Tissue Protection against Oxidative Damage in Rats. Rejuvenation Research 2008; 11(1): 43-62.

[67] Huang Y. Gerontology. Shanghai: Shanghai Science and Technology Press; 1989.

[68] Li GH. The Differentiation and Treatment of Parkinson's Disease According to Traditional Chinese Medicine. Journal of Chinese Medicine 1989; 30: 1- 4.

[69] Li XT, Zhang JJ, Chen WW. The effects of TCM Qi-invigorating, Qi-regulating Drugs and Polysaccharides on the Energy Charge of Rat Skeletal Muscle Cells. Journal of Beijing University of Traditional Chinese Medicine 2000; 23(5): 36–38.

[70] Leung HY, Ko KM. Herba Cistanche Extract Enhances Mitochondrial ATP Generation in Rat Hearts and H9c2 Cells. Pharmaceutical Biology 2008; 46: 418–424.

[71] Wong HS, Cheung WF, Tang WL, Ko KM. "Qi-Invigorating" Chinese Tonic Herbs (Shens) Stimulate Mitochondrial ATP Generation Capacity in H9c2 Cardiomyocytes *in Situ* and Rat Hearts *ex Vivo*. Chinese Medicine 2012; 3:101–105.

[72] Fink BD, Reszka KJ, Herlein JA, Mathahs MM, Sivitz WI. Respiratory Uncoupling by UCP1 and UCP2 and Superoxide Generation in Endothelial Cell Mitochondria. American Journal of Physiology-Endocrinology and Metabolism 2005; 288(1): 71–79.

[73] Bradford MM. A Rapid and Sensitive Method for the Quantation of Microgram Quantities of Protein Utilizing the Principle of Protein-dye Binding. Analytical Biochemistry 1976; 72(1-2): 248–254.

[74] Li XT, Chen R, Jin LM, Chen HY. Regulation on Energy Metabolism and Protection on Mitochondria of *Panax ginseng* Polysaccharide. The American Journal of Chinese Medicine 2009; 37(6): 1139–1152.

[75] Estabrook RW. Mitochondrial Respiratory Control and the Polarographic Measurement of ADP:O Ratios. Methods in Enzymology 1967; 10: 41–47.

[76] Kann O, Kovács R. Mitochondria and Neuronal Activity. American Journal of Physiology-Cell Physiology 2007; 292(2): C641–C657.

[77] Salt IP, Johnson G, Ashcroft SJ, Hardie DG. AMP-activated Protein Kinase is Activated by Low Glucose in Cell Lines Derived from Pancreatic beta Cells, and May Regulate Insulin Release. Biochemical Journal 1998; 335(3): 533–539.

[78] Shetty M, Loeb JN, Vikstrom K, Ismail-Beigi F. Rapid Activation of GLUT-1 Glucose Transporter Following Inhibition of Oxidative Phosphorylation in Clone 9 cells. Journal of Biological Chemistry 1993; 268(23): 17225–17232.

[79] Horton HR, Moran LA, Ochs RS, Rawn JD, Scrimgeour KG. Principles of Biochemistry (3rd ed.). New Jersey: Science Press and Pearson Education North Asia Limited; 2002.

[80] Hodgson E. A Textbook of Modern Toxicology (3rd ed). New Jersey: John Wiley and Sons Inc; 2004.

[81] Boudina S, Dale Abel E. Mitochondrial uncoupling: A key Contributor to Reduced Cardiac Efficiency in Diabetes. Physiology 2006; 21(4): 250–258.

[82] Mckee T, Mckee JR. Biochemistry: An Introduction (2nd ed.). New York: McGraw-Hill Companies Inc; 1999.

[83] Elahi MM, Kong YX, Matata BM. Oxidative Stress as a Mediator of Cardiovascular Disease. Oxidative Medicine and Cellular Longevity 2009; 2(5): 259–269.

[84] Lee HC, Wei YH. Oxidative Stress, Mitochondrial DNA Mutation, and Apoptosis in Aging. Experimental Biology and Medicine 2007; 232(5): 592–606.

Chapter 12

Network Pharmacology and Traditional Chinese Medicine

Qihe Xu, Fan Qu and Olavi Pelkonen

Additional information is available at the end of the chapter

http://dx.doi.org/10.5772/53868

1. Introduction

Traditional Chinese medicine (TCM), an age-old healthcare system derived from China, is a mainstream medicine in China and is also popular in many other parts of the world [1-3]. Due to historic reasons, the scientific base of TCM awaits consolidation but emerging evidence has begun to illustrate TCM as an area of important medical rediscoveries. For example, the 2011 Lasker-DeBakey Clinical Medical Research Award was awarded to Youyou Tu for the discovery of Chinese herb-derived artemisinin, a drug for malaria that has saved millions of lives across the globe [4,5] and the 7th Annual Szent-Györgyi Prize was awarded to Zhen-Yi Wang and Zhu Chen for their TCM research that led to the successful development of a new therapeutic approach to acute promyelocytic leukaemia. These award-winning projects were both conducted well before the human genome was decoded and when information technology was in infancy. What has TCM to offer in the post-genomic era and the Information Age? To address this important question, the GP-TCM project kicked in as the 1st EU-funded EU-China collaboration dedicated to applying emerging technologies to TCM research [6,7]. Besides the consensus that omics and systems biology approaches will likely play major roles in addressing the complexity of TCM [7-9], more than half GP-TCM consortium members who responded to a consortium survey also cast votes of confidence in network pharmacology in TCM research [7]. Then, what is network pharmacology? What is the state of the art of this technology in modern pharmacological and toxicological studies, and finally, what are its possible roles in TCM research?

2. What is network pharmacology?

Network could be used to refer to any interconnected things or people in a virtual or actual net-like structure. For example, in information technology, anatomy, systems biology and social science, it could refer to interconnect computers (e.g. intranet or internet), bodily structures (e.g. neurons and vessels), molecules (e.g. genes, mRNAs, proteins, metabolites), or an association of individuals having a common interest, formed to provide mutual assistance, helpful information, or the like (e.g. the FP7 GP-TCM consortium) [6,7], respectively. In network pharmacology, "network" doesn't mean that a group of scientists who share similar interests are interconnected, as the FP7 GP-TCM consortium and the famous Polymath Project of mathematicians do [7,10], nor does it refer to interconnected anatomical structures or computers. Instead, the concept is built on the belief that targeting multiple nodes in interconnected molecular systems, rather than individual molecules, could lead to better efficacy and fewer adverse effects [11,12]. It integrates polypharmacology [13,14] and computational pharmacology or *in silico* pharmacology [15] and is based on the principles and objectives of systems pharmacology [16,17]. Thus, network pharmacology could be regarded as the technical route to the ultimate ideal of systems pharmacology, in which drugs are designed to benefit a human being as an integrative system, taking into consideration the complex dynamics of interconnected organic and molecular systems.

In brief, network pharmacology is based on the principles of network theory and systems biology. Graph or network theory is a branch of mathematics, which is concerned with characteristics of networks ("webs") of interacting objects. Systems biology, as the name implies, deals with complex and comprehensive living systems involving a finite number of hierarchically ordered components, which form interacting networks affected by, and responding to, various perturbations within the system itself and from the environment [18]. Typical for the network's response to perturbations is the return of a system to a previous state or the adoption of a new homeostasis. 'Systems biology is an analytical approach to investigating relationships among system's components in order to understand its emergent, i.e. network-level properties' [19]. Emergent properties, e.g. homeostasis, are higher-level characteristics of complex systems, which are difficult to understand and predict just by studying a few components at a time in isolation. In medicine and pharmacology, when traditional approaches are mostly concerned with individual molecules or pathways, systems biology aims at integration of biological complexity at all levels of biological organisation, be it cell, organ, organism, or population.

Although polypharmacology and computational pharmacology have a relatively long history, network pharmacology and systems pharmacology are emerging new concepts that were only developed in the past 5-7 years. In October 2011, the Quantitative and Systems Pharmacology Working Group of the US National Institutes of Health published a white paper entitled *Quantitative and Systems Pharmacology in the Post-Genomic Era: New Approaches to Discovering Drugs and Understanding Therapeutic Mechanisms*, which provided a general report-level overview of the field from the perspectives of drug development and therapy and listed a number of important research goals for the future. It may be of interest to recapitulate one of the working definitions of the report:

"The goal of Quantitative and Systems Pharmacology is to understand, in a precise, predictive manner, how drugs modulate cellular networks in space and time and how they impact human pathophysiology."

---

http://dx.doi.org/10.5772/53868

3. Principles of systems biology and network pharmacology

Detailed descriptions of principles of networks in systems biology can be found in several articles and reviews [20-22]. Herein, only a short presentation of the most important features is provided. Some most important characteristics and their biological examples are shown in Table 1. Network is formed by nodes (basic building blocks), their connections ('edges') and modules (a collection of nodes with a higher number of connections with each other in comparison with the rest of the network), and is characterised by a number of topological features defining relationships between network objects. There is a hierarchy in the properties of nodes in that some of them ("hubs") are more central with a high number of connections to other nodes whereas the majority of nodes have only one or a few connections at the most with other nodes. Bridging nodes connect two other nodes or modules in the network. As a consequence of non-random nature of biological networks, these networks are called "scale-free" in the network theory; Barabasi & Oltvai also referred to them as 'scale-rich' [21].

Network characteristics	Definition and explanation	Biological entities and functions (examples)
Node	Basic component interacting (pair-wise) with other node(s)	• Small-molecular substrates (metabolic network) •Genes (genetic regulatory network) •Proteins (protein-protein network)
Edge (link, connection)	Connection between two nodes	• Connection may be physical, regulatory, genetic interaction; • Metabolic network: enzyme-catalysed reactions • Genetic regulatory network: expression data
Node degree or connectivity	Number of links to other nodes; "hubs" are nodes with a large number of connections, but there are only a few of them in any network	•Associated with topological robustness of biological networks, i.e. small degree nodes are more "disposable" than hubs
Path length	The average separation between arbitrarily chosen nodes	• Proximal and distal nodes in a functional module
Clustering coefficient	A measure of grouping tendency of the nodes	• Points to a motif and/or module
Motif and motif clusters	Recurring, significant patterns of interconnections	• Elementary building blocks (sub-networks) of biological networks
Network module	A set of nodes with high internal connectivity	• Subunits of a protein complex; dynamic functional unit, e.g. metabolic pathway, signalling cascade
Bridging node	A node bridging the shortest path between two other nodes or modules within a network	• A node linking two functional units ("crosstalk" point; a potential drug target), etc.
Bridging centrality	Measure for connectivity within a network for the measured node	

Table 1. Important network characteristics in biological and pharmacological networks [18,19,21]

Complex networks possess characteristics that are of considerable importance for the investigation of drug discovery and drug treatment. Emergent properties of networks have already been mentioned earlier. Recently, there has been some theoretical and experimental work on strong and weak emergent features of networks [23]. Network robustness is a very important feature, which refers to the ability of a network to respond to external or internal perturbations [21]. Biological networks demonstrate remarkable robustness, which is at least partially based on a scale-free assembly: failure of nodes with few connections (small degree nodes), which form the majority of nodes, does not affect the integrity of the network, whereas failure of a few key hubs disintegrates the network. This latter phenomenon also is the basis of vulnerability of a network, if key hubs are targets of disruptive influences.

It is perhaps fair to mention and emphasise that many network-level emergent properties are important concepts in physiology, which is a system-level discipline. Concepts such as homeostasis, set-points, regulation, feedback control and redundancy have been in physiology for a long time to explain and model the interactions between cells, organs, systems and organisms [24]. Many of these system-level concepts have direct correspondences or relatives in network systems biology.

4. How to build a network?

Building a network involves two opposite approaches: a bottom-up approach on the basis of established biological knowledge and a top-down approach starting from the statistical analysis of available data [18]. In a more detailed level, there are several ways to build and illustrate a biological network [25]. Perhaps the most versatile and general way is the *de novo* assembly of a network from direct experimental or computational interactions, e.g. chemical/gene/protein screens. For the broad screening, the application of known interactions to an omic data set either manually or by using pathway-analysis software (Ingenuity Pathway Analysis, MetaCore, etc) has been widely used for hypothesis building and for identifying crucial network components. The most direct way to employ time-honoured modelling and simulation practices and more restricted and focused experimental datasets is by reverse engineering to generate a subset of networks *ab initio*. Most biochemical and regulatory pathways have been built in the past via painstaking experimental work on a single or a few components of a system, which has become understandable *in toto* only later in the research process. Likewise, it has to be realised that the first assembly of a network is just the beginning of an iterative modelling-simulation-experimentation cycle and the final outcome may be quite different from the original network.

Building a biologically relevant network needs a lot of relevant information. Indeed, emergence of systems biology and network analysis has occurred alongside with, and made possible to a considerable extent by, the developments in various omic technologies, high-throughput platforms, high-content screens, bioinformatics, and large-scale data handling and storage [26]. Production of data on genes (genomics), transcripts (transcriptomics), proteins (proteomics), epigenetic changes, metabolites (metabolomics) has put forth the necessary raw material for building networks which encompass biologically relevant nodes (genes, proteins, metabolites), their connections (biochemical, regulatory), and modules (pathways, functional units), which through iterative process can become an increasingly relevant representation of real biological phenomena. On the other hand, the network analysis, once developed to a sufficient extent, offers a framework for data inclusion and interpretation by incorporating all pieces of information coming from earlier studies, current omics, high-content and high-throughput screening experiments, expected or unspecific findings, and these interpretations may lead to new experimental designs, both virtual and real.

Some experts envisage as a final goal the building of a virtual or *in silico* human [23]. Actually leading systems biologists signed the so-called Tokyo declaration in February 2008, with the aim for an *in silico* replica of a whole human body to be 90% complete by 2038. At the present, there are quite a number of simulation packages as spatiotemporal representations of various cellular functions [18].

5. Diseases as perturbations in biological networks

Many diseases, especially chronic ones, are initiated and perpetrated via dysregulation of multiple pathways, even if the primary reason is the mutation in a central gene associated with an endogenous or exogenous insult. The application of network analysis on human diseases, especially on those associated with polymorphisms, but increasingly also on diseases not primarily associated with structural mutations, has made it increasingly clear that chronic diseases demonstrate changes in expression of a large number of genes, proteins and metabolites, involve a large number of modules or functional units and show considerable overlap of important genes and network modules [27-31]. Obvious implications of this complexity are that single-target drugs may be completely inadequate to remedy a complex situation, and efficiency of any drug could be highly dependent on importance (centrality) of the target ("node" or "edge") in the disease network. In this respect, studies on drug-target networks suggest that many drugs developed earlier have rather peripheral targets in the disease-associated networks whereas many more novel drugs are interacting with targets closer to disease aetiology-linked components [32].

6. How to use network pharmacology in drug development?

Since the beginning of the genomic era, drug discovery process turned towards target based approaches for a deceptively simple reason: an ever efficient identification of a large number of potential targets for small and large molecules by the application of molecular biological and pharmacogenomics tools. Expectations have been large, but still costs have increased and the number of new medicinal entities stalled or decreased. Variable reasons for the increasing costs and a huge attrition even during clinical trials have been suggested, but many experts have begun to claim that the currently popular target-based approach is basically flawed as a guide for drug discovery process. Instead, many authors have argued that systems biology and polypharmacology encompassing network thinking should be adopted to remedy the current difficulties in drug discovery and development. However, because network pharmacology is a relatively new concept, there is not too much robust data to demonstrate its superiority in drug development process. Yet some pieces of information seem to point out that indeed network pharmacology is providing a new paradigm [12,33]. Some of the current suggestions based on network pharmacology are compiled in Table 2.

Target	Rationale	Example
Molecular target identification	Magic bullet aimed at target; if a target is a hub, the consequence may be too much toxicity	Current paradigm
Edgetic perturbation	Drug targeting towards a certain edge (connection) of an intended target	Inherited disorders seem to separate into node removal and edgetic-specific variants [34]
Motifs, modules	Drug targeting towards a common feature or a functional unit of importance to disease (symptom or aetiology)	Inhibitors of protein kinases with common structural motifs in the active site
Bridging nodes	A target resulting in a modulation of crosstalk between nodules, but not vital to cell function	No good example
Multi-targets	Multiple disease-associated nodes, which can be affected in an optimal manner without compromising vital cellular functions	Anti-psychotics on multiple transmitter-associated receptors

Table 2. Drug design, discovery, and repurposing potentialities of network pharmacology

Recently, Swinney & Anthony analysed preclinical discovery strategies that were used to identify potential drug candidates, which were ultimately approved by the US Food and Drug Administration (FDA) between 1999 and 2008 [35]. They classified strategies to target-based screening, phenotypic screening, modification of natural substances and biologic-based approaches, with an additional consideration on molecular mechanisms of action (MMOA). Out of the 259 agents that were approved, 75 were first-in-class drugs with new MMOAs, and out of these, 50 (67%) were small molecules and 25 (33%) were biologics. They claimed that the contribution of phenotypic screening to the discovery of first-in-class small-molecule drugs exceeded that of target-based approaches — with 28 and 17 of these drugs coming from the two approaches, respectively — in an era when the major focus was on target-based approaches. They postulated that a target-centric approach for first-in-class drugs, without consideration of an optimal MMOA, might contribute to the current high attrition rates and low productivity in pharmaceutical research and development. Instead, among follow-on drugs a vast majority were the outcomes of target-based approaches, which seem rather natural considering that for these drugs mechanism of action and many other crucial pieces of information could come much earlier and in more useful manner than for the first-in-class drugs. Actually the analysis of Swinney & Anthony concurs in many ways to the findings of Yildirim et al [32], in that many recent new drugs are interacting with novel targets thought to be more central in a corresponding disease aetiology, whereas follow-on molecules tend to stick to well-known, often more peripheral targets, which are more distal from core components of disease networks.

Although Swinney & Anthony did not specially mention network pharmacology (or corresponding) in their analysis, they refer to many crucial papers on network pharmacology. In their analysis phenotypic screening means the use of functional assays, which usually inform physiological parameters closer to real-life *in vivo* goals of drug therapy. Functional assays associated with the elucidation of the molecular mechanisms of action are much closer to the network analysis than the target-based screening. Intuitively it seems clear that functional assays are superior, at least from the drug discovery and development point of view, than target-based assays. However, in reality target-centred thinking has been dominant for more than a decade.

7. Properties of currently used drugs: Polypharmacology meets network pharmacology

Even if the current paradigm has been 'one target (or disease/symptom)-one drug', practising pharmacologists have always known that practically all drugs have multiple effects based on various known or unknown mechanisms, some desirable and others indifferent or harmful. A very good example is anti-psychotic drugs interacting with a large number of receptors and other targets. One target-one drug paradigm created a vision of a "magic bullet", which was eagerly adopted, although some scientists pointed out that even such "magic bullets" have pharmacokinetics-associated problems, e.g. potential drug-drug interactions, as well as structure-related problems such as allergic reactions. Now it is becoming increasingly apparent that biological systems are complex, redundant, homeostatic and resilient to perturbations and, consequently, most diseases are exhibiting much wider perturbations and variations than once thought. A new discipline, termed loosely as polypharmacology, has been gaining ground both conceptually and experimentally.

It seems highly likely that most current drugs are interacting with multiple targets. Current drug-protein interaction and chemogenomic studies have indicated that many drugs are interacting with two or more targets at reasonably close affinities. In these studies especially, the database of the FDA-approved drugs and their targets (effects) have been employed to create networks of drug-protein interactions [32,36] or to model similarities in chemical structure between drugs and potential ligands for the prediction of drug-target interactions [12, 37-38]. In Figure 1, a general approach to make use of the polypharmacology network is outlined [11]. In this approach the polypharmacology network is mapped onto the biological network, for example human disease-gene network, to reveal multiple actions of drugs on multiple targets and multiple diseases [30].

However, most of the studies on polypharmacology are based on computational and statistical associations, although some of the major findings have been studied further experimentally [37,38]. For example, a recent study demonstrated that unknown and unexpected "off-target" effects of many marketed drugs can be predicted by the computational analysis of ligand-target interaction; some predictions were experimentally confirmed [39]. Especially chemogenomic and chemoproteomic studies are based on direct or calculated affinities. It should be pointed out that affinity is not a reaction or other immediate outcome, e.g. antagonism, of an interaction and more distal functional or physiological consequences may or may not occur for various reasons even if a primary interaction has been demonstrated or predicted. Still clear evidence on functional consequences is required to be sure that an actual pharmacological significance is demonstrated for a substance.

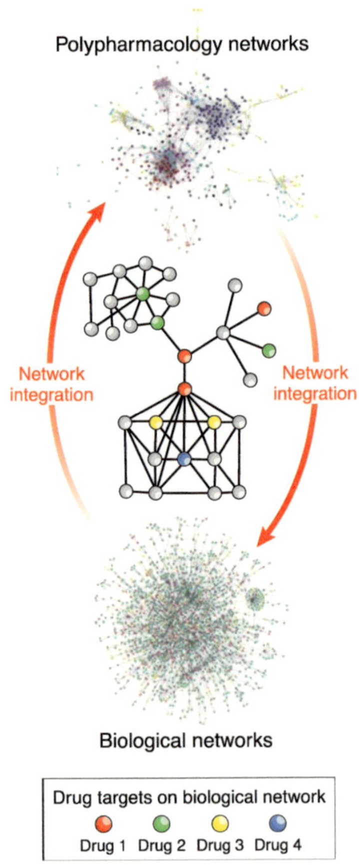

Figure 1. A network-centric view of drug action. Primary building blocks of network pharmacology are the drug-target network (above) and the biological network (below). The network in the centre is a part of the biological network in which proteins (nodes) targeted by the same drug are represented in the same colour. Consequently drug efficacy and toxicity can be understood by action at specific nodes and hubs. For the definition of nodes and hubs, see Table 1. The figure is reprinted by permission from Macmillan Publishers Ltd: [Nature Biotechnology] (11), copyright (2007).

Recently, a polypharmacological approach has been extended to include functional considerations. Simon et al [40] employed 1177 FDA-approved small molecular drugs by investigating interaction profiles based on *in silico* docking/scoring methods to a series of virtual non-target protein binding sites and contrasting these profiles with 177 major drug categories of the same series of FDA-approved drugs. Statistical analyses confirmed a close relationship between the studied effect categories and interaction profiles of small molecule drugs. On the basis of this relationship, the comprehensive effect profiles of drugs were apparent and furthermore, effects not previously associated with particular drugs could be predicted. A rather curious finding – which is not easily explained by classical pharmacological concepts – was that the prediction power was independent of the composition of the protein set used for interaction profile generation. Perhaps general chemical and physicochemical properties of molecules are of importance for potential interactions in general, whereas pharmacophores, i.e. specific stereochemical groups, are crucial for specific high-affinity interactions.

8. Systems toxicology

Network approach helps to understand and reveal on-target and off-target toxicity of pharmaceuticals, but it also helps to delineate the toxicities of any chemicals, be they industrial chemicals, agrochemicals, cosmetics, environmental pollutants, etc. Omic approaches provide voluminous information about time-dependent changes at various levels of biological complexity after the administration of a chemical and provide the so-called signatures of toxicity. On the other hand, the application of known and characterised toxicants has delineated a finite number of pathways of toxicity. Bringing this information together at the established network and systems level would create a 'systems toxicology' approach, analogous to systems pharmacology and polypharmacology [41].

9. Physiologically based pharmacokinetic (PBPK) modelling

A relatively isolated area in pharmacology and toxicology is the model building to describe the behaviour and disposition of drugs and other chemicals in the body [42]. Especially those models that make use of physiological principles resemble in many ways network pharmacology. Whole body PBPK models consist of absorption sites and manners, tissues with membranes drugs and their metabolites have to cross, with special reference to tissues which metabolise and excrete drugs and their metabolites, and so on. Concentrations of a studied chemical (and its important metabolites) in these various compartments could be equated to nodes. Connections are permeation and corresponding constants (for passive and active processes in the membranes and other cellular barriers, distribution coefficients, enzymatic reactions (clearance), and so on. Although the number of building blocks in pharmacokinetic models is finite and certainly much less than in most systems pharmacology networks, models have become quite complex, but still useful for predicting the behaviour of a drug in the body under various circumstances. Efforts to link PBPK models with *in vitro-in vivo* extrapolations under the systems pharmacology umbrella are underway [43].

Whole-body PBPK models illustrate also important challenges to, and potentialities of, network pharmacology. First of all, the framework for modelling is multi-scale [44], starting from enzymes and transporters (dealing with transformation and movement of drugs) and their quantitative functions (clearance, metabolite formation, membrane penetration) and their regulation and functions in the cells and tissues, kinetics of drugs and their metabolites throughout the body via circulation, distribution to different organs, elimination in urine, in bile, and integration of all processes into a dynamic model representing an individual (*in silico* human or animal, for that matter) and extending the modelling to evolution, development, environment, populations, diseases, etc. PBPK modelling is increasingly used in drug development and toxicity risk assessment with considerable success, probably because it is a rather restricted in dealing with behaviour of a single substance in the framework of a finite number of active players. On the other hand, pharmacodynamic models that have been developed for at least a couple of decades are closer to network building (*ab initio* models).

10. TCM network pharmacology & "network targets" for TCM drugs

In 2010, Liu & Du raised the concept of "TCM network pharmacology", linking the multiple components that play principal, complementary and assistant therapeutic roles in TCM formulae to principal, complementary and assistant targets in a disease network. They believed that such an approach to projecting a TCM drug component network onto a disease network offers a novel philosophical guide and technological route to designing and understanding mechanisms of action of TCM drugs and is thus likely proven important in modernisation of TCM [45]. Similarly, Li emphasised "network targets" of systems, connectivity and predictiveness features in studying TCM formulae and syndromes and the work of his team showed that the "network target" approach could facilitate discovery of effective compounds, understanding their interrelation, elucidating relationship between TCM formulae and diseases or TCM syndrome, developing rational TCM drug, as well as guiding integrated use of TCM and conventional drugs [46].

TCM network pharmacology heavily relies on omic platforms as well as algorithm- and network-based computational tools, which are elegantly summarised most recently by Leung et al [47]. In addition, TCM network pharmacology heavily relies on ever updating omics, pharmacological and TCM-related databases. While concerns about duplication of efforts, poor standardisation and low sustainability remain, many TCM databases have been developed, as recently reviewed by Barlow et al [48]. To mention a few, the Chem-TCM database developed by King's College London [49] has now been commercialised by TimTec LLC (http://www.chemtcm.com); the trial version of World Traditional & Natural Medicine Patent Database is currently being developed by Beijing East Linden Co. Ltd (http://www.east-linden.net/NewsShow.aspx?news_id=20081127102018850246); and the Herbal Ingredient Target database (HIT: http://lifecenter.sgst.cn/hit/) and the TCM Information Database

(TCM-ID: http://tcm.cz3.nus.edu.sg/group/tcm-id/tcmid_ns.asp) have been developed by academics based in China and Singapore [50,51].

11. Applications of TCM network pharmacology

In TCM, formulae are usually prescribed based on TCM syndrome patterns of a given patient, rather than a disease as defined in Western medicine. Thus, an important part of TCM network pharmacology is to establish links between network molecular targets and TCM syndrome patterns. Ma et al surveyed 4575 cases of Cold Syndrome patients and examined gene expression information of a typical Cold Syndrome pedigree by microarray. Results indicated that Cold Syndrome related genes played an essential role in energy metabolism, which were tightly correlated with the genes of neurotransmitters, hormones and cytokines in the neuro-endocrine-immune interaction network [52]. In TCM clinics, Cold Syndrome is treated by Warm formulae and Hot Syndrome is often treated by Cold formulae. Identification of the gene networks of Cold and Hot Syndromes [52, 53-55] should help understand nature of a condition and unravel mechanisms of its related TCM treatment [56].

In addition, Wang and colleagues (2011) proposed that network pharmacology could be applied to the following aspects of TCM studies:

11.1. "Disease-gene-target" network-based studies to identify targets and pathways affected by TCM drugs and to obtain fuller pictures of the efficacy and mechanisms of action of TCM drugs

Sun et al performed bioinformatic analysis of anti-Alzheimer's herbal medicines and found that ingredients of anti-Alzheimer's herbs not only bound symptom-relieving targets, but also interact closely with a variety of successful therapeutic targets related to other diseases, such as inflammation, cancer and diabetes, suggesting the possible cross-talk between these complicated diseases. Furthermore, the anti-Alzheimer's herbal ingredients densely targeted pathways of Ca^{2+} equilibrium maintaining upstream of cell proliferation and inflammation [57].

Wen et al used microarray and network analysis to establish that Si-Wu-Tang is an Nrf2 activator and phytoestrogen, thus suggesting its use as a nontoxic chemopreventive agent [58]. In fact, network analysis of all sorts of omic data can be used to explore the molecular targets and mechanisms of action of TCM drugs [59,60], as recently reviewed by Buriani et al [8]. In network pharmacology, roles for functional genes and proteins might vary in different stages of the same disease, thus the same disease could be treated differently, as emphasised in TCM; on the other hand, some functional proteins are "hubs" in the disease networks of more than one disease, thus different diseases could be treated similarly by targeting the same hubs [45]. Based on gene and phenotype information associated with the ingredient herbs of the classical Liu-wei-di-huang (LWDH) formula and LWDH-treated diseases, it was found that LWDH-treated diseases showed high phenotype similarity and identified certain "co-modules" enriched in cancer pathways and neuro-endocrine-immune pathways, which may be responsible for the action of treating different diseases by the same LWDH formula [61].

11.2. Construction of "TCM drugs-targets-diseases" network and elucidation of the scientific base of TCM drug formulation through network analysis

Zheng et al studied the interactions between 514 compounds contained in a Chinese herbal formula Jingzhi Tougu Xiaotong Granule (JZTGXTG) and 35 drug targets of relevance to osteoarthritis and the distribution of 514 compounds in drug-target space. By analysing parameters of the JZTGXTG compound-target interaction network and the drug-target interaction network including network heterogeneity and characteristic path length, the results illustrated the possible molecular mechanisms of JZTGXTG in the prevention and treatment of osteoarthritis at the network pharmacology level [62].

To predict multi-targets by multi-compounds found in Aconiti Lateralis Radix Praeparata, Wu et al constructed the corresponding multi-compound-multi-target network based on the drug-target relationship of FDA approved drugs. The predicted targets of 22 compounds of Aconiti Lateralis Radix Praeparata were validated by literature. Each compound in the established network was correlated with 16.3 targets on average, while each target was correlated with 4.77 compounds on average, which reflected the "multi-compound and multi-target" characteristic of TCM drugs [63].

A "network target" approach has been applied to virtual screening and established an algorithm known as network target-based identification of multicomponent synergy (NIMS) to prioritise synergistic combinations of agents in a high-throughput manner [64]. From a "network target" perspective, a method called distance-based mutual information model (DMIM) was established to identify useful relations among herbs in numerous herbal formulae and a novel concept of "co-module" across herb-biomolecule-disease multilayer networks was proposed to explore the potential mechanisms of herbal formulations [61]. DMIM, when used for retrieving herb pairs, achieved a good balance among the herb's frequency, independence, and distance in herbal formulae. A herb network constructed by DMIM from 3865 collaterals-related herbal formulae not only recovered traditionally defined herb pairs and formulae, but also generated novel anti-angiogenic herb ingredients and herb pairs with synergistic or antagonistic effects [61].

Li et al constructed a network of nine major active compounds from Fufang Danshen formula, their multi-targets and multiple related diseases. The nine compounds were tanshinone II A, salvianolic acid B, protocatechuic aldehyde, danshensu, cryptotanshinone, notoginsenoside R1, ginsenoside Rg1, ginsenoside Rb1 and borneol. Network analysis showed that these compounds could modulate 42 genes associated with cardiovascular diseases (e.g. PPARG, ACE, KCNJ11, KCNQ1 and ABCC8), which were related to 30 clinical conditions, including non-insulin-dependent diabetes mellitus, hyperinsulinaemic hypoglycaemia, hypertension and coronary heart disease [65].

http://dx.doi.org/10.5772/53868

11.3. Building "TCM drug properties-clinical indications-adverse effects" networks and illustrating the relationship between TCM drug properties and efficacy

Jia et al analysed 117 drug combinations and identified general and specific modes of action and highlighted the potential value of molecular interaction profiles in the discovery of novel multicomponent therapies [66].

Zhu et al performed network analysis of 2215 chemicals identified in 62 Chinese herbs indicated for patients with chronic kidney diseases, including 836 chemicals contained in 22 tonifying herbs and 1379 chemicals contained in 40 evil-expelling herbs, according to TCM theory, in comparison with 99 drugs used in conventional medicine. Interaction networks of tonifying herbs, evil-expelling herbs and drugs showed different patterns, regarding network parameters, especially network degree, average number of neighbours and characteristic path lengths and shortest paths [67].

Wu et al constructed a relational network of TCM decoction slices to discover and interpret the correlations between the natures and functions of decoction slices and their clinically indicated symptoms and channel tropism as defined in TCM. 3016 pairs of decoction slice-symptom correlation associated with 646 decoction slices were discovered [68].

11.4. Evaluation of the safety, efficacy and stability of TCM products through constructing network models and network analysis

Emerging studies have supported the potential for network pharmacology in quality control of TCM drugs [69], which can well interpret the mechanisms of action of TCM drugs [70], help understand how different constituents of a TCM formulation and how TCM and chemical drugs synergised through targeting different nodes in disease-related networks [71,72]. There is no regulatory requirement of omics-based data in any submitted dossier to any regulatory agency, including for TCM products. However, it has been acknowledged that such studies are being increasingly performed, and almost surely will eventually be included into regulatory submission dossiers, possibly initially as supplementary materials [9]. Such a prospect is likely also shared with systems and network pharmacology.

12. Inspirations and challenges that TCM has to offer to network pharmacology

12.1. More networks

In network pharmacology, "network" refers to the molecular network in a targeted organism, for instance the "network targets" in patients. In TCM network pharmacology, however, complex TCM drugs themselves become another important molecular network, which might be called "network bullets" that interact with "network targets" in order to help the body to regain balance. Importantly, some components of TCM drugs are not to target "network targets", but to target other drug components, so as to alleviate their side-effects, improve activity of the principal drug component, improve absorption and/or facilitate delivery of the principal drug to the targeted disease areas. Thus, TCM network pharmacology involves at least two networks to be considered in modelling and analysis.

In TCM, as guided by TCM theories, it is of paramount importance to choose a number of herbs (sometimes also zoological or mineral components) based on particular symptoms and characteristics of a patient. To assemble a formula or *fangji*, principal and enabling herbs are combined in order to optimise the effectiveness and minimise adverse effects. The principal herbs are known as the *jun* herbs, which treat the main cause or primary symptoms of a disease. The enabling herbs include the *chen* herbs, which serve to augment or broaden the effects of *jun* herbs and to relieve secondary symptoms; *zuo* herbs, which modulate the effects of *jun* and *chen* herbs and to counteract the toxic or side effects of these herbs; and the *shi* herbs, which function to facilitate absorption and delivery of active herbal components to the target organs. Thus, the combination of principal (*Jun*) and enabling (*Chen*, *Zuo* and/or *Shi*) components to form a drug network could form the basis for designing novel "network bullets" in the future application of network pharmacology.

12.2. More holistic

Network pharmacology aims to research and develop drugs holistically. However, the current model of network pharmacology that focuses on psychological and somatic diseases separately could be improved if it is to meet requirements of the psychosomatic model of health and ailments. Specifically, in addition to the well-known placebo effects of any interventions, the pathological damage of emotions to the internal organs is of primary concern of TCM practitioners. We propose that psychosomatic factors should be linked up in the next generation of network pharmacology and emotions should be included in the equations of future network analysis. By doing so, research might eventually help unravel and harness placebo effects and tackle psychosomatic ailments in a network pharmacological perspective.

12.3. More individualised

Personalised medicine is gaining momentum [73-75]. Network pharmacology needs to catch up with this trend as well. In TCM, individualisation goes beyond personalisation, because the same person at different ages, on different diets or living style, under different weather condition and at the different phases of the same disease could be diagnosed and treated differently. Can network pharmacology not only be personalised but also individualised, taking all the above variations into account?

13. Conclusions and perspectives

According to Paul Unschuld, a renowned German sinologist, cultural background has a great impact on the preferred directions of medical science. For example, both in ancient Greece and China philosophers came up with the idea of "relationist science" or "science of systematic correspondences" on the one hand and "analytical science" on the other. While in ancient Europe relationist science was soon marginalised and analytical science became the approach of choice, in ancient China the beginnings of an analytical perspective were not pursued further and relationist science became the approach of choice [76]. Nowadays, the post-genomic era is characterised by globalisation and digitalisation. While omic data represent the state of the art of the analytical power of Western science, these data could be meaningless "sacs of data" unless they are linked up functionally using a relationist approach. At this point, the dominant approaches in the West and East are integrated to relate pieces of fragmented omic data and their functions and this might well serve as a bridge of both medical traditions. Analyses of state-of-the-art modern and TCM pharmacological and toxicological research data appear to support the concept of network pharmacology, i.e. a systems network-based model can help better understand health, disease and how Western medicine, TCM drugs or integrated TCM and Western medicine work. It can be expected that this approach could play a more important role in research and development of new drugs and in helping understand the mechanisms of action of drugs, especially in TCM.

Acknowledgements

This manuscript is supported by the GP-TCM project funded by the European Commission under the FP7 grant agreement No. 223154. Dr. Qihe Xu is the Coordinator of the project; Professor Olavi Pelkonen is a member of the management and science committee. Both Professor Olavi Pelkonen and Dr. Fan Qu are non-beneficiary members.

Author details

Qihe Xu[1*], Fan Qu[2] and Olavi Pelkonen[3*]

*Address all correspondence to: qihe.xu@kcl.ac.uk

*Address all correspondence to: qihe.xu@kcl.ac.uk and olavi.pelkonen@oulu.fi

1 Department of Renal Medicine, King's College London, London, UK

2 Women's Hospital, Zhejiang University, Hangzhou, Zhejiang, China

3 Department of Pharmacology and Toxicology, University of Oulu, Oulu, Finland

References

[1] Normile D. Asian medicine. The new face of traditional Chinese medicine. Science 2003;299(5604): 188-90.

[2] Xue T., Roy R. Studying traditional Chinese medicine. Science 2003;300(5620): 740-1.

[3] Qiu J. Back to the future' for Chinese herbal medicines. Nature Reviews Drug Discovery 2007; 6: 506-507.

[4] Miller LH., Su X. Artemisinin: discovery from the Chinese herbal garden. Cell 2011;146(6): 855-8.

[5] Neill US. From branch to bedside: Youyou Tu is awarded the 2011 Lasker~DeBakey Clinical Medical Research Award for discovering artemisinin as a treatment for malaria. Journalof Clinical Investigation 2011;121(10): 3768-73.

[6] Uzuner H., Fan TP., Dias A., Guo DA., El-Nezami HS., Xu Q. Establishing an EU-China consortium on traditional Chinese medicine research. Chinese Medicine 2010;5: 42.

[7] Uzuner H., Bauer R., Fan TP., Guo DA., Dias A., El-Nezami H., Efferth T., Williamson EM., Heinrich M., Robinson N., Hylands PJ., Hendry BM., Cheng YC., Xu Q. Traditional Chinese medicine research in the post-genomic era: Good practice, priorities, challenges and opportunities. Journal of Ethnopharmacology 2012;140(3): 458-68.

[8] Buriani A., Garcia-Bermejo ML., Bosisio E., Xu Q., Li H., Dong X., Simmonds MS., Carrara M., Tejedor N., Lucio-Cazana J., Hylands PJ. Omic techniques in systems biology approches to traditional Chinese medicine research: present and future.Journal of Ethnopharmacology 2012;140(3): 535-44.

[9] Pelkonen O., Pasanen M., Lindon JC., Chan K., Zhao L., Deal G., Xu Q., Fan TP. Omics and its potential impact on R&D and regulation of complex herbal products. Journal of Ethnopharmacology 2012;140(3): 587-93.

[10] Gowers T., Nielsen M. Massively collaborative mathematics. Nature 2009;461(7266): 879-81.

[11] Hopkins AL. Network pharmacology. Nature Biotechnology 2007;25(10): 1110-1.

[12] HopkinsAL. Network pharmacology: The next paradigm in drug discovery. Nature Chemical Biology 2008;4(11): 682-90.

[13] Apsel B., Blair JA., Gonzalez B., Nazif TM., Feldman ME., Aizenstein B., Hoffman R., Williams RL., Shokat KM., Knight ZA. Targeted polypharmacology: discovery of dual inhibitors of tyrosine and phosphoinositide kinases. Nature Chemical Biology 2008;4(11): 691-9.

[14] Knight ZA., Lin H., Shokat KM. Targeting the cancer kinome through polypharmacology. Nature Reviews Cancer 2010;10(2):130-7.

[15] Ekins S., Mestres J., Testa B. In silico pharmacology for drug discovery: methods for virtual ligand screening and profiling. British Journal of Pharmacology 2007;152(1): 9-20.

[16] van der Greef J., McBurney RN. Innovation: Rescuing drug discovery: in vivo systems pathology and systems pharmacology. Nature Reviews Drug Discovery 2005;4(12): 961-7.

[17] Zhao S., Iyengar R. Systems pharmacology: network analysis to identify multiscale mechanisms of drug action.Annual Review of Pharmacology and Toxicology 2012;52: 505-21.

[18] Boerries M., Eils R., and Busch H. Systems Biology. In: Meyers RA. (ed.)Systems Biology.Boschstr: Wiley-VCH Verlag & Co. KGaA; 2012. p3-31.

[19] Arrell DK., Terzic A. Network systems biology for drug discovery. Clinical Pharmacology & Therapeutics 2010;88(1): 120-5.

[20] Barabasi AL., Albert R. Emergence of scaling in random networks. Science 1999; 286(5439): 509-12.

[21] Barabasi AL., Oltvai ZN. Network biology: understanding the cell's functional organization. Nature Reviews Genetics 2004;5(2): 101-13.

[22] Barabasi AL. Scale-free networks: a decade and beyond. Science 2009;325(5939): 412-3.

[23] Kolodkin A., Boogerd FC., Plant N., Bruggeman FJ., Goncharuk V., Lunshof J., Moreno-Sanchez R., Yilmaz N., Bakker BM., Snoep JL., Balling R., Westerhoff HV. Emergence of the silicon human and network targeting drugs. European Journalof Pharmaceutical Sciences 2012;46(4): 190-7.

[24] Joyner MJ. Physiology: alone at the bottom, alone at the top. Journal of Physiology 2011;589 (Pt 5): 1005.

[25] Merico D., Gfeller D., Bader GD. How to visually interpret biological data using networks. Nature Biotechnology 2009;27(10): 921-4.

[26] Westerhoff HV., Palsson BO. The evolution of molecular biology into systems biology. Nature Biotechnology 2004;22(10): 1249-52.

[27] Barabasi AL., Gulbahce N., Loscalzo J. Network medicine: a network-based approach to human disease. Nature Reviews Genetics 2011;12(1): 56-68.

[28] Barrenäs F., Chavali S., Holme P., Mobini R., Benson M. Network properties of complex human disease genes identified through genome-wide association studies. PLoS One 2009;4(11): e8090.

[29] Chavali S., Barrenas F., Kanduri K., Benson M. Network properties of human disease genes with pleiotropic effects. BMC Systems Biology 2010;4: 78.

[30] Goh KI., Cusick ME., Valle D., Childs B., Vidal M., Barabasi AL. The human disease network. The Proceedings of the National Academy of Sciences of the United States of America 2007;104(21): 8685-90.

[31] Schadt EE. Molecular networks as sensors and drivers of common human diseases. Nature 2009;461(7261): 218-23.

[32] Yildirim MA., Goh KI., Cusick ME., Barabasi AL., Vidal M. Drug-target network. Nature Biotechnology 2007;25(10): 1119-26.

[33] Hopkins AL., Mason JS., Overington JP. Can we rationally design promiscuous drugs? Current Opinion in Structural Biology 2006;16(1): 127-36.

[34] Zhong Q., Simonis N., Li QR., Charloteaux B., Heuze F., Klitgord N., Tam S., Yu H., Venkatesan K., Mou D., Swearingen V., Yildirim MA., Yan H., Dricot A., Szeto D., Lin C., Hao T., Fan C., Milstein S., Dupuy D., Brasseur R., Hill DE., Cusick ME., Vidal M. Edgetic perturbation models of human inherited disorders. Molecular Systems Biology2009;5: 321.

[35] Swinney DC., Anthony J. How were new medicines discovered? Nature Reviews Drug Discovery 2011;10(7): 507-19.

[36] Paolini GV., Shapland RH., van Hoorn WP., Mason JS., Hopkins AL. Global mapping of pharmacological space. Nature Biotechnology 2006;24(7): 805-15.

[37] Keiser MJ., Roth BL., Armbruster BN., Ernsberger P., Irwin JJ., Shoichet BK. Relating protein pharmacology by ligand chemistry. Nature Biotechnology 2007;25(2): 197-206.

[38] Keiser MJ., Setola V., Irwin JJ., Laggner C., Abbas AI., Hufeisen SJ., Jensen NH., Kuijer MB., Matos RC., Tran TB., Whaley R., Glennon RA., Hert J., Thomas KL., Edwards DD., Shoichet BK., Roth BL. Predicting new molecular targets for known drugs. Nature 2009;462(7270): 175-81.

[39] Lounkine E., Keiser MJ., Whitebread S., Mikhailov D., Hamon J., Jenkins JL., Lavan P., Weber E., Doak AK., Cote S., Shoichet BK., Urban L. Large-scale prediction and testing of drug activity on side-effect targets. Nature 2012;486(7403): 361-7.

[40] Simon Z., Peragovics A., Vigh-Smeller M., Csukly G., Tombor L., Yang Z., Zahoránszky-Kohalmi G., Végner L., Jelinek B., Hári P., Hetényi C., Bitter I., Czobor P., Málnási-Csizmadia A.Drug effect prediction by polypharmacology-based interaction profiling. Journal of Chemical Information and Modeling 2012;52(1): 134-45.

[41] Hartung T., van Vliet E., Jaworska J., Bonilla L., Skinner N., Thomas R. Food for thought ... systems toxicology. ALTEX - - Alternatives to Animal Experimentation2012;29(2): 119-28.

[42] Coecke S., Pelkonen O., Batista Leite S., Bernauer U., Bessems J., Bois F., Gundert-Remy U., Loizou G., Testai E., Zaldívar JM. Toxicokinetics as a key to the integrated toxicity risk assessment based primarily on non-animal approaches. Toxicology In Vitro 2012 Jul 4 [Epub ahead of print].

[43] Rostami-Hodjegan A. Physiologically Based Pharmacokinetics Joined With In Vitro-In Vivo Extrapolation of ADME: A Marriage Under the Arch of Systems Pharmacology. Clinical Pharmacology & Therapeutics 2012;92(1): 50-61.

[44] Vicini P. Multiscale modeling in drug discovery and development: Future opportunities and present challenges. Clinical Pharmacology & Therapeutics 2010;88(1): 126-9.

[45] Liu AL., Du GH. Network pharmacology: new guidelines for drug discovery. Yao Xue Xue Bao 2010;45(12): 1472–7.

[46] Li S. Network target: a starting point for traditional Chinese medicine network pharmacology. Zhongguo Zhong Yao Za Zhi. 2011;36(15):2017-20.

[47] Leung EL., Cao ZW., Jiang ZH., Zhou H., Liu L. Network-based drug discovery by integrating systems biology and computational technologies. Briefings in Bioinformatics 2012 Aug 9. [Epub ahead of print]

[48] Barlow DJ., Buriani A., Ehrman T., Bosisio E., Eberini I., Hylands PJ. In-silico studies in Chinese herbal medicines' research: evaluation of in-silico methodologies and phytochemical data sources, and a review of research to date.Journal of Ethnopharmacology 2012;140(3): 526-34.

[49] Ehrman TM., Barlow DJ., Hylands PJ. Phytochemical databases of Chinese herbal constituents and bioactive plant compounds with known target specificities.Journal of Chemical Information and Modeling 2007;47(2): 254-63.

[50] Chen X., Zhou H., Liu YB., Wang JF., Li H., Ung CY., Han LY., Cao ZW., Chen YZ. Database of traditional Chinese medicine and its application to studies of mechanism and to prescription validation. British Journalof Pharmacology 2006;149(8): 1092-103.

[51] Ye H., Ye L., Kang H., Zhang D., Tao L., Tang K., Liu X., Zhu R., Liu Q., Chen YZ., Li Y., Cao Z. HIT: linking herbal active ingredients to targets. Nucleic Acids Research 2011;39(Database issue): D1055-9.

[52] Ma T., Tan C., Zhang H., Wang M., Ding W., Li S. Bridging the gap between traditional Chinese medicine and systems biology: the connection of Cold Syndrome and NEI network. Molecular BioSystems 2010;6(4): 613-9.

[53] van Wietmarschen H., Yuan K., Lu C., Gao P., Wang J., Xiao C., Yan X., Wang M., Schroën J., Lu A., Xu G., van der Greef J. Systems biology guided by Chinese medicine reveals new markers for sub-typing rheumatoid arthritis patients. Journalof Clinical Rheumatology 2009;15(7): 330-7.

[54] Chen G., Lu C., Zha Q., Xiao C., Xu S., Ju D., Zhou Y., Jia W., Lu A. A network-based analysis of traditional Chinese medicine cold and hot patterns in rheumatoid arthritis. Complementary Therapies in Medicine2012; 20(1-2): 23-30.

[55] Jiang M., Xiao C., Chen G., Lu C., Zha Q., Yan X., Kong W., Xu S., Ju D., Xu P., Zou Y., Lu A. Correlation between cold and hot pattern in traditional Chinese medicine

and gene expression profiles in rheumatoid arthritis. Frontiers of medicine 2011;5(2): 219-28.

[56] Wang Y, Gao X, Zhang B, Cheng Y. Building methodology for discovering and developing Chinese medicine based on network biology.Zhongguo Zhong Yao Za Zhi 2011;36(2): 228-31.

[57] Sun Y., Zhu R., Ye H., Tang K., Zhao J., Chen Y., Liu Q., Cao Z. Towards a bioinformatics analysis of anti-Alzheimer's herbal medicines from a target network perspective. Briefings in Bioinformatics 2012 Aug 11. [Epub ahead of print].

[58] Wen Z, Wang Z, Wang S, Ravula R, Yang L, Xu J, Wang C, Zuo Z, Chow MS, Shi L, Huang Y. Discovery of molecular mechanisms of traditional Chinese medicinal formula Si-Wu-Tang using gene expression microarray and connectivity map. PLoS One 2011;6(3): e18278.

[59] Yue QX., Cao ZW., Guan SH., Liu XH., Tao L., Wu WY., Li YX., Yang PY., Liu X., Guo DA. Proteomics characterization of the cytotoxicity mechanism of ganoderic acid D and computer-automated estimation of the possible drug target network. Molecular & Cellular Proteomics 2008;7(5): 949-61.

[60] Gao X., Zheng X., Li Z., Zhou Y., Sun H., Zhang L., Guo X., Du G., Qin X. Metabonomic study on chronic unpredictable mild stress and intervention effects of Xiaoyaosan in rats using gas chromatography coupled with mass spectrometry. Journal of Ethnopharmacology 2011;137(1): 690-9.

[61] Li S., Zhang B., Jiang D., Wei Y., Zhang N. Herb network construction and co-module analysis for uncovering the combination rule of traditional Chinese herbal formulae. BMC Bioinformatics 2010;11(Suppl 11):S6.

[62] Zheng CS., Xu XJ., Liu XX., Ye HZ. Computational pharmacology of Jingzhi Tougu Xiaotong Granule in preventing and treating osteoarthritis. Acta Physico-Chimica Sinica 2010;26(3): 775-83.

[63] Wu L., Gao X., Wang L., Liu Q., Fan X., Wang Y., Cheng Y. Prediction of multi-target of Aconiti Lateralis Radix Praeparata and its network pharmacology. Zhongguo Zhong Yao Za Zhi. 2011;36(21): 2907-10.

[64] Li S., Zhang B., Zhang N. Network target for screening synergistic drug combinations with application to traditional Chinese medicine. BMC Systems Biology 2011; 5(Suppl 1): S10.

[65] Li X., Wu L., Fan X., Zhang B., Gao X., Wang Y., Cheng Y. Network pharmacology study on major active compounds of Fufang Danshen formula.Zhongguo Zhong Yao Za Zhi 2011;36(21): 2911-5.

[66] Jia J., Zhu F., Ma X., Cao Z., Li Y., Chen YZ. Mechanisms of drug combinations: interaction and network perspectives. Nature Reviews Drug Discovery 2009;8(2): 111-28.

[67] Zhu W., Qiu XH., Xu XJ., Lu CJ. Computational network pharmacological research of Chinese medicinal plants for chronic kidney disease. Science China Chemistry 2010; 53(11): 2337-42.

[68] Wu L., Gao X., Cheng Y., Wang Y., Zhang B., Fan X. Symptom-based traditional Chinese medicine slices relationship network and its network pharmacology study. Zhongguo Zhong Yao Za Zhi 2011;36(21):2916-9.

[69] Tilton R., Paiva AA., Guan JQ., Marathe R., Jiang Z., van Eyndhoven W., Bjoraker J., Prusoff Z., Wang H., Liu SH., Cheng YC. A comprehensive platform for quality control of botanical drugs (PhytomicsQC): a case study of Huangqin Tang (HQT) and PHY906. Chinese Medicine 2010;20;5:30.

[70] Lam W., Bussom S., Guan F., Jiang Z., Zhang W., Gullen EA., Liu SH., Cheng YC. The four-herb Chinese medicine PHY906 reduces chemotherapy-induced gastrointestinal toxicity. Science Translational Medicine 2010;2(45): 45ra59.

[71] Wang E., Bussom S., Chen J., Quinn C., Bedognetti D., Lam W., Guan F., Jiang Z., Mark Y., Zhao Y., Stroncek DF., White J., Marincola FM., Cheng YC. Interaction of a traditional Chinese Medicine (PHY906) and CPT-11 on the inflammatory process in the tumor microenvironment. BMC Medical Genomics 2011;4: 38.

[72] Wang L., Zhou GB., Liu P., Song JH., Liang Y., Yan XJ., Xu F., Wang BS., Mao JH., Shen ZX., Chen SJ., Chen Z. Dissection of mechanisms of Chinese medicinal formula Realgar-Indigo naturalis as an effective treatment for promyelocytic leukemia.The Proceedings of the National Academy of Sciences of the United States of America 2008;105(12): 4826-31.

[73] Chen R., Mias GI., Li-Pook-Than J., Jiang L., Lam HY., Chen R., Miriami E., Karczewski KJ., Hariharan M., Dewey FE., Cheng Y., Clark MJ., Im H., Habegger L., Balasubramanian S., O'Huallachain M., Dudley JT., Hillenmeyer S., Haraksingh R., Sharon D., Euskirchen G., Lacroute P., Bettinger K., Boyle AP., Kasowski M., Grubert F., Seki S., Garcia M., Whirl-Carrillo M., Gallardo M., Blasco MA., Greenberg PL., Snyder P., Klein TE., Altman RB., Butte AJ., Ashley EA., Gerstein M., Nadeau KC., Tang H., Snyder M. Personal omics profiling reveals dynamic molecular and medical phenotypes. Cell 2012;148(6): 1293-307.

[74] DeFrancesco L. Omics gets personal. Nature Biotechnology 2012;30(4): 332.

[75] Vaidyanathan G. Redefining clinical trials: the age of personalized medicine. Cell 2012;148(6): 1079-80.

[76] Unschuld PU. What is Medicine? Western and Eastern Approaches to Healing. 1st Edition, Berkeley: University of California Press; 2009.

بہت تیز بخار

تیز بخار جلد ہی کم نہ کیا جائے تو خطرناک ہوسکتا ہے۔ اس سے تشنج کے دورے پڑ سکتے ہیں اور دماغ کو مستقل نقصان (فالج، ذہنی سستی، مرگی وغیرہ) پہنچ سکتا ہے۔ تیز بخار چھوٹے بچوں کے لیے سب سے زیادہ خطرناک ہے۔

بخار بہت تیز ہوجائے (140 درجے فارن ہائیٹ/ 40 درجے سینٹی گریڈ سے اوپر) تو اسے فوراً کم کرنے کی کوشش کرنی چاہیے:

1۔ مریض کو ٹھنڈی جگہ پر لٹائیں۔

2۔ تمام کپڑے اتار دیں۔

3۔ پنکھا جھلیں۔

4۔ اس پر ٹھنڈا (بالکل یخ نہیں) پانی ڈالیں یا ٹھنڈے پانی میں بھگوئے ہوئے کپڑے کی پٹیاں سینے اور ماتھے پر رکھیں۔ پٹیوں پر پنکھا جھلیں اور انہیں ٹھنڈا رکھنے کے لیے بدلتے رہیں۔ جب تک بخار کم نہ ہوجائے (101 درجے فارن ہائیٹ/ 38 درجے سینٹی گریڈ سے نیچے) یہ عمل کرتے رہیں۔

5۔ اسے پینے کے لیے بہت سا ٹھنڈا (بالکل یخ نہیں) پانی دیں۔

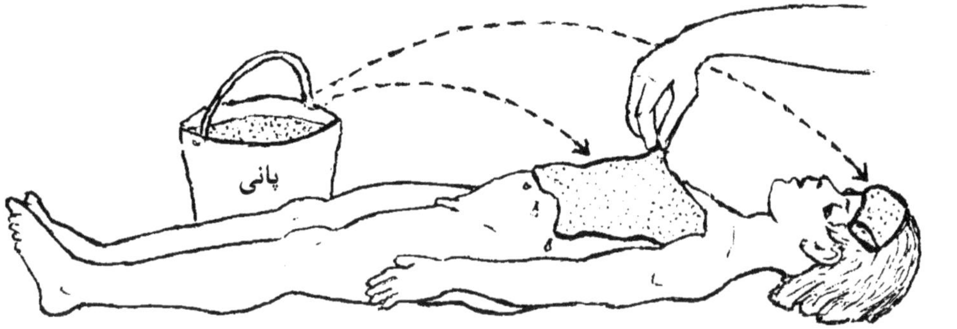

6۔ بخار کم کرنے کے لیے دوا دیں۔ اسپرین یا اسیٹامائینوفین مفید ہوتی ہے۔

خوراک: اسپرین یا اسیٹامائینوفین کی خوراک (بالغ افراد کے لیے 300 ملی گرام کی گولیوں کی شکل میں ملتی ہے)

12 سال سے زیادہ عمر کے افراد کے لیے: 2 گولیاں ہر 4 گھنٹے بعد

6 سے 12 سال کے بچوں کے لیے: 1 گولی ہر 4 گھنٹے بعد

3 سے 6 سال کے بچوں کے لیے: $\frac{1}{2}$ (آدھی) گولی ہر 4 گھنٹے بعد

3 سال سے کم عمر بچوں کے لیے: $\frac{1}{4}$ (چوتھائی) گولی ہر 4 گھنٹے بعد

نوٹ: 12 سال سے کم عمر بچے کے لیے، جسے زکام، فلو یا خسرہ ہو اسیٹامائینوفین اسپرین سے زیادہ محفوظ ہوتی ہے (دیکھیں صفحہ 379)۔

اگر بخار میں مبتلا فرد گولیاں نہیں نگل سکتا تو انہیں پیس کر پوڈر بنالیں، پوڈر میں کچھ پانی ملائیں اور بغیر سوئی کی سرنج سے یا انیما کے طور پر مقعد (پاخانے کی جگہ) میں داخل کریں۔

اگر تیز بخار جلد کم نہیں ہوتا یا اگر تشنج کے دورے پڑنا شروع ہوجاتے ہیں تو پانی سے ٹھنڈا کرنے کا عمل جاری رکھیں اور فوری طور پر طبی امداد حاصل کریں۔

شاک یا صدمہ

شاک یا صدمہ ایک جان لیوا کیفیت ہے جو بہت زیادہ جلنے، خون ضائع ہونے، سخت بیماری، پانی کی کمی یا شدید الرجک ردعمل سے ہوسکتی ہے۔ شاک، جسم کے اندر بہت زیادہ خون بہنے سے، چاہے وہ نظر نہ آرہا ہو، بھی ہوسکتا ہے۔

صدمے کی علامات:

- کمزور اور تیز نبض (100 فی منٹ سے زیادہ)
- ٹھنڈے پسینے، جلد کا پیلا، ٹھنڈا اور نم پڑ جانا
- خون کا دباؤ (بلڈ پریشر) خطرناک حد تک گر جانا
- ذہنی الجھن، کمزوری یا بے ہوشی۔

صدمے کی روک تھام یا علاج کے لیے کیا کیا جائے:

صدمے کی پہلی علامت پر، یا اگر صدمے کا خطرہ ہو...

- مریض کو یوں لٹائیں کہ پیر سر کے مقابلے میں کچھ اوپر ہوں، اس طرح:

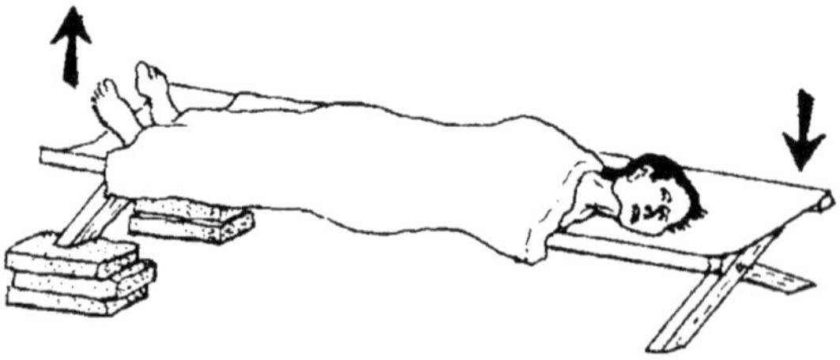

تاہم اگر اس کے سر پر شدید زخم ہے تو اسے نیم دراز (کچھ لیٹے کچھ بیٹھے) حالت میں لائیں (صفحہ 91)۔

- خون بہہ رہا ہو تو روکیں۔
- مریض کو سردی لگ رہی ہو تو کمبل اوڑھائیں۔
- اگر وہ ہوش میں ہے اور پی سکتا ہے تو پانی یا کوئی اور مشروب چسکیوں میں پلائیں۔ اگر اس میں پانی کی کمی محسوس ہورہی ہو تو بہت سا پانی اور دوسرے مشروبات پلائیں اور نمکول دیں (صفحہ 152)۔
- زخم ہوں تو ان کا علاج کریں۔
- اگر اسے درد ہو تو اسپرین یا درد کی کوئی اور دوا دیں لیکن کوڈین جیسی کوئی سکون آور دوا نہ دیں۔
- اسے پرسکون رکھیں اور تسلی دیں۔

اگر مریض بے ہوش ہے تو:

- اسے کروٹ کے بل لٹائیں، سر نیچے، پیچھے ڈھلکا ہوا اور ایک طرف کو رکھیں (اوپر کی تصویر دیکھیں)۔ اگر اس کی سانس رکتی ہوئی محسوس ہورہی ہے تو انگلی سے اس کی زبان آگے کھینچیں۔
- اگر اسے الٹی آئی ہے تو اس کا منہ فوراً صاف کریں۔ اس کا سر نیچے، پیچھے ڈھلکا ہو اور ایک طرف کو ہونا چاہیے تاکہ سانس کے ساتھ قے پھیپھڑوں میں نہ جائے۔
- جب تک وہ ہوش میں نہ آجائے کھانے پینے کی کوئی چیز نہ دیں۔
- اگر آپ کو یا آپ کے آس پاس موجود کسی شخص کو ڈرپ (نارمل سیلائن) لگانا آتا ہے تو تیز ڈرپ کے ساتھ دیں۔
- جلد طبی امداد حاصل کریں۔

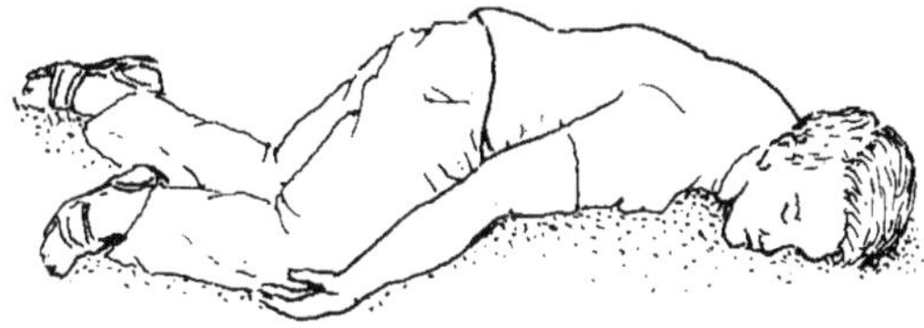

بے ہوشی

بے ہوشی کی عام وجوہات یہ ہیں:

- نشے میں دھت ہونا
- سر پر ضرب لگنا
- شاک یا صدمہ (صفحہ 77)
- جھٹکوں کے دورے (صفحہ 178)
- زہر پھیل جانا (صفحہ 103)
- غشی (خوف، کمزوری وغیرہ سے)
- لو لگنا (صفحہ 81)
- فالج (صفحہ 327)
- دل کا دورہ (صفحہ 325)

اگر کوئی شخص بے ہوش ہے اور آپ کو وجہ معلوم نہیں تو **فوراً مندرجہ ذیل چیزیں دیکھیں:**

1۔ کیا وہ **ٹھیک سے سانس** لے رہا ہے؟ اگر ایسا نہیں، تو اس کا سر پیچھے ڈھلکائیں اور جبڑے اور زبان کو آگے کھینچیں۔ اگر اس کے حلق میں کوئی چیز پھنسی ہے تو باہر نکالیں۔ اگر وہ سانس نہیں لے رہا تو فوراً منہ کے ذریعے مصنوعی سانس دلائیں (دیکھیں صفحہ 80)۔

2۔ کیا اس کا بہت **خون ضائع ہو رہا ہے؟** اگر ایسا ہے تو خون روکیں (دیکھیں صفحہ 82)۔

3۔ کیا وہ صدمے میں ہے (گیلی، پیلی جلد، کمزور اور تیز نبض)؟ اگر ایسا ہے تو اسے اس طرح لٹائیں کہ سر، پیر کی سطح سے نیچے ہو اور کپڑے ڈھیلے کر دیں (دیکھیں صفحہ 77)۔

4۔ کیا لو لگ گئی ہے (پسینہ نہیں آ رہا، تیز بخار، گرم سرخ جلد)؟ اگر ایسا ہے تو اسے دھوپ سے بچائیں، سر کو پیروں سے اوپر بلند سطح پر رکھیں اور ٹھنڈے (ممکن ہو تو برف کے) پانی میں بھگو دیں اور پنکھا جھلیں (دیکھیں صفحہ 81)۔

بے ہوش شخص کو کس حالت میں لٹایا جائے:

بہت پیلی جلد:
(شاک، غشی وغیرہ)

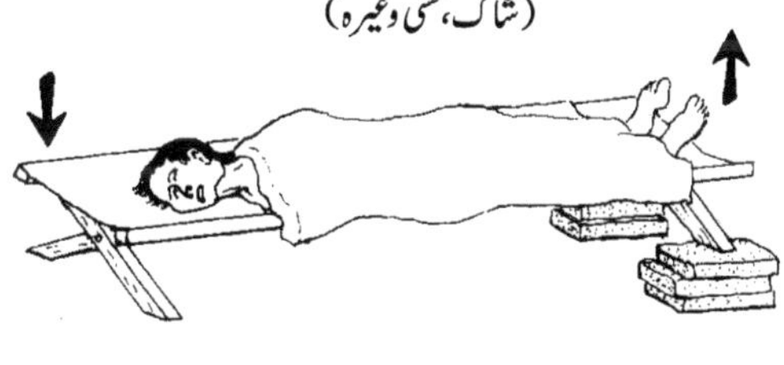

سرخ یا معمول کی رنگت کی جلد:
(لو لگنا، فالج، دل کی تکلیف، سر کا زخم)

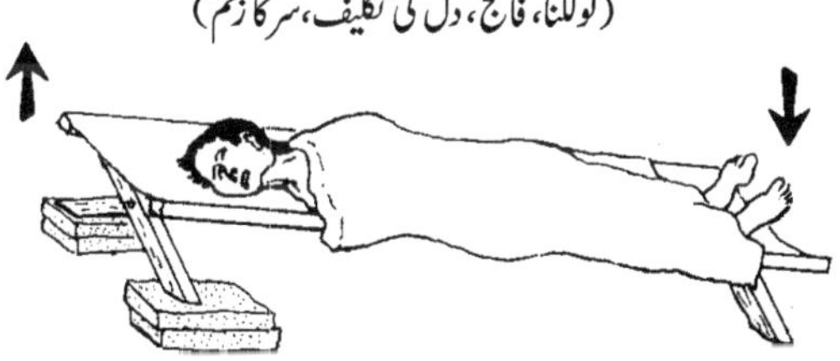

اگر اندیشہ ہے کہ بے ہوش شخص سخت زخمی ہے:

جب تک وہ ہوش میں نہیں آتا اسے ہلانا جلانا مناسب نہیں۔ اگر ہلانا ضروری ہو تو بہت احتیاط سے ایسا کریں کیونکہ اگر گردن یا ریڑھ کی ہڈی ٹوٹی ہوئی ہے تو پوزیشن میں کسی تبدیلی سے زخم بڑھ سکتا ہے (دیکھیں صفحہ 100)۔

دیکھیں کہ کوئی زخم یا ٹوٹی ہوئی ہڈی تو نہیں لیکن بے ہوش شخص کو جہاں تک ممکن ہو کم سے کم ہلائیں۔ اس کی پیٹھ یا گردن نہ موڑیں۔

بے ہوش شخص کو ہرگز کوئی چیز کھلانے پلانے کی کوشش نہ کریں۔